Neoplastic Hematopathology

Guest Editor

RANDY D. GASCOYNE, MD

HEMATOLOGY/ONCOLOGY CLINICS OF NORTH AMERICA

www.hemonc.theclinics.com

August 2009 • Volume 23 • Number 4

SAUNDERS an imprint of ELSEVIER, Inc.

W.B. SAUNDERS COMPANY
A Division of Elsevier Inc.

1600 John F. Kennedy Blvd. ● Suite 1800 ● Philadelphia, PA 19103-2899

http://www.theclinics.com

HEMATOLOGY/ONCOLOGY CLINICS OF NORTH AMERICA Volume 23, Number 4
August 2009 ISSN 0889-8588, ISBN 13: 978-1-4377-1226-1, ISBN 10: 1-4377-1226-6

Editor: Kerry Holland
Developmental Editor: Donald Mumford

Hematology/Oncology Clinics (ISSN 0889-8588) is published bimonthly by Elsevier Inc., 360 Park Avenue South, New York, NY 10010-1710. Months of issue are February, April, June, August, October, and December. Business and Editorial Offices: 1600 John F. Kennedy Blvd., Suite 1800, Philadelphia, PA 19103-2899. Customer Service Office: 11830 Westline Industrial Drive, St. Louis, MO 63146. Periodicals postage paid at New York, NY and additional mailing offices. Subscription prices are $283.00 per year (domestic individuals), $439.00 per year (domestic institutions), $141.00 per year (domestic students/residents), $321.00 per year (Canadian individuals), $537.00 per year (Canadian institutions) $382.00 per year (international individuals), $537.00 per year (international institutions), and $191.00 per year (international and Canadian students/residents). International air speed delivery is included in all *Clinics* subscription prices. All prices are subject to change without notice. **POSTMASTER:** Send address changes to *Hematology/Oncology Clinics of North America*, 11830 Westline Industrial Drive, St. Louis, MO 63146. Customer Service (orders, claims, online, change of address): Elsevier Periodicals Customer Service, 11830 Westline Industrial Drive, St. Louis, MO 63146. Tel: 1-800-654-2452 (U.S. and Canada). Fax: 314-523-5170. E-mail: journalscustomerservice-usa@elsevier.com (for print support); journalsonlinesupport-usa@elsevier.com (for online support).

Reprints. For copies of 100 or more, of articles in this publication, please contact the Commercial Reprints Department, Elsevier Inc., 360 Park Avenue South, New York, New York 10010-1710; Tel.: 212-633-3813, Fax: 212-462-1935, E-mail: reprints@elsevier.com.

Hematology/Oncology Clinics of North America is covered in *MEDLINE/PubMed (Index Medicus), EMBASE/ Excerpta Medica, and BIOSIS.*

Printed and bound by CPI Group (UK) Ltd, Croydon, CR0 4YY

Transferred to Digital Print 2011

Contributors

GUEST EDITOR

RANDY D. GASCOYNE, MD
Clinical Professor of Pathology, Department of Pathology and Advanced Therapeutics, British Columbia Cancer Agency, British Columbia Cancer Research Centre, Vancouver, British Columbia, Canada

AUTHORS

JOHN ANASTASI, MD
Associate Professor, Department of Pathology, University of Chicago, Chicago, Illinois

DANIEL A. ARBER, MD
Professor of Pathology; and Associate Chair for Clinical Services, Stanford University Medical Center, Stanford, California

LAURENCE DE LEVAL, MD, PhD
Professor of Clinics, Department of Pathology, C.H.U. Sart Tilman, Institute of Pathology, Liège, Belgium

KATHRYN FOUCAR, MD
Professor, Department of Pathology, Health Sciences Center, University of New MexicoTriCore Reference Laboratory, Albuquerque, New Mexico

RANDY D. GASCOYNE, MD
Clinical Professor of Pathology, Department of Pathology and Advanced Therapeutics, British Columbia Cancer Agency, British Columbia Cancer Research Centre, Vancouver, British Columbia, Canada

DAVID J. GOOD, MD
Department of Pathology and Laboratory Medicine, British Columbia Cancer Agency, Vancouver, British Columbia, Canada

ROBERT PAUL HASSERJIAN, MD
Associate Professor, Department of Pathology, Massachusetts General Hospital, Boston, Massachusetts

AMY HEEREMA-McKENNEY, MD
Clinical Assistant Professor, Department of Pathology, Stanford University Medical Center, Stanford, California

ERIC D. HSI, MD
Section Head, Section of Hematopathology, Department of Clinical Pathology, Cleveland Clinic, Cleveland, Ohio

DRAGAN JEVREMOVIC, MD, PhD
Division of Hematopathology, Department of Laboratory Medicine and Pathology, Mayo Clinic, Rochester, Minnesota

PAUL J. KURTIN, MD
Consultant, Division of Hematopathology; and Professor, Department of Laboratory Medicine and Pathology, Mayo Clinic, Rochester, Minnesota

PEI LIN, MD
Associate Professor, Department of Hematopathology, University of Texas-MD Anderson Cancer Center, Houston, Texas

WILLIAM R. MACON, MD
Professor, Mayo College of Medicine; Consultant and Head of Lymph Node Working Group, Division of Anatomic Pathology, Department of Laboratory Medicine and Pathology; and Consultant, Division of Hematopathology, Department of Laboratory Medicine and Pathology, Mayo Clinic, Rochester, Minnesota

PHUONG L. NGUYEN, MD
Associate Professor, Division of Hematopathology, Department of Laboratory Medicine and Pathology, Mayo Clinic, Rochester, Minnesota

MIHAELA ONCIU, MD
Associate Member, Department of Pathology, St. Jude Children's Research Hospital, Memphis, Tennessee

BERTRAM SCHNITZER, MD
Professor of Pathology, Department of Pathology, University of Michigan, Ann Arbor, Michigan

DAVID S. VISWANATHA, MD
Division of Hematopathology, Department of Laboratory Medicine and Pathology, Mayo Clinic, Rochester, Minnesota

QIAN-YUN ZHANG, MD, PhD
Associate Professor, Department of Pathology, Health Sciences Center, School of Medicine, University of New Mexico, Albuquerque, New Mexico

Contents

> The evolution of acute myeloid leukemia (AML) classification reflects greater understanding of the AML pathogenesis. The 2008 World Health Organization classification incorporated cytogenetic and molecular genetic findings and introduced important prognostic correlations. In this article, the authors discuss the different types of AML and their diagnoses.

> Acute lymphoblastic leukemia and lymphoblastic lymphoma constitute a family of genetically heterogeneous lymphoid neoplasms derived from B- and T-lymphoid progenitors. Diagnosis is based on morphologic, immunophenotypic, and genetic features that allow differentiation from normal progenitors and other hematopoietic and nonhematopoietic neoplasms. Current intensive chemotherapy regimens have accomplished overall cure rates of 85% to 90% in children and 40% to 50% in adults, with outcomes depending on the genetic subtype of disease and clinical features at presentation. Therapy is optimized using minimal residual disease studies that employ flow cytometric and molecular methodologies, and are important determinants of prognosis. Genetic analyses currently underway are likely to provide insight into biology, mechanisms of relapse, pharmacogenetics, and new potential therapeutic targets, which should aid in further improvement of outcome in this disease.

> Myelodysplastic syndromes (MDS) are a heterogeneous group of bone marrow disorders that affect mostly the elderly and have a variable probability of progression to acute leukemia. The diagnosis of MDS rests largely on a critical morphologic review of blood and bone marrow slides, with careful correlation with other clinical and essential laboratory data, including cytogenetics. This article discusses the epidemiology and clinical and pathologic features of MDS and pertinent diagnostic and prognostic classifications, with a brief overview of treatment options. Other considerations in the differential diagnosis are also briefly outlined.

The lymphomas of small B lymphocytes are a biologically diverse group of B cell derived neoplasms that includes B cell small lymphocytic lymphoma/chronic lymphocytic leukemia; mantle cell lymphoma; follicular lymphoma; nodal, splenic and extranodal marginal zone lymphomas; and lymphoplasmacytic lymphoma. They are distinguished from one another on clinical, morphological, phenotypic and genetic grounds. This article reviews the essential diagnostic and biologic features of these clinically indolent B cell malignancies.

Diffuse large B-cell lymphomas (DLBCLs) and Burkitt lymphoma (BL) account for the majority of aggressive lymphomas in adults and children. DLBCLs exhibit marked biological heterogeneity and variable clinical presentation and clinical course. Conversely, BL is genetically relatively homogeneous but associated with variable clinicopathological features. In this article, the authors summarize the recent advances pertaining to these B-cell neoplasms, following the latest World Health Organization classification and focusing on changes introduced since the previous edition. These changes include the addition of variants and subgroups of DLBCLs and "borderline" categories for high-grade B-cell neoplasms that show features intermediate between DLBCL and classical Hodgkin lymphoma, or between DLBCL and BL. In particular, the diagnostic and therapeutic problems related to neoplasms with features intermediate between DLBCL and BL will be discussed.

Peripheral T-cell lymphomas (PTCLs) are malignancies of immunologically mature T-cells that arise in peripheral lymphoid tissues such as lymph nodes, spleen, gastrointestinal tract, and skin. These lymphomas are uncommon as compared with the incidence of B-cell lymphomas, and they comprise only 5% to 10% of non-Hodgkin lymphomas in North America and Western Europe. A variety of specific disease entities have been recognized among PTCLs, and they tend to have lymph node, extranodal/cutaneous, or mixed leukemic/lymphomatous presentations. Most PTCLs have an aggressive clinical course. The clinicopathologic features of the various PTCLs are described herein.

The leukemias of mature B cells and T cells are a limited set of diseases in which blood and bone marrow are the primary sites of involvement.

Although they may superficially resemble one another, they have distinct clinical and pathologic features and must be distinguished from one another. In this article, the major clinical, morphologic, phenotypic, and molecular genetic features of the mature B- and T-cell leukemias are reviewed, and differential diagnostic considerations are discussed.

Bone marrow evaluation plays a critical role in staging and predicting prognosis in patients with Hodgkin lymphoma or non-Hodgkin lymphoma. Bone marrow can be the initial site of detection of lymphoma in patients with unexplained symptoms or cytopenias. A comprehensive evaluation of bone marrow includes complete blood counts, blood morphology, bone marrow aspirate, and generous core biopsy sections. Specialized testing should be used in a logical fashion on a case by case basis.

This chapter summarizes the significance and molecular diagnostic detection of genetic abnormalities commonly associated with hematolymphoid neoplasms. Methodologic aspects of laboratory diagnosis are presented, as well as discussion of multiparameter genotyping of tumors for prognosis and the role of minimal residual disease monitoring in specific neoplasms.

THE CLINICS ARE NOW AVAILABLE ONLINE!

Access your subscription at:
www.theclinics.com

Preface

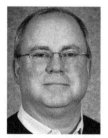

Randy D. Gascoyne, MD
Guest Editor

The field of neoplastic hematopathology is constantly evolving, and the rate of change has accelerated recently. High-throughput genomic strategies are allowing the generation of new data at a rapid pace, and these new findings are adding texture to the current classification schemes used in the new World Health Organization (WHO) classification of tumors of the hematopoietic and lymphoid tissues. Both myeloid and lymphoid tumors are the paradigm of diseases wherein morphologic, immunopheno-typic, cytogenetic, and molecular findings are intricately woven together to establish accurate diagnoses and to facilitate the recognition of new subentities. For these reasons, the field is in constant flux.

In 2001, the WHO classification of tumors of the hematopoietic and lymphoid tissues listed 89 separate International Classification of Diseases for Oncology (ICD-O) codes, including a number of provisional entities. The 2008 edition of the WHO book lists 145 distinct ICD-O codes, and it is 88 pages longer than the previous edition. Several of the authors of articles in this issue of *Hematology/Oncology Clinics of North America* made contributions to the current WHO book and thus are considered experts in the field. Most of the major disease categories of the latest classification are covered in this issue of *Clinics*. Emphasis is placed on key diagnostic features used in daily practice, and therefore most articles contain helpful tables that list key differential features that allow one to distinguish between different entities. In addition, this issue covers several overarching topics, including molecular diagnostics in hematopathology and specific diagnostic features and patterns of involvement of the bone marrow in lymphoid neoplasms. The article on molecular hematopathology covers the gamut of diagnostic tests used for both myeloid and lymphoid diseases. Moreover, topics such as minimal residual disease monitoring and the detection of single nucleotide variants are discussed. This article also includes a section on where the field is likely to go in the near future. The article on lymphomatous bone-marrow involvement in hematopathol-ogy is extremely useful, succinctly covering a wealth of helpful diagnostic features that would otherwise require an entire textbook to adequately address. There is also an article devoted to diseases that may mimic lymphoma, and it discusses the histo-logic, immunophenotypic, and molecular features that can be used to distinguish these entities from true lymphoid tumors.

Hematol Oncol Clin N Am 23 (2009) xi–xii
doi:10.1016/j.hoc.2009.06.001
0889-8588/09/$ – see front matter © 2009 Elsevier Inc. All rights reserved.
hemonc.theclinics.com

This issue of *Hematology/Oncology Clinics of North America* is beautifully illustrated, with numerous high-quality photomicrographs highlighting key diagnostic features, and all are in color. These images, together with informative line diagrams and concise descriptions of most of the major disorders that encompass lymphoid and myeloid diseases, should make this a cherished resource for all who are interested in neoplastic hematopathology.

Randy D. Gascoyne, MD
Department of Pathology and Advanced Therapeutics
British Columbia Cancer Agency
British Columbia Cancer Research Centre
675 W. 10th Avenue, Room 5-113
Vancouver, BC V5Z 4E6, Canada

E-mail address:
rgascoyn@bccancer.bc.ca (R.D. Gascoyne)

Acute Myeloid Leukemia

Amy Heerema-McKenney, MD[a], Daniel A. Arber, MD[b],*

KEYWORDS

- Acute myeloid leukemia • WHO 2008 classification
- Recurrent genetic abnormalities
- Myelodysplasia-related changes
- Therapy-related myeloid neoplasms

The evolution of acute myeloid leukemia (AML) classification reflects greater understanding of the AML pathogenesis. The French-American-British (FAB) cooperative group classification of AML provided a useful common terminology, but it was limited in biologic, prognostic, and therapeutic significance. The 2001 World Health Organization (WHO) classification incorporated cytogenetic and molecular genetic findings and introduced important prognostic correlations. The 2008 WHO classification (**Box 1**) expanded the number of entities with recurrent chromosomal translocations and included two provisional entities characterized by gene mutations, AML with cytoplasmic/mutated *NPM1* and AML with *CEBPA* mutations.[1] It retains FAB-like terminology for a morphologic classification of AML not otherwise specified (AML-NOS),[2] but only a subset of cases fall into this category. The diagnosis of myelodysplasia or myelodysplastic syndrome (MDS)-related disease has been further refined, with specification of a history of prior MDS, MDS-associated cytogenetic abnormalities, or severe multilineage dysplasia.[3] Therapy-related AML remains a category with important biologic and clinical features.[4] Myeloid proliferations of Down syndrome are now separately classified.[5]

A diagnosis of AML requires the presence of 20% blasts enumerated from all nucleated cells in the blood or bone marrow in most cases. In myelomonocytic and monocytic leukemias, promonocytes are considered comparable to blasts. The blast count should be obtained from at least a 200-cell count of all nucleated cells in the blood and a 500-cell count of all nucleated cells in the bone marrow. Detection of a t(8;21), inv(16), t(16;16), or t(15;17) is diagnostic of their respective acute leukemias even when blasts are less than 20%. Similarly, the presence of a myeloid sarcoma is diagnostic of AML even if blasts are not significantly elevated in the blood or bone marrow. A morphologic–genetic correlation is now recognized for certain AML subtypes;

a Department of Pathology, Stanford University Medical Center, 300 Pasteur Drive, Lane Building, Room 235, Stanford, CA 94305, USA
b Stanford University Medical Center, 300 Pasteur Drive, H1507C- M/C5627, Stanford, CA 94305-5627, USA
* Corresponding author.
E-mail address: darber@stanford.edu (D.A. Arber).

Hematol Oncol Clin N Am 23 (2009) 633–654
doi:10.1016/j.hoc.2009.04.003
0889-8588/09/$ – see front matter © 2009 Elsevier Inc. All rights reserved.

Box 1
2008 WHO classification of AML

AML with recurrent genetic abnormalities

    AML with t(8;21)(q22;q22); (*RUNX1-RUNX1T1*)

    AML with inv(16)(p13.1q22) or t(16;16)(p13.1;q22); (*CBFB-MYH11*)

    Acute promyelocytic leukemia (APL) with t(15;17)(q22;q12); (*PML-RARA*)

    AML with t(9;11)(p22;q23); (*MLLT3-MLL*)

    AML with t(6;9)(p23;q34); (*DEK-NUP214*)

    AML with inv(3)(q21q26.2) or t(3;3)(q21;q26.2); (*RPN1-EVI1*)

    AML (megakaryoblastic) with t(1;22)(p13;q13); (*RBM15-MKL1*)

    Provisional entity: AML with mutated *NPM1*

    Provisional entity: AML with mutated *CEBPA*

AML with MDS-related changes

Therapy-related myeloid neoplasms

AML-NOS

    AML with minimal differentiation

    AML without maturation

    AML with maturation

    Acute myelomonocytic leukemia

    Acute monoblastic/monocytic leukemia

    Acute erythroid leukemias

        Pure erythroid leukemia

        Erythroleukemia, erythroid/myeloid

    Acute megakaryoblastic leukemia

    Acute basophilic leukemia

    Acute panmyelosis with myelofibrosis

Myeloid sarcoma

Myeloid proliferations related to Down syndrome

    Transient abnormal myelopoiesis

    AML associated with Down syndrome

Courtesy of the World Health Organization; with permission.

---

however, a spectrum of blast morphologies exists within these categories and even within any given case.

All patients evaluated for acute leukemia must have bone marrow cytogenetic studies performed. Molecular studies are an integral part of WHO classification for AML lacking one of the recognized cytogenetic abnormalities and are recommended for risk stratification of other subtypes. Risk stratification of AML into favorable, intermediate, and poor prognostic groups is based on cytogenetics and gene mutation status (*FLT3, KIT, NPM1,* and *CEBPA*) and is used to identify which patients benefit from allogeneic stem cell transplantation (allo-SCT).[6] Some schema may include other factors, such as timing of attainment of complete remission (CR) and white blood cell

(WBC) count at presentation. HLA-matched sibling donor allo-SCT seems most beneficial for patients with intermediate- and poor-risk AML, improving disease-free survival and overall survival. Younger patients with poor-risk disease may benefit from matched, unrelated donor allo-SCT. Patients with favorable-risk disease, specifically core-binding factor leukemias, do not appear to benefit from allo-SCT. Some schema require a WBC of less than 20×10^9/L and the absence of additional unfavorable cytogenetic abnormalities for a designation of "favorable." Two newer additions to the favorable-risk category include patients with normal karyotype and mutated *NPM1*, without *FLT3* internal tandem duplication (*FLT3*-ITD), and patients with normal karyotype and mutated *CEBPA*.

ACUTE MYELOID LEUKEMIA WITH BALANCED TRANSLOCATIONS/INVERSIONS

The seven subtypes of leukemia in this category have characteristic morphologic, clinical, and prognostic features in addition to specific cytogenetic and molecular genetic findings. The 2008 WHO classification introduces three rarer balanced abnormalities in addition to the more common abnormalities from the WHO 2001 classification.[1]

Acute Myeloid Leukemia with t(8;21)(q22;q22)

AML with t(8;21) is common in children and adults, accounting for approximately 8% of the cases of AML. The translocation results in a fusion product involving the *RUNX1* gene (also known as core-binding factor alpha and *AML1*) on chromosome 21 and the *RUNX1T1* (also known as *ETO*) gene on chromosome 8. The presence of this genetic abnormality is diagnostic of AML regardless of the blast count. Cases of AML with t(8;21) share a common morphology and immunophenotype.[1] The blasts are large with a background of myeloid maturation (FAB M2). In the bone marrow, blasts have cytoplasmic hofs, occasional Auer rods, and occasional large, salmon-colored granules (**Fig. 1**). The maturing neutrophils are commonly dysplastic. Background eosinophilia is variably present. Immunophenotypically, blasts express CD34, CD13, CD33, and myeloperoxidase (MPO), with typical aberrant weak CD19 expression. Other B lineage antigens may be found, such as PAX5, CD79a, and TdT. These do not warrant a designation of B/myeloid mixed phenotype acute leukemia in the presence of a t(8;21)(q22;q22).[1]

Core-binding factor leukemias are associated with a favorable prognosis in children and adults, especially when treated with repetitive cycles of high-dose cytarabine postremission.[7] Mutations of *KIT* in core-binding factor AML are common (20%–25%). In adults, *KIT* mutations in exons 8 and exon 17 appear to worsen prognosis. It is unclear if they have a similar prognostic effect in children or whether t(8;21) AML with *KIT* mutation benefits from allo-SCT in first remission.[8–10] Mutations in *FLT3* are rare in core-binding factor leukemia. Additional cytogenetic abnormalities are present in most cases of t(8;21) AML, most commonly including loss of a sex chromosome or partial deletion of the long arm of chromosome 9. The presence of an unfavorable additional cytogenetic abnormality, such as monosomy 7, may adversely impact prognosis. After therapy, reverse transcription polymerase chain reaction (RT-PCR) may detect *RUNX1-RUNX1T1* transcripts in the absence of any clinical disease. Quantitative PCR measuring the kinetics of *RUNX1-RUNX1T1* transcripts appears more useful for monitoring minimal residual disease.[7]

Acute Myeloid Leukemia with inv(16)(p13;q22) or t(16;16)(p13;q22)

AML with an inv(16)(p13;q22) or t(16;16) (p13;q22) comprises 10% of adult AML and approximately 6% of childhood AML. The genes at the breakpoint junction are the

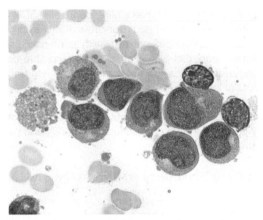

Fig. 1. AML with t(8;21)(q22;q22) *RUNX1-RUNX1T1*. Blasts show distinct perinuclear hofs and salmon-colored cytoplasmic granules.

beta subunit of the core-binding factor (*CBFB*) at 16q22 and a gene encoding smooth muscle myosin heavy chain (*MYH11*) at 16p13. Because this disorder and AML with t(8;21) disrupt the core-binding factor necessary for normal hematopoiesis, both are often referred to as the core-binding factor leukemias. The presence of this genetic abnormality is diagnostic of AML, regardless of the blast count.[1] AML with inv(16) or t(16;16) has a characteristic morphology of acute myelomonocytic leukemia with abnormal eosinophils in the bone marrow(FAB-M4Eo). Typical myeloblasts, monoblasts, and promonocytes are seen in the peripheral blood and marrow, with increased and dysplastic eosinophils seen in the bone marrow (**Fig. 2**). The dysplastic eosinophils have abundant and large basophilic granules. Flow cytometry immunophenotyping typically reveals multiple populations, including an immature blast population expressing CD34 and/or CD117 and groups of cells exhibiting granulocytic (CD13, CD33, CD15, MPO) or monocytic (CD4, CD11b, CD11c, CD14, CD64,

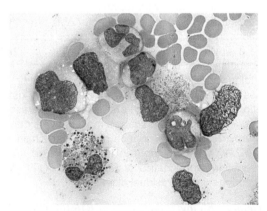

Fig. 2. AML with inv(16)(p13.1q22) *CBFB-MYH11*. Blasts show myeloid and monocytic differentiation and are accompanied by abnormal eosinophils with large, dark, basophilic granules.

CD36, lysozyme) differentiation. Aberrant coexpression of CD2 has been described but is not specific for this subtype of AML.

The incidence of extramedullary disease is higher than for most types of AML, with a high incidence of central nervous system relapse. Similar to AML with t(8;21), this core-binding factor leukemia has a favorable prognosis. *KIT* mutations are present in approximately 30% of cases and negatively impact prognosis in adults. It is not clear if AML with inv(16) or t(16;16) and mutated *KIT* benefits from allo-SCT or tyrosine kinase inhibitor therapy. Levels of the *CBFB/MYH11* transcript by RT-PCR decrease slowly after therapy; patients may continue to test positive in early CR. Molecular remissions are possible and correlate well with long-term remission.[7]

Acute Promyelocytic Leukemia with t(15;17) (q22;q12)

Acute promyelocytic leukemia (APL) usually presents with an abrupt onset and comprises 5% to 8% of cases of AML. It is most common in young adults with a diminishing incidence after age 60 years.[1] Prompt recognition of the diagnosis is essential because of the high frequency of life-threatening disseminated intravascular coagulation (DIC). The t(15;17)(q22;q21) results in fusion of the promyelocytic gene (*PML*) on chromosome 15 with the retinoic acid receptor (*RARA*) gene on chromosome 17. Detection of this abnormality is diagnostic of APL regardless of the blast count. The blasts are highly sensitive to anthracycline-based chemotherapy and differentiate in response to all-*trans*-retinoic acid treatment (ATRA). Two morphologic variants (hypergranular and hypogranular) are recognized to have distinct immunohistochemical and genetic features.[11–14]

Hypergranular or "typical" APL represents 60% to 70% of cases and usually presents with a lower white blood cell count. The abnormal promyelocytes (**Fig. 3**) have numerous large red to purple cytoplasmic granules, often obscuring the nuclear contours. Most cases have cells containing multiple Auer rods. The abnormal promyelocytes are considered comparable to blasts for the purpose of diagnosing APL because typical myeloblasts may not be significantly increased. Flow cytometry immunophenotyping shows increased side scatter and the combined lack of expression of HLA-DR and CD34, with bright CD33, bright cytoplasmic MPO, and variable expression of CD13. CD117 and CD64 are commonly expressed, and CD15 is typically absent. The CD34, HLA-DR negative immunophenotype is not specific to APL

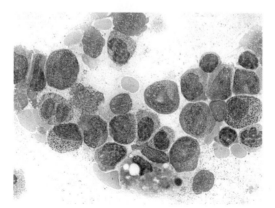

Fig. 3. APL with t(15;17)(q22;q12) *PML-RARA*, Hypergranular variant. The abnormal promyelocytes show dense eosinophilic granules, often obscuring nuclear detail, with frequent Auer rods.

because it is also observed in some cases of cytogenetically normal AML without differentiation, often with cup-like nuclear invaginations.[15,16]

Hypogranular or "microgranular" APL typically presents with leukocytosis with numerous circulating abnormal promyelocytes. The two forms have abnormal reniform or bilobed nuclei. In the microgranular variant of APL, the blood leukocyte count is elevated; in some cases, it is markedly elevated. The leukemic cells have fine granulation and bilobed or "butterfly" shaped nuclei (**Fig. 4**). Cells containing multiple Auer rods are less abundant than in typical hypergranular APL. The MPO and Sudan black B reactions are strong and diffuse in the abnormal cells of both variants. The hypogranular variant shows CD13, CD33, and MPO expression similar to the hypergranular variant but may show dim HLA-DR and dim CD34. Cases may exhibit CD64 expression, and caution is warranted not to misdiagnose a hypogranular APL as AML with monocytic differentiation. Aberrant expression of CD2 is more commonly observed in hypogranular APL.[14] CD56 expression is described in 15% to 20% of all APL patients and has been associated with shorter CR and poorer overall survival in some studies.[17] Three breakpoint regions are described on the *PML* gene at band q22 of chromosome 15. Two (bcr1, bcr2) lead to long transcripts, and the third (bcr3) leads to the short transcript. The short transcript is more common to the hypogranular variant.

Cytogenetic analysis, fluorescent in situ hybridization (FISH), or RT-PCR is necessary for genetic confirmation of the *PML-RARA* fusion. FISH, RT-PCR, and immunofluorescence for the microspeckled nuclear distribution of the *PML* protein may aid in rapid diagnosis. RT-PCR is the only technique that can identify the *PML-RARA* isoform useful for minimal residual disease monitoring.[12] Atypical promyelocytes may persist in the marrow for up to several weeks after induction chemotherapy, as may detection of *PML-RARA* by karyotype, FISH, or RT-PCR. These findings do not necessarily indicate resistant disease. Detection of *PML-RARA* by RT-PCR post-induction does not impact subsequent clinical outcome. However, detection of *PML-RARA* after CR is obtained strongly predicts risk for relapse.

FLT3 mutations are common in APL and are present in approximately 40% of patients, with the majority being internal tandem duplication (ITD) mutations.

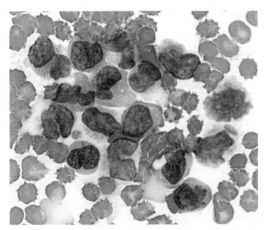

Fig. 4. APL with t(15;17)(q22;q12) *PML-RARA*, Hypogranular variant. The abnormal promyelocytes show characteristic bilobed or "butterfly-shaped" nuclei with only fine, indistinct cytoplasmic granularity.

FLT3-ITD in APL is strongly associated with the hypogranular subtype, with high WBC counts in peripheral blood and the bcr3 breakpoint in *PML*. In a retrospective study, patients with mutant *FLT3* had a higher rate of death during the period of induction chemotherapy but no significant difference in relapse rate or 5-year overall survival.[11]

The PML-RARA fusion protein mediates a block in myeloid differentiation, which can be overcome using ATRA therapy and arsenic trioxide . In most instances, a remission can be achieved with ATRA alone, but relapse invariably occurs. Standard induction chemotherapy with high-dose anthracyclines is therefore generally given in addition to ATRA. In adult patients that achieve a CR, the prognosis is better than for any other category of AML. The diagnosis of APL must be rapid. Initiation of therapy should not wait for genetic confirmation when clinical, morphologic, or flow cytometric findings, or rapid molecular pathology results suggest a diagnosis of APL.[12]

Acute Promyelocytic Leukemia with Variant RARA Translocations

Uncommonly, a case with many of the morphologic, immunophenotypic, and clinical features of promyelocytic leukemia has a variant cytogenetic translocation that involves the *RARA* gene on chromosome 17 but not the *PML* gene on 15. The most common variant rearrangements include t(11;17)(q23;q12) *ZBTB16-RARA* (formerly *PLZF-RARA*), t(11;17)(q13;q12) *NUMA1-RARA*, t(5;17)(q35;q12) *NPM1-RARA,* and t(17; 17)(q11.2;q12) *STAT5B-RARA*.[1,12] The t(11;17) (q23;q12) *ZBTB16-RARA* is best described. The morphology differs from hypergranular or microgranular APL in that the majority of nuclei are round to oval, Auer rods are usually absent, and pelgeroid neutrophils may be seen. Patients with variant *RARA* translocations often experience DIC. These cases are important to recognize, because although they have many of the features of typical APL, some variants, including *ZBTB16-RARA* and *STAT5B-RARA,* do not respond to ATRA therapy.[1,11–13]

Acute Myeloid Leukemia with t(9;11)(p22;q23)

Translocations involving the *MLL* gene on chromosome 11q23 are found in approximately 6% of cases of AML and are associated with more than 50 different partner genes. In addition to AML, *MLL* rearrangements are common to therapy-related myeloid proliferations, acute lymphoblastic leukemia (ALL), and acute leukemias of ambiguous lineage. The 2008 WHO classification now recognizes only t(9;11) (p22;q23) (*MLLT3-MLL*) as a specific entity in the category of AML with recurrent genetic abnormalities.[1] The t(9;11) (*MLLT3-MLL*) AML typically occurs in children, with an intermediate prognosis. Extramedullary disease of the gingiva and skin and presentation with DIC have been described. The blasts typically have a monocytic or myelomonocytic morphology, although occasionally they may lack differentiation (**Fig. 5**). Cases morphologically consisting mostly of monoblasts and promonocytes are typically MPO negative by cytochemistry. In children, AML with t(9;11) typically expresses CD33, CD4, CD65, and HLA-DR, with minimal to no CD13, CD14, and CD34 expression. In adults, AML with 11q23 translocations often show monocytic morphologic differentiation and may express multiple monocytic antigens, including CD14, CD64, CD11b, CD11c, and CD4. CD34 is often negative, with variable CD117 and CD56 reactivity.

AML with balanced rearrangements of 11q23 other than t(9;11)(p22;q23) are diagnosed as AML-NOS, with the rearrangement stated in the diagnosis line, with exception of those occurring after cytotoxic therapy (which would be considered as therapy-related AML) or the t(11;16)(q23;p13.3) and t(2;11)(p21;q23), which are MDS-associated genetic abnormalities and would be considered AML with

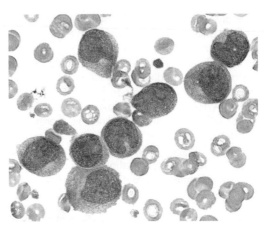

Fig. 5. AML with t(9;11)(p22;q23) *MLLT3-MLL*. Blasts show early monocytic differentiation with relatively abundant cytoplasm and some nuclear folds.

MDS-related changes.[1,3,4] In addition to t(9;11)(p22;q23), the most common *MLL* translocations in AML include t(10;11) (p12;q23) *MLL-MLLT10* (*AF10*), t(11;19)(q23;p13.1) *MLL-ELL*, t(6;11)(q27;q23) *MLL-MLLT4* (*AF6*), and t(11;19)(q23;p13.3) *MLL-MLLT1* (*ENL*). Of these, only the t(11;19)(q23;p13.1) *MLL-ELL* has not been associated with ALL.[18,19]

Gene mutations in *KIT* or *FLT3*-ITD are uncommon in AML with 11q23 translocations. Approximately 20% of AML with t(9;11) have activating loop domain point mutations in *FLT3*, but these are of uncertain prognostic significance.[20] Pediatric AML with t(9;11) has an intermediate prognosis, whereas leukemias associated with a different chromosome 11q23 translocation, in general, have a poorer prognosis. Overexpression of ectopic virus integration-1 (EVI1) has been described in multiple variant translocations of 11q23 and has been associated with a poor prognosis.[21]

Acute Myeloid Leukemia with t(6;9)(p23;q34)

AML with t(6;9) is a rare subtype of AML comprising approximately 1% of cases in children and adults. The median age in adults for this subtype of AML is young (35 years).[1,22–24] The blasts of t(6;9) AML may show occasional Auer rods and may exhibit monocytic features. Dyspoiesis of all three lineages may be evident on the peripheral smear and bone marrow aspirate (**Fig. 6**). Basophilia (>2% marrow or blood basophils) is present in roughly half of reported cases. By flow cytometry, blasts typically express CD45, CD13, CD33, HLA-DR, and intracytoplasmic MPO, with variable expression of CD34, CD15, and CD11c. TdT may be positive in some cases by flow cytometry or immunohistochemistry. *FLT3*-ITD mutations are common in this type of AML, with a reported frequency of 70%. Although the majority of patients with t(6;9) AML may achieve CR, survival rates are poor with conventional chemotherapy. Patients may benefit from allo-SCT. The presence of fewer than 20% blasts in a patient with the t(6;9)(p23;q34) is not considered diagnostic of AML, and patients should be followed closely for progression.

Acute Myeloid Leukemia with inv(3)(q21q26.2) or t(3;3)(q21;q26.2)

AML with inv(3)(q21q26.2) or t(3;3)(q21;q26.2) *RPN1-EVI1* occurs primarily in adults, representing 1% to 2% of cases of AML. Rare cases are reported in children in association with monosomy 7.[1,25] Patients typically present with anemia, and sometimes

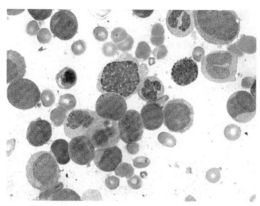

Fig. 6. AML with t(6;9)(p23;q34) *DEK-NUP214*. Myeloid blasts are accompanied by dysery-thropoiesis and basophilia in the bone marrow.

thrombocytosis, with or without prior MDS. Hepatosplenomegaly may be present. In addition to blasts, the peripheral blood may show dysplastic neutrophils and platelets. Circulating megakaryocyte naked nuclei may be seen. The bone marrow blasts may show multiple morphologies, including FAB M1, M4, and M7 types. Myeloperoxidase activity is often low. Megakaryocytes may be normal or increased in number , usually with small unilobated and bilobated forms or other dysplastic features. Dyserythropoiesis and/or dysmyelopoiesis are commonly present (**Fig. 7**). The core biopsy may show decreased cellularity and occasionally fibrosis. Few studies describe flow cytometry in this disease. Blasts typically express CD34, CD13, CD33, and HLA-DR, with aberrant CD7 expression in some cases. Cases with megakaryocytic differentiation may express CD41 and CD61.

EVI1 is abnormally expressed in AML with inv(3)(q21q26.2) or t(3;3)(q21;q26.2). High expression of EVI1 is a poor prognostic indicator independent of 3q26 rearrangement.[6] Cytogenetics may fail to identify cryptic rearrangements of 3q26 detectable by FISH.[21] Secondary karyotypic abnormalities are present in most cases, including most of those with poor prognosis, MDS-associated abnormalities of -7, -5q, and

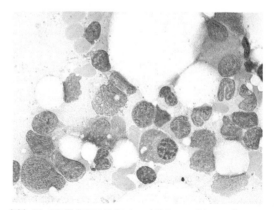

Fig. 7. AML with inv(3)(q21q26.2) *RPN1-EVI1*. In addition to blasts, the marrow shows a proliferation of small, bilobed megakaryocytes.

complex aberrant karyotypes. *FLT3*-ITD mutations are found in a small subset of patients (13%). Patients with AML with inv(3) or t(3;3) typically have short survival. Age greater than 60 years appears to be an independent risk factor for poor overall survival.[26] Patients able to tolerate allo-SCT may benefit from this approach to therapy. Patients with inv(3) or t(3;3) may present with less than 20% blasts and should be closely monitored for the development of AML.

AML (Megakaryoblastic) with t(1;22)(p13;q13)

Acute megakaryoblastic leukemia (AMkL) with t(1;22) is a rare form of infantile AML.[1,27,28] The median age at diagnosis is 4 months, and 80% of cases are diagnosed in the first year of life. AMkL with t(1;22) composes approximately 1% of childhood AML. The clinical presentation commonly masquerades as a solid tumor with hepatosplenomegaly and/or skeletal lesions (bilaterally symmetric periostitis and osteolytic lesions), sometimes without involvement of the bone marrow.[29] Biopsy of the lesions may show cohesive nests of small round blue cells also suggestive of a childhood solid tumor, leading to a misdiagnosis. The complete blood count may show anemia and thrombocytopenia. Blasts in the blood and/or bone marrow show typical features of megakaryoblasts with a small amount of agranular cytoplasm typically with budding or blebs (**Figs. 8 and 9**). Marrow fibrosis may be so extensive as to yield an aparticulate, hemodilute aspirate. Multilineage dysplasia is not described. Micromegakaryocytes are reportedly common. Few cases have a reported flow cytometry immunophenotype. CD45 and CD34 may be negative, and the myeloid antigens CD13 and CD33 are inconsistently expressed, as is HLA-DR. Immunoreactivity for megakaryocytic antigens, CD41 and CD61, is commonly seen, and some cases may express CD56. Immunohistochemically, the cells are often negative for CD45, although they commonly express CD43. Markers of megakaryocytic differentiation, such as von Willebrand factor, may be positive. The diagnosis of a myeloid sarcoma AMkL with t(1;22) may not be obvious until cytogenetics reveals the presence of the translocation. "Older" patients (greater than 6 months of age) commonly have

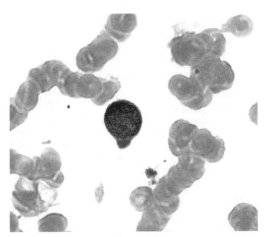

Fig. 8. AML (megakaryoblastic) with t(1;22)(p13;q13) *RBM15-MKL1*. Rare megakaryoblasts are seen on this mostly hemodilute aspirate, with typical dense nuclei and basophilic cytoplasmic projections.

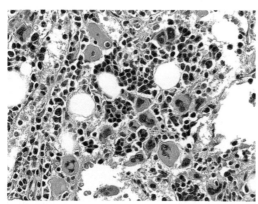

Fig. 9. AML (megakaryoblastic) with t(1;22)(p13;q13) *RBM15-MKL1*. The bone marrow core biopsy shows clusters of megakaryoblasts and a proliferation of small megakaryocyte.

complex additional karyotypic abnormalities. The frequency of *FLT3* mutations is unclear, given the rarity of AMkL with t(1;22). AMkL with t(1;22) was associated with poor survival in earlier studies, but more recent studies suggest that they respond well to intensive AML therapy. Cases commonly present with less than 20% blasts in the blood and/or marrow, but the presence of myeloid sarcoma is diagnostic of AML regardless of the marrow blast count.

ACUTE MYELOID LEUKEMIA WITH GENE MUTATIONS

The current model of myeloid leukemogenesis recognizes two genetic hits.[30] Type I mutations confer proliferation and cell survival advantages to the clone, and type II mutations impair cellular differentiation. Receptor tyrosine kinase mutations are common type I mutations. Of these, mutations in fms-like tyrosine kinase (*FLT3*) and *KIT* are most often used in clinical risk stratification. FLT3 is normally expressed on hematopoietic progenitors. Activation through ligand binding or constituitive activation from *FLT3* mutations leads to cell proliferation and survival.

As is evident from the diagnostic categories detailed above, *FLT3* and *KIT* mutations do not define exclusive categories of AML and are present in many subtypes. *FLT3* abnormalities include internal tandem duplications (*FLT3*-ITD), tyrosine kinase domain point mutations, and the rare juxtamembrane domain mutations. *FLT3*-ITD mutations are associated with shorter CR duration and overall survival. The ratio of mutant *FLT3* to wild type allele can identify patients with poor outcomes. *KIT* mutations appear to have the most clinical relevance in core-binding factor leukemias, particularly in adults. In contrast, *FLT3* internal tandem duplications are rare in core-binding factor leukemias.[1,8,11,20,31]

Chromosomal translocations provide the most significant AML prognostic information at diagnosis; however, up to half of adults with AML will have a normal karyotype. Among cytogenetically normal AML (CN-AML), *FLT3* mutations are present in roughly one-third of cases.[31,32] The morphology spans the spectrum of FAB subtypes, with the most common subtype being AML without differentiation (FAB M1). The myeloblasts have frequent expression of CD7.[33] Cup-like nuclear invaginations are described, as is the lack of expression of CD34 and HLA-DR, with strong expression of CD123 (**Fig. 10**).[16] Optimal treatment for patients with CN-AML and mutated *FLT3* is not clear; some studies demonstrate a benefit of allo-SCT in first remission, whereas

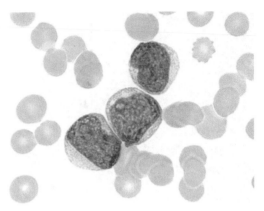

Fig.10. AML with cup-like nuclear inclusions. This case of cytogenetically normal AML lacked expression of CD34 and HLA-DR by flow cytometry. This morphology and immunophenotype are frequently associated with *FLT3* and/or *NPM1* mutations.

others failed to demonstrate improved survival with allo-SCT. The use of small molecule FLT3 inhibitors with chemotherapy is currently under investigation.

Mutations in nucleophosmin (*NPM1*) and CCAAT/enhancer binding protein-alpha (*CEBPA*) also tend to occur in cases of AML with normal cytogenetics and define unique clinico-biologic entities with favorable prognoses in the absence of *FLT3* abnormalities. These are provisional diagnostic categories in the WHO 2008 classification.

Acute Myeloid Leukemia with Mutated NPM1

The *NPM1* gene at chromosome 5q35 encodes a molecular chaperone, shuttling molecules from the nucleus to the cytoplasm, in addition to multiple other roles. The native product appears to have oncogenic and tumor suppressor capabilities and is typically located in nucleoli. Mutations in exon 12 create a nuclear export motif, with resultant dislocation of NPM to the cytoplasm. AML with mutated *NPM1* is found in approximately 50% of adult AML patients with a normal karyotype and 20% of pediatric AML patients with a normal karyotype.[1,34,35] *NPM1* mutations of exon 12 may be identified by RT-PCR. Alternatively, the mutation may be inferred by cytoplasmic localization of NPM1 by immunohistochemistry (**Fig. 11**). Approximately 40% of *NPM1* mutated patients are also *FLT3*-ITD positive. *NPM1* mutation in CN-AML is associated with a favorable prognosis in the absence of an *FLT3*-ITD mutation, similar to core-binding factor leukemias. *NPM1* mutations are rarely reported in association with 11q23 abnormalities or other recurring cytogenetic abnormalities.

In adults, most of the *NPM1* mutated cases show monocytic differentiation (FAB M5b), whereas all FAB subtypes except M3, M4Eo, and M7 have been observed. In children, *NPM1* mutated cases most commonly show FAB M1, M2, or M4 morphologies. Adult cases of AML with mutated *NPM1* are predominantly CD34 negative. Among cases with FAB M1 morphology are those demonstrating cup-like nuclear inclusions and lacking CD34 and HLA-DR expression, also described in cases with *FLT3*-ITD mutations.[15,16] It is not clear if the two gene mutations always occur together in this morphologic subtype. Because of the prognostic importance of *FLT3* mutations in this provisional AML subtype, it is imperative that *FLT3* mutations be studied with *NPM1* in all cases.

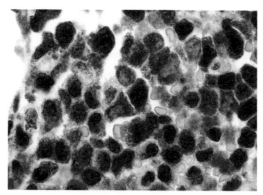

Fig. 11. AML with mutated/cytoplasmic NPM1. Immunohistochemistry for NPM1 demonstrates abnormal localization of the protein in the leukemic cell cytoplasm. Occasional non-neoplastic cells with nuclear localization are present.

Acute Myeloid Leukemia with CEBPA Mutations

C/EBPα is a differentiation-inducing transcription factor involved in granulocytic differentiation and other diverse processes. Point mutations of the *CEBPA* gene at chromosome 19q31.1 are detected in 13% of CN-AML cases in adults and 17% to 20% of CN-AML cases in children.[1,31,32,36–38] More than 100 different nonsilent mutations have been described, most often leading to production of a smaller dominant negative isoform inhibiting wild type C/EBPα function. *FLT3* abnormalities are uncommon in AML with *CEBPA* mutations. In the absence of adverse prognostic factors, AML with *CEBPA* mutations has a favorable prognosis not likely to benefit from allo-SCT, although further study is needed to address optimal postremission therapy, because the number of cases studied is too small to be definitive.

The morphologic subtypes of myeloblasts described in AML with *CEBPA* mutations are most commonly FAB M1 and M2, with fewer cases of M4 and M5 described. *CEBPA* mutations are rarely described in therapy-related AML, which should be diagnosed as therapy-related AML, with comment on the detection of a *CEBPA* mutation. Approximately 70% of AML patients with *CEBPA* mutations have a normal karyotype. Approximately 10% have a single karyotypic abnormality, and only rare cases have a complex karyotype. No specific immunophenotype of AML with *CEBPA* mutations has been described.

ACUTE MYELOID LEUKEMIA WITH MDS-RELATED CHANGES

The category of AML with multilineage dysplasia from the 2001 WHO classification has been expanded to now incorporate historical and cytogenetic criteria into the diagnosis (**Box 2**). AML with MDS-related changes (AML-MRC) may present as a de novo disease or may evolve from an earlier (MDS) or myelodysplastic/myeloproliferative disorder (MDS/MPD). The significance of morphologic multilineage dysplasia independent of the cytogenetic abnormalities common to AML has long been debated, leading to the changes in the new classification to "AML with myelodysplasia-related changes." The category now includes patients with any of the following: (1) AML arising from a previous MDS or MDS/MPD, (2) AML with a specific MDS-associated cytogenetic abnormality, and/or (3) AML with multilineage dysplasia. Cases may meet any one or all three of the defining criteria but should not have a history of prior

---

Box 2
Criteria for diagnosis of AML-MRC

1. Greater than 20% blasts in the blood or bone marrow

2. No history of prior cytotoxic therapy for other disease

3. Absence of a chromosomal rearrangement recognized as a recurrent genetic abnormality

   and one or more of the following features:

1. Previous history of MDS or MDS/MPD

2. Multilineage dysplasia (dyspoiesis in at least 50% of the elements from two or more lineages)

3. Presence of an MDS-associated cytogenetic abnormality, defined as the following:

   -Complex karyotype (three or more unrelated abnormalities)

   -Unbalanced abnormalities

      -7/del(7q)

      -5/del(5q)

      i(17q)/t(17p)

      -13/del(13q)

      del(11q)

      del(12p)/t(12p)

      del(9q)

      idic(X)(q13)

   -Balanced abnormalities

      t(11;16)(q23;p13.3)

      t(3;21)(q26.2;q22.1)

      t(1;3)(p36.3;q21.1)

      t(2;11)(p21;q23)

      t(5;12)(q33;p12)

      t(5;7)(q33;q11.2)

      t(5;17)(q33;p13)

      t(5;10)(q33;q21)

      t(3;5)(q25;q34)

---

cytotoxic therapy and should not have one of the recurring cytogenetic abnormalities of AML with recurrent genetic abnormalities.

AML-MRC is more common in elderly patients. The diagnosis of AML-MRC may approach 50% of cases of adult AML with the new definition. Although it is reportedly rare in children, more children are likely to be recognized as having AML-MRC, given the cytogenetic criteria.[3,39,40]

The blast count must be 20% or more in the blood or marrow. The morphologic criteria for AML-MRC are similar to the 2001 WHO descriptions for multilineage dysplasia (evidence of dysplasia in 50% or more of developing cells in two or more lineages) (**Fig. 12**). Blasts of AML may have FAB M2, M4, M5, M6, or M7 morphologies. Multilineage dysplasia is common to therapy-related AML and some of the AML with recurrent genetic abnormalities; these cases are excluded from the

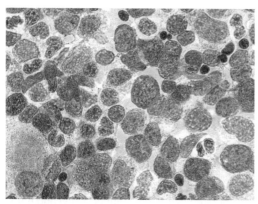

Fig. 12. AML with MDS-related changes. Blasts exceed 20% of all nucleated cells and are associated with multilineage dysplasia, evident here as a normoblast with nuclear budding, a small hypolobated megakaryocyte, and hypogranular mature neutrophils.

designation AML-MRC and classified as therapy-related AML or according to the recurrent cytogenetic abnormality.[1,4] The incorporation of MDS-associated cytogenetic abnormalities or the history of MDS, MDS/MPD as diagnostic criteria now allows correct classification of cases with high percentages of blasts and only minimal discernible evidence of multilineage dysplasia. These changes also help distinguish AML-MRC from AML-NOS, acute erythroleukemia or AML-NOS, AMkL in many cases, many of which are not classified as AML-MRC, allowing for a more prognostically meaningful classification.

Consistent with the varied blast morphologies, no consistent immunophenotype is found in AML-MRC. Aberrant expression of CD7, CD10, and CD56 may occur. The frequent morphologic monocytic differentiation is reflected in common expression of CD4 and CD14. Cases with abnormalities of chromosomes 5 and 7 may show "aberrant" expression of TdT and CD7 along with CD34.

MDS-associated chromosomal abnormalities are commonly high-risk changes. The complex karyotype, defined as three or more unrelated clonal abnormalities, is universally considered unfavorable. Unbalanced structural abnormalities leading to a loss of genetic material are the most common aberrations. Monosomy 7 has long been recognized as a high-risk subtype of pediatric AML.[25] Although trisomy 8, del(20q), and loss of chromosome Y are each common in MDS, they are not considered sufficient in isolation for a diagnosis of AML-MRC. Autosomal monosomies are now recognized to be particularly deleterious. Recent data suggest that autosomal monosomies are a better marker of poor prognosis than complex karyotype alone.[41] The "monosomal karyotype" is defined as either two autosomal monosomies in the karyotype or one autosomal monosomy in the presence of one or more structural chromosomal abnormalities (excluding core-binding factor abnormalities). It appears that most AML cases with the "monosomal karyotype" would be grouped with AML-MRC because they almost all have complex karyotypes, but not all cases of AML with complex karyotypes have the "monosomal karyotype". In this one study at least, the monosomal karyotype patients have a worse prognosis than those with a complex karyotype, nonmonosomal. Monosomy 7 appears to be most frequent, but the dismal prognosis seems to be independent of which particular autosomal chromosome was monosomic. Potentially, some patients with the monosomal karyotype not including -7, -5, or -13 and not harboring three or more of the defining cytogenetic abnormalities of AML-MRC would not be captured in the diagnostic category of AML-MRC. Some might harbor a recurrent genetic abnormality, such as inv3 or t(6;9), already recognized as poor prognosis. It is not yet clear how many patients with a monosomal karyotype would potentially be classified as having AML-NOS, but this number is likely small.

All of the nine balanced cytogenetic rearrangements of AML-MRC are also seen in therapy-related myeloid proliferations. If a history of cytotoxic therapy for another neoplasm is present, the case should be diagnosed as therapy-related AML and not AML-MRC.[4] Four of the nine rearrangements involve 5q33, often with activation of the platelet-derived growth factor receptor B (PDGFRB) at that locus. Imatinib is approved for treatment of MDS and chronic myelomonocytic leukemia with translocations involving 5q33, but efficacy in AML-MRC with this rearrangement is unclear.[42] Two rearrangements involve the MLL locus at 11q23, and they should be diagnosed as AML-MRC (MDS-associated cytogenetic abnormality) and not AML with 11q23 rearrangement (which is now restricted to t[9;11]). Two rearrangements involve 3q26 (EVI1 locus) and 3q21 (RPN1 and GATA2 loci); both are involved in the recurrent genetic abnormality AML with inv(3) or t(3;3).[1,43] The MDS-associated rearrangement t(3;5)(q25;q35) NPM/MLF1 cases of AML-MRC occur in young patients (third and fourth decades of life) and may show a male predominance. In addition to multilineage dysplasia, there is often an erythroid hyperplasia that may fulfill criteria for acute erythroid leukemia; cases should not be classified as AML-NOS or acute erythroleukemia because this is a less clinically relevant diagnosis. Auer rods are frequently seen with the genetic abnormality, even in the cases of MDS with lower blast cell counts. The morphologic and immunophenotypic features of these cases are otherwise nonspecific. Although early studies of this leukemia type suggested a poor prognosis, recent studies suggest a more favorable prognosis with allo-SCT.

Multilineage dysplasia may not be detected in up to half of the cases with MDS-associated cytogenetic abnormalities. It has been observed that patients with MDS-associated cytogenetic abnormalities have a worse prognosis than those with multilineage dysplasia lacking the cytogenetic abnormalities.[3] The morphologic designation seems to be useful; however, patients with a normal or intermediate-risk karyotype and multilineage dysplasia have worse outcomes compared with AML-NOS.[39]

Some patients with AML-MRC characterized by multilineage dysplasia may have normal cytogenetic findings or a cytogenetic abnormality not related to the AML-MRC category or recurrent genetic abnormality diagnosis. These patients may have mutations of FLT3, NPM1, or CEBPA that may affect their prognosis. The presence of these mutations, in addition to the designation of AML-MRC (multilineage dysplasia), should be included in the diagnosis.

The prognosis of AML-MRC is typically unfavorable. In patients with lower blast counts and multilineage dysplasia (20%–29% blasts), disease progression may behave more like MDS; this is especially true in children, who show a slower course of disease progression. Patients with MDS-associated cytogenetic abnormalities have a more consistently poor prognosis, especially those with a monosomal karyotype.[3,25,41] Patients with normal cytogenetic findings, mutated NPM1, and wild type FLT3 may have a more favorable course, although the data on this combination of mutations in this category are limited. Some larger studies of these gene mutations in cytogenetically normal AML included small numbers of patients with secondary AML, although the analyses did not account for these patients separately.[31] The basis for categorization as AML-MRC should be stated in the diagnosis, eg, "AML with myelodysplasia-related changes (multilineage dysplasia and myelodysplasia-associated cytogenetic abnormality)," as should the presence of gene mutations in *NPM1*, *CEBPA,* or *FLT3*. The blast count should be clearly stated in the report so that patients with lower blast counts may be closely followed for progression.

THERAPY-RELATED MYELOID NEOPLASMS

Therapy-related AML and MDS (t-AML/MDS) remain in a separate category, with the additional recognition of myelodysplastic/myeloproliferative overlap syndromes that can occur after cytotoxic therapy. t-AML/MDS are no longer subtyped by causative agent (alkylating therapy vs topoisomerase II inhibitors), because numerous agents are now implicated and many patients receive combination therapy.[4] Therapy-related myeloid neoplasms comprise roughly 10% of AML and 20% of MDS cases. The incidence is increasing as more patients survive cancer.[44] Given the impossibility of distinguishing the natural evolution of an MPD to AML from therapy-related development of AML in this setting, this scenario is excluded from this category of disease.

The longer latency cases (5–7 years after therapy) are classically associated with alkylating agents. They usually present with MDS with typical cytopenias and morphologic multilineage dysplasia. The bone marrow may be hypercellular, normocellular, or hypocellular, and may have associated fibrosis. Blast counts are variable; approximately half of the t-MDS patients will have fewer than 5% blasts. Some patients will have features of a myelodysplastic/myeloproliferative overlap disorder, hence the expansion of this disease category to "therapy-related myeloid neoplasms." No specific immunophenotypic profile is associated with therapy-related disease. Aberrant CD7 and CD56 expression can be seen, similar to AML-MRC. Longer latency cases are commonly associated with chromosomal losses, often of chromosomes 5 and 7, in a setting of a complex karyotype, similar to AML-MRC.

Shorter latency cases arise 1 to 3 years after therapy and comprise 20% to 30% of t-AML/MDS. These cases are usually associated with topoisomerase II inhibitor therapy and often have chromosomal translocations involving the *MLL* gene at 11q23 or *RUNX1* at 21q22. The morphologic features are similar to de novo AML, with frequent FAB morphologic subtypes of M2, M4, and M5 AML, with or without multilineage dysplasia. Some patients may have karyotypic changes identical to de novo AML, including favorable prognosis core-binding factor leukemias or acute promyelocytic leukemia. In contrast to the dismal prognosis of most t-AML, cases with t(15;17) or inv(16) may behave more similarly to their de novo counterparts.

The prognosis of therapy-related myeloid neoplasms is poor in general, with overall survival reported at less than 10%. Patients with monosomy 5 and/or 7 karyotypes have a particularly dismal prognosis, with a median survival of less than 1 year, regardless of the blast percentage.[4] Treatment is limited by toxicities of prior treatment and drug resistance mechanisms in the neoplastic cells. *FLT3* mutations have been observed in t-AML, but their contribution to prognosis is unknown. There are few data on *NPM1* or *CEBPA* mutations in t-AML/MDS. Intensive and low-dose chemotherapy regimens have been tried with variable success. Treatment-related mortality is very high for intensive therapy. Allo-SCT may be the patient's best chance for a cure, but with significant short- and long-term mortality.[44,45]

ACUTE MYELOID LEUKEMIA, NOT OTHERWISE SPECIFIED

FAB-like terminology is retained for morphologic description of cases lacking a recognized recurrent genetic abnormality, criteria for AML-MRC, a history of prior therapy, or Down syndrome.[2] The epidemiology and clinical prognosis of these categories in the modern classification is unknown, because good and poor prognostic groups have been removed from the earlier, more expansive FAB categories.

Minimally differentiated AML is an acute leukemia with uniform blast cells without cytoplasmic granules, with no Auer rods, and negative blast cell cytochemical reactions for MPO, Sudan black B, and nonspecific esterase (NSE). The blast cell lineage is only recognizable by immunophenotyping methods, which usually show the blast cells to be CD13 and CD33 positive, and some may be MPO positive by immunophenotyping. The blasts should not express lymphoid specific antigens but may be TdT positive. Without immunophenotyping, these cases may be misdiagnosed as ALL based on the negative cytochemical reactions.

AMLs that are MPO positive and NSE negative by cytochemistry that show less than 10% bone marrow cells with maturation to or beyond the promyelocyte level of differentiation are designated AML-NOS without maturation. AML-NOS with maturation is defined as cytochemically similar to AML without maturation, but with 10% or more bone marrow cells showing maturation to or beyond the promyelocyte level.

Acute myelomonocytic leukemia consists of a blast cell proliferation with folded nuclei, and some blast cells may have cytoplasmic granules and Auer rods. A subset of the blast cells are MPO positive, but the strong positivity of virtually all cells seen in the microgranular variant of APL, which may mimic AML-NOS and acute myelomonocytic leukemia, is not usually present. The blast cells of acute myelomonocytic leukemia are also NSE positive, reflecting monocytic differentiation, with 20% to 80% of bone marrow blast cells positive by definition. Double staining for chloroacetate esterase and NSE may show dual positive cells in some cases. Cases with abnormal eosinophils are excluded from the AML-NOS classification because the feature almost always correlates with AML with inv(16) or t(16;16).

When more than 80% of blast cells are NSE positive, a diagnosis of AML-NOS, acute monocytic, or monoblastic leukemia is made. These cases may be MPO negative but differ from minimally differentiated AML by their positivity for NSE. The blasts of acute monocytic or monoblastic leukemia have abundant, often agranular cytoplasm that may contain vacuoles. The blast nuclei may be round and uniform or folded. Cases with more immature nuclear feature in the bone marrow are termed acute monoblastic leukemia, whereas those with evidence of monocytoid maturation in the bone marrow are termed acute monocytic leukemia.

AML-NOS, erythroleukemia, or erythroid/myeloid leukemia of the WHO differs somewhat from FAB M6. One form is a myeloid blast cell proliferation that occurs in association with erythroid hyperplasia. By definition, erythroid precursors must represent 50% or more of the bone marrow cells, and blast cells are 20% or more of the non-erythroid elements for this diagnosis. Cases with very high bone marrow erythroid precursor numbers and low blast cell counts might be diagnosed as acute leukemia. Many of these cases are now more precisely classified as AML-MRC when total marrow blasts are 20% or more. Pure erythroid leukemia is a second type of acute erythroid leukemia in the WHO AML-NOS category. It is defined as a bone marrow proliferation of more than 80% neoplastic, immature erythroid cells without a significant myeloblast component. AML-NOS and AMkL are probably uncommon because it would not include AMkL with t(1;22), AML of Down syndrome, AML with inv(3) or t(3;3), or cases meeting criteria for AML-MRC. The WHO defines AMkL as an acute leukemia in which 50% or more of the blasts are of megakaryocytic lineage. The morphologic and immunophenotypic features are those of the megakaryoblasts described in the aforementioned entities, with detection of CD41 and CD61 expression being the most common means of defining megakaryocytic lineage. These cases are commonly associated with marked marrow fibrosis and a "dry tap," making diagnosis difficult in many cases.

The AML-NOS group includes acute basophilic leukemia, defined as an AML with differentiation to basophils. Whether this represents a distinct entity remains unclear, because some specific AML types are associated with basophilia and should not be placed in this category, such as t(9;22) AML, blast crisis of CML, t(6;9) AML, t(3;6) AML, and AMLs with 12p abnormalities. In addition, cases of AML with the abnormal eosinophils of inv(16) and cases of mast cell leukemia may be mistaken for basophilic leukemias. The true entity of acute basophilic leukemia is likely rare. Every attempt should be made to diagnose cases with increased basophils or basophil-like cells into more specific disease categories.

Acute panmyelosis with myelofibrosis is defined by the WHO as an acute panmyeloid proliferation with accompanying bone marrow fibrosis. Similar features are seen in fibrotic phases of chronic myeloproliferative neoplasms and in AMkL, and such designations should be used when appropriate. Acute panmyelosis with myelofibrosis should only be diagnosed in mixed proliferations of myeloid, erythroid, and megakaryocytic precursors without a history of a chronic myeloproliferative neoplasm or that meet the criteria for AML-MRC.

Myeloid sarcoma is its own diagnostic category in the WHO 2008 classification, defined as an extramedullary proliferation of myeloid blasts. Correlation with cytogenetics and molecular genetic status is essential to provide the most clinically meaningful diagnosis, because extramedullary presentations of AML with t(8;21), inv(16), t(1;22), and some 11q23 translocations are not uncommon.

REFERENCES

1. Arber DA, Brunning RD, LeBeau MM, et al. Acute myeloid leukaemia with recurrent genetic abnormalities. In: Swerdlow SH, Campo E, Harris NL, et al, editors. WHO classification of tumours of haematopoietic and lymphoid tissues. 4th edition. Lyon: IARC Press; 2008. p. 110–23.

2. Arber DA, Brunning RD, Orazi A, et al. Acute myeloid leukaemia, not otherwise specified. In: Swerdlow SH, Campo E, Harris NL, et al, editors. WHO classification of tumours of haematopoietic and lymphoid tissues. 4th edition. Lyon: IARC Press; 2008. p. 130–9.

3. Arber DA, Brunning RD, Orazi A, et al. Acute myeloid leukaemia with myelodysplasia-related changes. In: Swerdlow SH, Campo E, Harris NL, et al, editors. WHO classification of tumours of haematopoietic and lymphoid tissues. 4th edition. Lyon: IARC Press; 2008. p. 124–9.

4. Vardiman JW, Arber DA, Brunning RD, et al. Therapy-related myeloid neoplasms. In: Swerdlow SH, Campo E, Harris NL, et al, editors. WHO classification of tumours of haematopoietic and lymphoid tissues. 4th edition. Lyon: IARC Press; 2008. p. 127–9.

5. Baumann I, Niemeyer CM, Brunning RD, et al. Myeloid proliferations related to Down syndrome. In: Swerdlow SH, Campo E, Harris NL, et al, editors. WHO classification of tumours of haematopoietic and lymphoid tissues. Lyon: IARC Press; 2008. p. 142–4.

6. Lowenberg B. Acute myeloid leukemia: the challenge of capturing disease variety. Hematology Am Soc Hematol Educ Program 2008;2008:1–11.

7. Paschka P. Core binding factor acute myeloid leukemia. Semin Oncol 2008;35: 410–7.

8. Boissel N, Leroy H, Brethon B, et al. Incidence and prognostic impact of c-Kit, FLT3, and Ras gene mutations in core binding factor acute myeloid leukemia (CBF-AML). Leukemia 2006;20:965–70.
9. Goemans BF, Zwaan CM, Miller M, et al. Mutations in KIT and RAS are frequent events in pediatric core-binding factor acute myeloid leukemia. Leukemia 2005; 19:1536–42.
10. Shimada A, Taki T, Kubota C, et al. N822 mutation of KIT gene was frequent in pediatric acute myeloid leukemia patients with t(8;21) in Japan: a study of the Japanese childhood AML cooperative study group. Leukemia 2007;21:2218–9.
11. Gale RE, Hills R, Pizzey AR, et al. Relationship between FLT3 mutation status, biologic characteristics, and response to targeted therapy in acute promyelocytic leukemia. Blood 2005;106:3768–76.
12. Lo-Coco F, Ammatuna E, Montesinos P, et al. Acute promyelocytic leukemia: recent advances in diagnosis and management. Semin Oncol 2008;35:401–9.
13. Sainty D, Liso V, Cantu-Rajnoldi A, et al. A new morphologic classification system for acute promyelocytic leukemia distinguishes cases with underlying PLZF/RARA gene rearrangements. Group Francais de Cytogenetique Hematologique, UK Cancer Cytogenetics Group and BIOMED 1 European Coomunity-Concerted Acion Molecular Cytogenetic Diagnosis in Haematological Malignancies. Blood 2000;96:1287–96.
14. Lin P, Hao S, Medeiros LJ, et al. Expression of CD2 in acute promyelocytic leukemia correlates with short form of PML-RARalpha transcripts and poorer prognosis. Am J Clin Pathol 2004;121:402–7.
15. Chen W, Rassidakis GZ, Li J, et al. High frequency of NPM1 gene mutations in acute myeloid leukemia with prominent nuclear invaginations ("cuplike" nuclei). Blood 2006;108:1783–4.
16. Kussick SJ, Stirewalt DL, Yi HS, et al. A distinctive nuclear morphology in acute myeloid leukemia is strongly associated with loss of HLA-DR expression and FLT3 internal tandem duplication. Leukemia 2004;18:1591–8.
17. Ito S, Ishida Y, Oyake T, et al. Clinical and biological significance of CD56 antigen expression in acute promyelocytic leukemia. Leuk Lymphoma 2004;45:1783–9.
18. Meyer C, Schneider B, Jakob S, et al. The MLL recombinome of acute leukemias. Leukemia 2006;20:777–84.
19. Shih LY, Liang DC, Fu JF, et al. Characterization of fusion partner genes in 114 patients with de novo acute myeloid leukemia and MLL rearrangement. Leukemia 2006;20:218–23.
20. Meshinchi S, Alonzo TA, Stirewalt DL, et al. Clinical implications of FLT3 mutations in pediatric AML. Blood 2006;108:3654–61.
21. Lugthart S, van Drunen E, van Norden Y, et al. High EVI1 levels predict adverse outcome in acute myeloid leukemia: prevalence of EVI1 overexpression and chromosome 3q26 abnormalities underestimated. Blood 2008;111:4329–37.
22. Alsabeh R, Brynes RK, Slovak ML, et al. Acute myeloid leukemia with t(6;9) (p23;q34): association with myelodysplasia, basophilia, and initial CD34 negative immunophenotype. Am J Clin Pathol 1997;107:430–7.
23. Chi Y, Lindgren V, Quigley S, et al. Acute myelogenous leukemia with t(6;9)(p23;q34) and marrow basophilia: an overview. Arch Pathol Lab Med 2008;132:1835–7.
24. Slovak ML, Gundacker H, Bloomfield CD, et al. A retrospective study of 69 patients with t(6;9)(p23;q34) AML emphasizes the need for a prospective, multi-center initiative for rare 'poor prognosis' myeloid malignancies. Leukemia 2006; 20:1295–7.

25. Hasle H, Alonzo TA, Auvrignon A, et al. Monosomy 7 and deletion 7q in children and adolescents with acute myeloid leukemia: an international retrospective study. Blood 2007;109:4641–7.
26. Weisser M, Haferlach C, Haferlach T, et al. Advanced age and high initial WBC influence the outcome of inv(3) (q21q26)/t(3;3) (q21;q26) positive AML. Leuk Lymphoma 2007;48:2145–51.
27. Bernstein J, Dastugue N, Haas OA, et al. Nineteen cases of the t(1;22)(p13;q13) acute megakaryblastic leukaemia of infants/children and a review of 39 cases: report from a t(1;22) study group. Leukemia 2000;14:216–8.
28. Hama A, Yagasaki H, Takahashi Y, et al. Acute megakaryoblastic leukaemia (AMKL) in children: a comparison of AMKL with and without Down syndrome. Br J Haematol 2008;140:552–61.
29. Athale UH, Kaste SC, Razzouk BI, et al. Skeletal manifestations of pediatric acute megakaryoblastic leukemia. J Pediatr Hematol Oncol 2002;24:561–5.
30. Gilliland DG. Molecular genetics of human leukemias: new insights into therapy. Semin Hematol 2002;39:6–11.
31. Schlenk RF, Dohner K, Krauter J, et al. Mutations and treatment outcome in cyto-genetically normal acute myeloid leukemia. N Engl J Med 2008;358:1909–18.
32. Baldus CD, Mrozek K, Marcucci G, et al. Clinical outcome of de novo acute myeloid leukaemia patients with normal cytogenetics is affected by molecular genetic alterations: a concise review. Br J Haematol 2007;137:387–400.
33. Rausei-Mills V, Chang KL, Gaal KK, et al. Aberrant expression of CD7 in myelo-blasts is highly associated with de novo acute myeloid leukemias with FLT3/ITD mutation. Am J Clin Pathol 2008;129:624–9.
34. Brown P, McIntyre E, Rau R, et al. The incidence and clinical significance of nucleophosmin mutations in childhood AML. Blood 2007;110:979–85.
35. Falini B, Mecucci C, Saglio G, et al. NPM1 mutations and cytoplasmic nucleo-phosmin are mutually exclusive of recurrent genetic abnormalities: a comparative analysis of 2562 patients with acute myeloid leukemia. Haematologica 2008;93:439–42.
36. Ho P, Alonzo TA, Gerbing R, et al. Prevalence and prognostic implications of CEBPA mutations in pediatric AML, 2009: a report from the Children's Oncology Group. Seattle (WA): Children's Oncology Group; 2009.
37. Leroy H, Roumier C, Huyghe P, et al. CEBPA point mutations in hematological malignancies. Leukemia 2005;19:329–34.
38. Liang DC, Shih LY, Huang CF, et al. CEBPalpha mutations in childhood acute myeloid leukemia. Leukemia 2005;19:410–4.
39. Weinberg OK, Seetharam M, Ren L, et al. Clinical characterization of acute myeloid leukemia with myelodysplasia-related changes as defined by the 2008 WHO classification system. Blood 2009;113(9):1906–8.
40. Raimondi SC, Chang MN, Ravindranath Y, et al. Chromosomal abnormalities in 478 children with acute myeloid leukemia: clinical characteristics and treatment outcome in a cooperative pediatric oncology group study-POG 8821. Blood 1999;94:3707–16.
41. Breems DA, Van Putten WL, De Greef GE, et al. Monosomal karyotype in acute myeloid leukemia: a better indicator of poor prognosis than a complex karyotype. J Clin Oncol 2008;26:4791–7.
42. Kantarjian H, O'Brien S, Cortes J, et al. Therapeutic advances in leukemia and myelodysplastic syndrome over the past 40 years. Cancer 2008;113:1933–52.
43. Lahortiga I, Vazquez I, Agirre X, et al. Molecular heterogeneity in AML/MDS patients with 3q21q26 rearrangements. Genes Chromosomes Cancer 2004;40:179–89.

44. Rund D, Ben-Yehuda D. Therapy-related leukemia and myelodysplasia: evolving concepts of pathogenesis and treatment. Hematology 2004;9:179–87.
45. Rund D, Krichevsky S, Bar-Cohen S, et al. Therapy-related leukemia: clinical characteristics and analysis of new molecular risk factors in 96 adult patients. Leukemia 2005;19:1919–28.

Acute Lymphoblastic Leukemia

Mihaela Onciu, MD

KEYWORDS

- Acute leukemia • Acute lymphoblastic leukemia
- Lymphoblastic lymphoma • Cytogenetics • Genes

Acute lymphoblastic leukemia (ALL) encompasses a group of lymphoid neoplasms that morphologically and immunophenotypically resemble B-lineage and T-lineage precursor cells. These neoplasms may present predominantly as a leukemic process, with extensive involvement of the bone marrow and peripheral blood or may be limited to tissue infiltration, with absent or only limited (less than 25%) bone marrow involvement. The latter cases are typically designated as lymphoblastic lymphomas (LBLs). ALL and LBLs appear to constitute a biologic continuum, although they may show distinct clinical features. The current World Health Organization Classification of hematopoietic neoplasms designates these disorders as B- or T-lymphoblastic leukemia/lymphoma.[1]

EPIDEMIOLOGY

Most ALL cases occur in children, with an incidence of 3 to 4/100,000 in patients 0 to 14 years of age and ~1/100,000 in patients older than 15 years, in the United States.[2] In children, ALLs represent 75% of all acute leukemias (which in turn represent 34% of all cancers in this age group), with a peak incidence at 2 to 5 years of age.[3] This percentage is much lower in adults, in whom acute myeloid leukemias (AMLs) and chronic lymphocytic leukemias are more common.[3,4] There is a slight male predominance in all age groups and a significant excess incidence among white children.[2]

ALL presents primarily as de novo disease, with only rare cases occurring as secondary neoplasms.[5] A variety of genetic and environmental factors have been related to ALL. It occurs with increased frequency in patients with Down syndrome, Bloom syndrome, neurofibromatosis type I, and ataxia-telangiectasia.[6] In addition, exposure in utero to ionizing radiation, pesticides, and solvents has also been related to an increased risk for childhood leukemia.[6] Leukemia-specific fusion genes or immunoglobulin (Ig) and clonal Ig gene rearrangements have been identified in neonatal spot (Guthrie) cards of patients who later developed ALL.[7,8]

Department of Pathology, St. Jude Children's Research Hospital, MS#250, 262 Danny Thomas Place, Memphis, TN 38105, USA
E-mail address: mihaela.onciu@stjude.org

Hematol Oncol Clin N Am 23 (2009) 655–674
doi:10.1016/j.hoc.2009.04.009
0889-8588/09/$ – see front matter © 2009 Elsevier Inc. All rights reserved.

hemonc.theclinics.com

CLINICAL PRESENTATION

The clinical onset of ALL is most often acute, although a small percentage of cases may evolve insidiously over several months.[9] The presenting symptoms and signs correlate with the leukemic cell burden and the degree of marrow replacement, leading to cytopenias. The most common symptoms include fever (caused by leukemia or a secondary infection secondary to neutropenia), fatigue and lethargy (as a result of anemia), bone and joint pain, and a bleeding diathesis (related to thrombocytopenia). Patients with precursor T-cell ALL/LBL often present with a mediastinal mass with or without associated pleural effusions, which may lead to respiratory distress and other signs of superior vena cava syndrome. Common extramedullary sites of involvement include lymph nodes, liver, spleen, and meninges, whereas less commonly, ALL may infiltrate orbital tissues, testes, tonsils, and adenoids. Rare patients presenting with B-LBL may show skin lesions of lymphadenopathy in the head and neck area or discrete bone lesions.[10] The most common laboratory abnormalities in ALL include anemia, thrombocytopenia, neutropenia, and leucopenia or leukocytosis, with hyperleukocytosis ($>100 \times 10^9$/L) present in approximately 15% of the pediatric patients.[9] Other common laboratory abnormalities include elevated serum uric acid and lactose dehydrogenase levels, correlating with the tumor burden and degree of tumor lysis.

PATHOLOGIC DIAGNOSIS
Morphology

The classic morphologic features of ALL have been well described in the literature and are best summarized by the categories outlined by the first classification of ALL, the French-American-British (FAB) system, which was based primarily on the microscopic appearance of the leukemic cells, as seen on Wright-Giemsa–stained smears.[11,12] The FAB classification outlined three morphologic groups of ALL, designated as L1, L2, and L3 (**Fig. 1**). Most commonly, ALL blasts are small to intermediate in size, with scanty cytoplasm, condensed nuclear chromatin, and indistinct or absent nucleoli (FAB L1 subtype). Less commonly, ALL cells may be larger, with moderate amounts of pale basophilic cytoplasm, finely dispersed nuclear chromatin, and prominent nucleoli (FAB L2 subtype). Very rarely, ALL may present as the FAB L3 subtype, which consists of large blasts, with abundant deeply basophilic and occasional vacuolated cytoplasm, coarsely clumped nuclear chromatin, and variably prominent nucleoli. Most of the cases presenting with this morphology are Burkitt lymphomas, a subtype of high-grade mature B-cell lymphoma. However, a small subset of precursor B-cell neoplasms, often associated with hypodiploidy, may also present with FAB L3 features (see **Fig. 1**).

When seen in hematoxylin and eosin-stained histologic sections of bone marrow biopsies and tissue infiltrates, the neoplastic lymphoblasts of ALL/LBL may show features that correspond to the FAB categories. The most characteristic appearance is that of a neoplasm with diffuse growth pattern, sometimes with a partial starry-sky appearance, expanding the interfollicular area in subtotally replaced lymphoid organs (such as lymph nodes or tonsils). The blasts are small, with finely granular chromatin and small pinpoint nucleoli. In rare cases, the blasts may have prominent nucleoli (such as in the L2 subtype) or may resemble large-cell lymphoma cells (see **Fig. 1**). Occasional cases of ALL may present with variable degrees of marrow necrosis or associated marrow fibrosis.[13]

Various morphologic variants of ALL have been described, none of which has prognostic significance. The leukemic blasts may contain vacuoles,[14] pale pink or

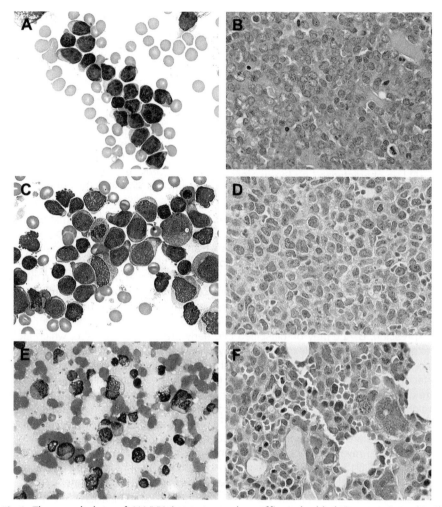

Fig. 1. The morphology of ALL/LBL in smears and paraffin-embedded tissue sections. (*A, B*) ALL L1. (*C–D*) ALL L2. (*E, F*) Morphologic findings in a case of precursor B-ALL with hypodip-loidy, resembling a high-grade, mature B-cell lymphoma (*A, C, E,* Wright-Giemsa stain) (*B, D, F,* hematoxylin-eosin; original magnification 60x oil immersion).

azurophilic granules ("granular ALL"),[15–17] or giant inclusions.[18,19] In some cases, the blasts may show eccentric cytoplasmic uropod-like projections ("hand-mirror cell ALL").[20] Some cases of ALL may show prominent associated eosinophilia (and even hypereosinophilic syndrome),[21] which relates to a specific genetic lesion (See later section).

Cytochemistry

Cytochemical staining has been used with decreasing frequency in the diagnosis of ALL due to the availability of immunophenotyping. The leukemic cells of ALL are uniformly negative for myeloperoxidase (MPO), Sudan Black-B, chloroacetate esterase, and nonspecific esterases.[22] A notable exception is that of granular ALL, which frequently shows nonspecific esterase staining localized to the granules and may also show light gray staining with Sudan Black-B.[1,23] The blasts of ALL are often (75%) positive for PAS and may also be positive for acid phosphatase, more frequently seen in T-cell ALL.[22]

Immunophenotype

Immunophenotypic studies are an essential component of the diagnostic workup of ALL/LBL. As opposed to the morphologic features, the lineage of ALL established in this manner subdivides this disease into two broad, clinically and biologically meaningful categories: precursor B-cell ALL (B-ALL) and precursor T-cell ALL (T-ALL).

B-ALL is characterized by the expression of a variety of B-cell–specific antigens, which often include PAX-5 (B-cell–specific activator protein), CD19, CD20, CD22 (surface and cytoplasmic), CD24, and CD79a (cytoplasmic). Notably, CD20, a marker of mature B cells, may be expressed only partially and weakly by the leukemic lymphoblasts or may be entirely negative in B-ALL. A large proportion of B-ALL also express CD10 (common acute lymphocytic leukemia antigen), an antigen consistently expressed by normal B-cell progenitors. Most B-ALL show dim expression of CD45 (leukocyte common antigen), and a subset of these leukemias, most common in children, may be CD45 negative. Other antigens often expressed by the leukemic blasts include progenitor markers often seen in early-stage B-cell precursors, including CD34 and terminal deoxynucleotidyl transferase (Tdt). Depending on their pattern of Ig expression, B-ALL may be classified into early pre-B (or pro-B) ALL, which lacks Ig expression, pre–B-ALL (expression of cytoplasmic μ chains, without Ig light chain expression or restriction), and transitional pre–B-ALL (with cytoplasmic and weak surface expression of μ chains, without Ig light chain expression or restriction).[1] Rare cases of precursor B-ALL may show surface expression of complete IgM with light chain restriction,[24,25] sometimes associated with other features of mature B cells (such as lack of CD34 and Tdt expression).[24] Such cases should be carefully differentiated from mature B-cell neoplasms. Most cases of B-ALL also show expression of one or several myeloid-associated antigens, most often CD13 and CD33 and less often CD11b, CD15, and CD66c. The pattern of immunophenotypic aberrancies correlates to some extent with the underlying genetic lesion in B-ALL (see later section).

T-ALL is characterized by expression of T-lineage–associated antigens (CD2, CD3, CD4, CD5, CD7, CD8) as well as CD1a, CD10, CD34, CD99, HLA-DR, and Tdt. The pattern of antigen expression may be used to subclassify T-ALLs according to the stages of normal thymocyte development that they resemble[1,26] (**Table 1**). A subset of T-ALL, typical of the cortical subtype, may show coexpression of weak CD79a.[27] Notably, some T-ALL/LBL may be negative for Tdt,[28] which may raise the differential diagnosis with mature T-cell lymphomas, particularly difficult in cases that are also

Table 1
Subclassification of T-ALL according to stages of normal thymocyte maturation

T-ALL Subtype	CD1a	CD2	cCD3	sCD3	CD4	CD5	CD7	CD8	CD34
Pro-T	−	−	+	−	−	−	+	−	+
Pre-T	−	+	+	−	−	±	−	−	±
Cortical T	+	+	+	−	+	±	+	+	−
Medullary T	−	+	+	+	±[a]	±	+	±	−

[a] Medullary stage T-ALL shows either CD4 or CD8 expression.

negative for HLA-DR and CD34. T-ALL may frequently express myeloid antigens, including CD11b, CD13, CD15, and CD33. Rare cases express CD117 (c-kit). This latter feature is seen most often in association with a recently described subset of T-ALL that appear to resemble early T-cell precursors recently migrated from the bone marrow to the thymus.[29] These genetically heterogeneous cases share a CD1a-, CD8-, CD5 weakly+, CD117+, CD34+, HLA-DR+, CD13+, CD33+, CD11b+, or CD65+ immunophenotype and appear to invariably correlate with a poor response to therapy, including remission induction failure and/or hematologic relapse. Therefore, an aggressive therapeutic approach, including hematopoietic stem cell transplantation, is warranted in these patients.

GENETICS OF ACUTE LYMPHOBLASTIC LEUKEMIA

Although relatively homogeneous at the morphologic and immunophenotypic level, ALL/LBLs show significant heterogeneity at the genetic level. Their genetic lesions define disease subsets with distinct biology and response to therapy and are used in the risk stratification schemas for most current treatment protocols.

Genetics of Precursor B-cell Acute Lymphoblastic Leukemia

Genetic Subgroups
B-ALLs include several cytogenetic subgroups with distinct biologic and pharmaco-logic features[1] that are very important in the current risk stratification of these patients. These subgroups account for ~60% to 80% of cases in children and adults and can be identified by conventional cytogenetics, molecular diagnostics (reverse transcrip-tase polymerase-chain reaction), flow cytometry (cell cycle analysis/DNA index),[9,30,31] and, currently in preclinial trials, gene expression profiling using oligonucleotide arrays. The remaining ALL cases are still characterized only on the basis of the morphologic and immunophenotypic features. Gene expression profiling studies have shown that these cytogenetic subgroups, although extensively overlapping in morphology and immunophenotype, have distinct gene expression signatures.[32,33] and in vitro sensitivities to drugs,[34–36] which correlate with different patterns of drug-metabolizing enzyme gene expression.[37] Genome-wide genetic analyses, using single nucleotide polymorphism arrays and genomic DNA sequencing, have found that these cytogenetic subgroups also contain distinct alterations in genes encoding principal regulators of B-lymphocyte development and differentiation.[38] These high-throughput methodologies have provided a starting point for a much more detailed molecular characterization of these genetic subgroups.[39–42] The clinicopathologic and molecular features of the main genetic subtypes of B-ALL are summarized in **Table 2**.

Genetics of T-cell Acute Lymphoblastic Leukemia

Although extensive molecular studies combined with gene expression profiling have uncovered a wealth of information regarding the molecular biology of T-ALL, none of this data is currently used in therapy decisions in this disease, likely due to the smaller numbers of cases available for evaluation in this less common form of ALL. However, since some of these genetic alterations appear to correlate with outcome, it is likely that at least some of them will enter the clinical realm in the near future.

Recurrent chromosomal abnormalities in T-ALL often include reciprocal transloca-tions that disrupt developmentally important transcription factor genes, as a result of rearrangements to loci for the T-cell receptor (*TCR*) genes, most commonly *TCRα* (14q11.2) and *TCRβ* (7q35). Common examples include the t(1;14) (p32;q11) (3% of

Table 2
Cytogenetic subtypes of precursor B-ALL and their clinicopathologic features

Cytogenetic Subgroup	Frequency (%)	Cytogenetic Abnormality	Fusion Gene	Unique Morphologic Features	Unique Immunophenotypic Features	Additional Molecular Abnormalities	Pharmacologic Features	Prognostic Category
Hyperdiploid ALL	27–29 (P) 6–8 (A)	51–65 chromosomes (+4, +14, +21, +X)	NA	NA	NA	Uncommon BCDG mutations (13%), FLT3 mutations (21%–25%)	Higher sensitivity to MTX, MP	Favorable/ low risk (P) Unfavorable (A)
ALL with t(12;21)	22–25 (P) 1–2 (A)	t(12;21) (p13;q22)	TEL/AML1 (ETVXI RUNX1)	NA	Early pre– B-ALL, My+	Monoallelic PAX5 deletions (28%)	Higher sensitivity to asparaginase	Favorable/ low risk (P)
ALL with t(1;19)	3–6 (P) 5–7 (A)	t(1;19) (q23;p13)	E2A (TCF3)/ PBX1	NA	Pre–B-ALL, CD34-/dim+, CD20-, CD9++	NA	NA	Standard risk (P) Unfavorable (A)
Philadelphia+ ALL	2–3 (P) 20–30 (A)	t(9;22) (q34;q11.2)	BCR/ABL (P190, P210)	ALL L1, sometimes granular blasts	NA	IKZF1 (Ikaros) deletions, BCDG mutations in 66%	NA	Unfavorable/ high risk (P,A)

ALL with t(v;11q23); MLL rearranged	2–3 (P) 5–7 (A)	t(4;11) (q21;q23) t(19;11) (p13;q23)	*AF4/MLL ENL/MLL*	NA	Early pre-B, CD10-, CD15+, sCD22-, CD65+, NG2+	FLT3 mutations (18%) Increased expression of *HOX* genes	Higher sensitivity to cytarabine	Unfavorable/ high risk (P,A)
Hypodiploid ALL	5%–6% (P) NA (A)	<46 chromosomes (typically near haploid or low hypodiploid)	NA	NA	NA	BCDG mutations in 100%	NA	Unfavorable/ High risk
ALL with eosinophilia	<1	t(5;14 q31;q32)	*IL3/IGH*	Increased dysplastic eosinophils	NA	NA	NA	NA

Abbreviations: A, % in adults; BCDG, B-cell development genes (eg, PAX5, EBF1, IKZF1, LEF1, TCF3, BLNK); FLT3, fms-related tyrosine kinase 3; MP, mercaptopurines; MTX, methotrexate; My, myeloid antigens; NA, not applicable, not known; P, % in pediatric patients.

cases), involving the TAL/SCL1 gene (1p32), the t(10;14) (q24;q11.2) disrupting the *HOX11* transcription factor gene (10q24),[43,44] the translocation t(5;14) (q35;q32), with rearrangements of the *HOX11L2* gene,[45,46] and the t(11;14) and t(7;11) involving the *LMO1*(11p15) and *LMO2*(11p13) oncogenes, respectively.[47] Less common translocations that do not involve the *TCR* genes include the t(9;17) and the t(10;11) (p12;q14), leading to the *AF10-CALM* fusion gene.[48,49] The latter is associated with a mature or immature TCR $\gamma\delta$ phenotype and in limited studies, is associated with a poor prognosis for the subset of patients with immature TCR $\gamma\delta$ leukemia.[50,51]

T-ALL may also harbor molecular lesions present without detectable cytogenetic abnormalities. Up to 50% of T-ALL contains activating mutations of *TAL1/SCL*, independent of detectable translocations. These mutations correlate with leukemias arrested at the late cortical stage of thymocyte maturation, which express TCR$\alpha\beta$, and appear to have an inferior prognosis.[52,53] Approximately 30% of T-ALL contain *HOX11(TLX1)*, more common in adults than in children. These cases correspond to an early cortical thymocyte phenotype expressing TCR$\alpha\beta$ and appear to have a superior survival.[52–54] *LYL1* mutations are present in up to 22% of pediatric T-ALL, and they correlate with the double-negative early thymocyte stage of differentiation[52] and with an inferior survival. *MLL* gene mutations are present in 4% to 8% of T-ALLs, are associated with maturation arrest at early thymocyte stages and expression of TCR$\gamma\delta$, and have no impact on prognosis.[53] Activating mutations of the *NOTCH1* gene are present in more than 50% of T-ALL.[55]

Limited studies have suggested a correlation between these genetic abnormalities present in T-ALL blasts and the patient age, possibly corresponding to different stages of thymic development and involution.[56]

Immunoglobulin and T-Cell Receptor Gene Rearrangements in Acute Lymphoblastic Leukemia

Rearrangements of *Ig* and/or *TCR* genes are present in most ALL/LBL. These rearrangements are not always lineage specific, as B-ALL may contain *TCR* rearrangements,[57,58] and T-ALL may contain *Ig* rearrangements,[59] possibly due to continuous recombinase activity in the malignant hematopoietic cells.[60]

Ig and TCR rearrangements in B-cell acute lymphoblastic leukemia

Most B-ALLs (97%) contain *IG* gene rearrangements, involving the heavy chain gene (*IgH*) (>95%), kappa light chain gene (*IgK*) (30%), or lambda light chain gene (*IgL*) (20%).[59] These rearrangements are often oligoclonal (multiple *IgH* rearrangements present in 30%–40%, multiple *IgK* rearrangements in 5%–10%).[61] B-ALL may also contain *TCR* rearrangements and/or deletions, involving the *TCR* β, γ, and/or δ genes (in 35%, 55%, and 90% of the cases, respectively).[58] These may be biclonal or oligoclonal (*TCRβ* in 3%, *TCRγ* in 10%).[59] The oligoclonality seen in these neoplasms may be due to continuing rearrangements[60] and secondary rearrangements, which may account for changes in patterns of *Ig* and *TCR* gene rearrangements often seen in B-ALL at relapse.[58]

Ig and TCR rearrangements in T-cell acute lymphoblastic leukemia

T-ALL/LBLs typically contain *TCR* gene rearrangements (95%–100%). A lower frequency is observed in rare pro-T ALLs, where *TCR* genes are in germline configuration in about 10% of the cases.[59] TCR$\alpha\beta$+ T-ALLs contain *TCRβ* (100%) and *TCRγ* (100%) gene rearrangements and have at least one deleted *TCRδ* allele, whereas deletion of the second allele is seen in 65% of the cases. TCR$\gamma\delta$+ T-ALLs have *TCRδ* and *TCRγ* rearrangements (100% of the cases for each) and typically also contain *TCRβ* rearrangements (95%). In contrast to B-ALL, lineage-inappropriate *Ig* gene rearrangements are encountered only in ~20% of T-ALL, typically as incomplete *IgH* (D_H-J_H) rearrangements. In addition, oligoclonality is seen only rarely in diagnostic T-ALL samples.[62] Relapsed T-ALL may show secondary *TCRγ* and *TCRβ* rearrangements in 15% to 20% of the cases.[62]

Differential Diagnosis

ALL/LBL may overlap morphologically and immunophenotypically with a variety of benign and malignant entities.

BENIGN PROLIFERATIONS

Expansions of benign B-cell precursors ("hematogones") and normal thymocytes may enter the differential diagnosis of B-ALL/LBL and T-ALL/LBL, respectively, due to their close morphologic and immunophenotypic resemblance to their neoplastic counterparts.

Benign precursor B cells (hematogones) are normal precursor B cells found primarily in the bone marrow but also in small numbers in extramedullary sites, such as peripheral blood, lymph nodes, and tonsils.[63–66] They may increase in numbers (sometimes to a significant proportion of the normal cells) in bone marrows from patients of any age but most often in children and young adults,[67] in a variety of reactive or regenerative conditions. These include viral infections and marrow recovery after infection, chemotherapy, and bone marrow transplantation.[67] Morphologically, hematogones include cells that resemble ALL L1-type lymphoblasts and immature and mature small lymphocytes. There is also an immunophenotypic range of maturation, which can be summarized in several distinct stages.[68,69] Typically, Stage I hematogones (CD34+, Tdt+ cells) represent a very minor component of the reactive hematogone expansions. However, in certain settings, especially recovery postchemotherapy, this subset may become more prominent (or even predominant), raising the differential diagnosis with recurrent leukemia.[70] Flow cytometric analysis is often essential for this distinction, as in most cases B-ALL will show immunophenotypic aberrancies not expected in benign hematogone expansions.[68]

Normal cortical thymocytes are important in the differential diagnosis of precursor T-ALL/LBL, in samples obtained from mediastinal lesions, which may contain normal or hyperplastic thymic cortex, in addition to neoplastic tissue, and from cervical lesions, which may contain ectopic thymic tissue or ectopic thymoma. The morphologic distinction is typically clear, primarily based on the presence of the characteristic thymic architecture and the more mature-appearing thymocyte features. However, significant overlap may occur at the immunophenotypic level. Therefore, findings of Tdt+, CD34+, and CD1a+ precursor T-cells on flow cytometry of mediastinal or cervical masses (especially in children and young adults) should always be correlated with the morphologic findings. Similar to hematogones, when examined immunophenotypically, normal thymocytes show a characteristic sequence of maturation, whereas T-ALL/LBLs show immunophenotypic aberrancies in all cases, which should be useful in the differential diagnosis.[68]

Malignant Neoplasms

A variety of malignant neoplasms with overlapping morphologic and immunophenotypic features may enter the differential diagnosis of ALL/LBL.

Other Blastic Hematopoietic Neoplasms may include AML, mixed-lineage leukemias, plasmacytoid dendritic cell (DC2) leukemias, and, especially in adults, blastic mantle cell lymphoma. *AML* may present as a tissue infiltrate (termed myeloid or monoblastic sarcoma) with or without an associated leukemic process and is often considered in the differential diagnosis of ALL/LBL, especially in cases with larger blasts and prominent nucleoli. In some cases, myeloid sarcoma may be associated with immature eosinophilic elements. Extensive immunophenotyping by flow cytometry typically allows for an easy distinction. However, in paraffin-embedded tissue samples, only a more limited panel of immunohistochemical markers can be applied, rendering this differential diagnosis more difficult. A panel of markers including those for MPO, lysozyme, Tdt, PAX5, and CD3 typically suffices. Notably, AML with t(8;21) may be occasionally challenging in this context, as it may express CD19, CD79a, and PAX5, in addition to MPO.[71] Tdt expression may also be encountered in other types of AML.[72] *Acute mixed-lineage leukemias* (particularly acute biphenotypic leukemias) may be considered in the differential diagnosis of ALL in cases expressing several myeloid antigens. Scoring systems devised for this purpose should be applied in such cases. *DC2 leukemia* is a rare type of leukemia (<1% of all leukemias)[73] thought to derive from a subtype of antigen-presenting cells, the plasmacytoid DC2 cells. Morphologically they may resemble ALL L2 or may show ample cytoplasm, with pseudopodia and cytoplasmic vacuoles lined along the cell outlines like a "string or pearls." The leukemic cells express CD4, CD56, HLA-DR, as well as the DC2-specific antigens CD123, BDCA-2, and BDCA-4. Some cases may express lymphoid and myeloid antigens of low specificity (such as CD2, CD22, Tdt, and CD33), but they are typically negative for other myeloid antigens, CD3, TCR, CD79a, and CD34.[73,74] At present, these leukemias are treated similar to ALL. *Blastic mantle cell lymphoma* may rarely enter the differential diagnosis of ALL/LBL. The characteristic immunophenotype of this lymphoma, CD5+, CD10-, CD20+, Tdt-, and cyclin D1+, should allow for easy differentiation.[75]

Burkitt lymphoma/leukemia

Typically, the distinction relies on the distinctive morphologic appearance of Burkitt lymphoma, combined with a mature B-cell immunophenotype, CD10+, CD20+, surface Ig positive with light chain restriction, CD34-, Tdt-, and negative for myeloid antigens. This distinction may be difficult in the setting of so-called "precursor B or atypical Burkitt lymphoma," which contains the classic Burkitt-associated chromosomal translocations but has immunophenotypic features closer to precursor B-cell neoplasms.[76,77] The immunophenotype includes features of precursor B cells (eg, expression of Tdt and CD34, dim CD20) and of mature B cells (surface IgM with light chain restriction). In the setting of such combinations of features, ALL should be diagnosed with caution, and findings should be correlated with cytogenetics, because in the presence of the t(8;14) or its variants, the patients are treated according to Burkitt lymphoma protocols.[77]

Peripheral T-Cell lymphoma

A variety of mature (or peripheral) T-cell lymphomas may present with leukemic involvement of the bone marrow and /or peripheral blood, which may morphologically mimic T-ALL. These include T-cell prolymphocytic leukemia, adult T-cell leukemia/lymphoma, Sézary syndrome, and rarely anaplastic large-cell lymphoma (ALCL).[78] The differential diagnosis depends on a combination of morphologic features, clinical presentation, and the finding of a mature T-cell immunophenotype in the latter lymphomas. Certain immunophenotypic features, such as expression of CD30 and the ALK protein, can also be used to exclude T-ALL. In this context, one should also remember that some mature T-cell lymphomas, especially ALCL, may express myeloid antigens, such as CD33, a feature typically associated with T-ALL.[79] Last, the presence of genetic lesions such as the t(2;5) for ALCL would further exclude ALL.

Non-hematopoietic neoplasms

A variety of blastic small blue-cell tumors of childhood may enter the differential diagnosis of ALL/LBL in the pediatric age group. *Ewing sarcoma* is the childhood nonhematopoietic neoplasm most likely to be considered in the differential diagnosis of LBL, especially in small samples. It is typically composed of small blastic cells without prominent nucleoli, which are CD45- and CD99+, similar to a subset of precursor B-cell ALL.[80] On further evaluation, Ewing sarcoma is always negative for B-lineage markers and Tdt, which should be included in diagnostic panels for small blue-cell tumors of children. *Merkel cell carcinoma*, most often seen in adults, may show immunophenotypic overlap with B-ALL/LBL, as both PAX-5 and Tdt expression have been reported in this tumor.[81,82] Notably, PAX-5 expression, although largely specific for B-lineage in hematopoietic neoplasms, may be seen in a variety of other nonhematopoietic tumors, such as neuroendocrine carcinomas, and a variety of other subtypes of carcinomas.[82–85] In all of these entities, correlation with clinical presentation and morphology and applying the appropriate panels of immunohistochemical stains allow for accurate distinction from ALL/LBL.

PROGNOSIS AND TREATMENT
Prognosis

The prognosis of ALL has improved dramatically over the past several decades as a result of adapting therapy to the level of risk for relapse, improvements in supportive care, and optimization of the existing chemotherapy drugs. The outcome of pediatric ALL has evolved from an overall survival of less than 10% in the 1960s to approximately 75% to 80% at present.[9] However, adult patients have a less optimistic outlook. The remission rates have reached 85% to 90%, with overall survival rates of only 40% to 50%.[86] About 75% of the patients present with poor risk features and have a disease-free survival of 25%, and only 25% present with standard risk features that confer disease-free survival greater than 50%.[30] ALL patients are stratified and treated according to algorithms that integrate the presenting features (patient age, leukocyte counts, the presence or absence of central nervous system [CNS], or testicular involvement), leukemia features (lineage, genetic subgroup), and of early therapy response (measuring the dynamic of disease clearance in the first 1–2 weeks of therapy).[9,30] Patients at low risk for relapse are treated primarily with antimetabolite therapy. Pediatric patients presenting with high-risk features or showing induction failure or persistent minimal residual disease (MRD) after the first 2 weeks of induction receive more aggressive therapy and are considered for allogeneic hematopoietic stem-cell transplantation. All the remaining cases are classified as standard risk for relapse and are treated with intensive multiagent chemotherapy regimens.

Therapy of acute lymphoblastic leukemia

In most centers, the treatment of ALL involves short-term intensive chemotherapy (with high-dose methotrexate, cytarabine, cyclophosphamide, dexamethasone or prednisone, vincristine, L-asparaginase, and/or an anthracyclin).[9,30] This is followed by intensification or consolidation therapy to eliminate residual leukemia, prevent or eradicate CNS leukemia, and ensure continuation of remission. Radiation may be used for patients showing evidence of CNS or testicular leukemia, although this approach is controversial at the current time, especially in children.[9] In adult patients, the use of growth factors such as granulocyte colony-stimulating factor that accelerate hematopoietic recovery has greatly improved the success rate of ALL therapy.[87]

Pharmacogenetics of acute lymphoblastic leukemia

Increasing numbers of pharmacogenetic studies have shown that germline polymorphisms and mutations present in ALL patients may affect the levels of expression and functionality of drug-metabolizing genes. They may lead to an increase in the likelihood of leukemia in their carriers, may influence the response of leukemic blasts to specific chemotherapy agents, and may also increase the probability of developing secondary (treatment-related) malignancies.[88,89] Such genes are those encoding for thiopurine methyltransferase, glutathione S-transferase, cytochrome P450 3A4, and methylene-tetrahydrofolate reductase. Furthermore, leukemic blasts with various chromosomal abnormalities (such as hyperdiploid ALL) and therefore additional copies of the wild-type genes for drug-metabolizing enzymes may differ from the somatic cells with respect to their production of these enzymes, leading to altered resistance to the related drugs.[90] Thus, chemotherapy regimens need to be tailored not only to the specific features of each acute leukemia but also to the patients' individual genetic background.

MINIMAL RESIDUAL DISEASE STUDIES IN ACUTE LYMPHOBLASTIC LEUKEMIA

The utility of MRD studies has been well documented in the management of children with ALL[91] and in further stratification of adults with standard-risk ALL.[92] They include several types of techniques that can detect amounts of residual leukemia that cannot be identified reliably using morphologic examination or conventional flow cytometry ("submicroscopic disease"). The technical approaches currently used for the detection and quantification of MRD include flow cytometry and molecular analysis (polymerase-chain reaction [PCR]) for leukemia-specific *Ig* and *TCR* gene rearrangements or fusion transcripts. Although generally there is good correlation between these methodologies in most cases, the use of both techniques is the ideal approach for adequate MRD monitoring in all patients.

Flow cytometric detection of MRD (FC-MRD) is based on the presence of an aberrant leukemia-associated immunophenotype, distinct from that of normal (benign) lymphoid precursors present in the bone marrow and peripheral blood. For T-ALL, the detection of cells coexpressing T-lineage antigens and Tdt or CD34 in peripheral blood or marrow is sufficient to support the presence of MRD, since normal T-cell precursors are not normally encountered outside the thymus. For B-ALL, the distinction is much more difficult, because, as previously discussed, normal precursor B cells (hematogones) can be encountered at all anatomic sites, and more refined analyses are required to differentiate these cells from leukemic B lymphoblasts. Additionally, benign progenitor cells occurring in the postchemotherapy or post-transplantation settings may have immunophenotypic features distinct from those encountered in reactive conditions. In addition, leukemic cells may show immunophenotypic shifts during therapy and between initial diagnosis and relapse.[93] These factors have to be considered when constructing panels of markers adequate for MRD monitoring and analyzing the data in this setting. Aberrant leukemia-associated immunophenotypes can be identified in 95% of pediatric ALL.[94,95] Markers typically included in FC-MRD panels include myeloid antigens commonly expressed in B-cell leukemia (e.g. CD13, CD15, CD33, CD65, CD66c) as well as markers often expressed inappropriately for stage of maturation in ALL (CD21, normally only coexpressed on mature B cells; CD38, lower than normal cells; CD58, higher than normal cells). The sensitivity of FC-MRD in routine clinical samples is typically 1 in 10^4 cells.[96] Under ideal experimental conditions and when leukemic cells have a very distinct immunophenotype and at least 1×10^7 cells are available, the sensitivity may be as high as 1 in 10^5 cells.[96]

Advantages of FC-MRD detection (as opposed to PCR) include the possibility of direct quantitation and that of excluding dying cells and cellular debris from analysis. Disadvantages include a lower sensitivity and the difficulties resulting from immunophenotypic shifts in the leukemic cells, with possible disappearance of some of the aberrancies used to identify MRD in a specific case.[96] FC-MRD detection can be applied in a different manner to peripheral blood and bone marrow samples, depending on the lineage of ALL.[97] In T-ALL, monitoring MRD levels using peripheral blood is an acceptable substitute for bone marrow samples, as the MRD levels at the two locations always match. For B-ALL, bone marrow residual disease may be found without peripheral blood involvement, and often the levels of MRD found in the bone marrow significantly exceed those found in the blood. The prognostic value of FC-MRD has been demonstrated in retrospective and prospective studies.[95] At the current time, it is hoped that high-throughput methodologies for genetic analysis in ALL will lead to the discovery of new leukemia-associated markers that can be used in FC-MRD studies.[95]

PCR for Ig or TCR gene rearrangements. If using PCR with consensus primers (including heteroduplex and GeneScan strategies), the detection limit of MRD is 1% to 5% depending on the number of polyclonal B- or T-lymphocytes present in the sample.[59] Since this sensitivity is comparable to the use of morphologic and immunophenotypic evaluation, alternative approaches have been employed. The sensitivity attained by using patient-specific, junctional region–specific oligonucleotide probes is more suitable for MRD detection. These probes are generated through sequencing of the junctional regions of the rearranged *Ig* and/or *TCR* genes found in the leukemic cells of each patient at the time of initial diagnosis.[98,99] They are then used in real-time quantitative PCR (RQ-PCR) assays in follow-up samples. Through this approach, the sensitivity of MRD detection has increased to 10^{-4} to 10^{-6} (ie, 1–100 leukemic cells among 10^6 normal cells).

PCR for leukemia-specific fusion transcripts. This methodology detects and quantifies fusion transcripts that correspond to the leukemia-associated translocations such as t(9;22), t(4;11), t(1;19), or t(12;21) (See **Table 2**), typically via reverse transcriptase RQ-PCR assays.[91] It can only be applied to less than 50% of ALLs, which contain such fusion genes. The sensitivity of this methodology is as high as 10^{-4}, depending of the amount and quality of the RNA available in the sample.[91,100] Due to its high sensitivity and lack of patient specificity, a major pitfall is related to false-positive results due to cross-contamination.[91] Although this modality appears to correlate well with the other two methodologies in most patients,[100] its use in the prediction of outcome in ALL remains to be established.[59]

RELAPSED ACUTE LYMPHOBLASTIC LEUKEMIA

The overall frequency of relapse in ALL is approximately 25% in children and 50% in adults, with a rate that is highly dependent on the immunophenotypic and genetic subtype or otherwise-defined risk category of ALL.[9,30,87] Recent insights have identified additional genetic predictors of relapse, such as deletions of the *IKZF1 (Ikaros)* gene.[101] The genetic subgroup also determines the characteristics of the relapse and the prognosis of these patients. For instance, relapse in patients with Philadelphia-positive ALL, representing approximately 10% of the relapsed ALL (rALL) in some studies, typically occurs following a short complete remission (CR) and correlates with an extremely poor prognosis, as a second CR cannot be induced in many of these patients. ALLs with *TEL/AML1* most often relapse following a long first CR, and a second CR is relatively easy to induce and maintain, often for long periods of time. Most ALLs relapse in the first 3 to 5 years from diagnosis. Only a very small percentage relapse more than 5 years from diagnosis, and relapses may occur 10 to 20 years later in a minority of patients.[102] rALL may involve the bone marrow or extramedullary tissues (most often at "sanctuary sites," such as CNS, testis, ovary) or both. The isolated bone marrow relapses appear to correlate with a less favorable prognosis than the isolated extramedullary or combined relapses.[9]

The morphologic and immunophenotypic features of rALL are often largely similar to those seen at the time of initial diagnosis. However, variable immunophenotypic shifts may also be observed, whereby some antigens (most often Tdt, CD10, HLA-DR, myeloid antigens) may increase or decrease in intensity or even be lost at relapse.[93,103] Such variations may be found in 34% to 73% of pediatric B-ALL and 15% of pediatric T-ALL.[93,103] The most extreme variations consist of lineage switch, from B-ALL to T-ALL, or from ALL to AML or biphenotypic leukemia. Conventional cytogenetics and molecular analysis typically identify the translocations and fusion transcripts present at the time of initial diagnosis. In addition, cytogenetic analysis often (75%) identifies newly acquired abnormalities.[22] Very rarely, an entirely different karyotype may be identified, suggesting the possibility of a second de novo ALL. Molecular studies document shifts in the pattern of *Ig* and *TCR* gene rearrangements and even acquisition of new fusion genes.[104] In rare cases (0.5%–1.5%), detailed molecular studies may support a new (second) ALL, distinct from the previous disease.[104] It appears that a combination of immunophenotypic and molecular studies may distinguish three categories of ALL relapse: rALL similar to the leukemia present at initial diagnosis, rALL clonally derived from the initial leukemia, and, rarely, a second de novo ALL.[104] Recent high-throughput genomic studies using SNP arrays and comparing diagnostic and relapse ALL samples correlate with these findings.[105] In these latter studies, a minority (8%) of rALL were similar to the initial diagnostic samples, a third (34%) were consistent with clonal evolution of the cells predominant at diagnosis, and half (52%) were shown to have derived by clonal evolution from minor clones present at the time of diagnosis that appeared to precede the dominant clones in the sequence of genetic lesions ("ancestral clones"). About 6% of rALL were completely genetically distinct from the diagnostic samples, suggesting *de novo* disease.

SUMMARY

Although relatively homogeneous at the morphologic and immunophenotypic level, ALL/LBLs encompass a family of extremely heterogeneous disorders when examined at the genetic level. This heterogeneity is reflected in the outcome of pediatric and adult patients in the context of contemporary therapies. High-throughput analysis methodologies have begun to characterize this heterogeneity and, although only in their early stages, have begun to uncover new clinically significant disease subsets, previously unidentified markers useful for MRD monitoring, mechanisms and predictors of disease relapse, germline polymorphisms important in individualized therapy, and new attractive therapeutic targets. These insights are likely to further improve the treatment outcome of patients with ALL.

REFERENCES

1. Swerdlow SH, Campo E, Harris NL, et al, editors. WHO classification of tumours of haematopoietic and lymphoid tissues. Lyon, France: IARCPress; 2008. p. 157–78.
2. National Cancer Institute. SEER Cancer Statistics Review, 1975–2006. Available at: http://seer.cancer.gov/csr/1975_2006/. Accessed January 23, 2009.

3. Gurney JG, Severson RK, Davis S, et al. Incidence of cancer in children in the United States. Sex-, race-, and 1-year age-specific rates by histologic type. Cancer 1995;75(8):2186–95.
4. American Cancer Society. Cancer facts and figures 2008. Available at: http://www.cancer.org. Accessed January 23, 2009.
5. Shivakumar R, Tan W, Wilding GE, et al. Biologic features and treatment outcome of secondary acute lymphoblastic leukemia–a review of 101 cases. Ann Oncol 2008;19(9):1634–8.
6. Spector LG, Ross JA, Robison LL, et al. Epidemiology and etiology. In: Pui CH, editor. Childhood leukemias. New York: Cambridge University Press; 2006. p. 48–66.
7. Gale KB, Ford AM, Repp R, et al. Backtracking leukemia to birth: identification of clonotypic gene fusion sequences in neonatal blood spots. Proc Natl Acad Sci U S A 1997;94(25):13950–4.
8. Taub JW, Konrad MA, Ge Y, et al. High frequency of leukemic clones in newborn screening blood samples of children with B-precursor acute lymphoblastic leukemia. Blood 2002;99(8):2992–6.
9. Pui CH. Acute lymphoblastic leukemia. In: Pui CH, editor. Childhood leukemias. New York: Cambridge University Press; 2006. p. 439–72.
10. Kahwash SB, Qualman SJ. Cutaneous lymphoblastic lymphoma in children: report of six cases with precursor B-cell lineage. Pediatr Dev Pathol 2002; 5(1):45–53.
11. Bennett JM, Catovsky D, Daniel MT, et al. Proposals for the classification of the acute leukaemias. French- American-British (FAB) co-operative group. Br J Haematol 1976;33(4):451–8.
12. Bennett JM, Catovsky D, Daniel MT, et al. The morphological classification of acute lymphoblastic leukaemia: concordance among observers and clinical correlations. Br J Haematol 1981;47(4):553–61.
13. Lorsbach RB, Onciu M, Behm FG. Bone marrow reticulin fiber deposition in pediatric patients with acute lymphoblastic leukemia. Mod Pathol 2002;15(1): 1048.
14. Lilleyman JS, Hann IM, Stevens RF, et al. Blast cell vacuoles in childhood lymphoblastic leukaemia. Br J Haematol 1988;70(2):183–6.
15. Darbyshire PJ, Lilleyman JS. Granular acute lymphoblastic leukaemia of childhood: a morphological phenomenon. J Clin Pathol 1987;40(3):251–3.
16. Dyment PG, Savage RA, McMahon JT. Anomalous azurophilic granules in acute lymphoblastic leukemia. Am J Pediatr Hematol Oncol 1982;4(2):207–11.
17. Stein P, Peiper S, Butler D, et al. Granular acute lymphoblastic leukemia. Am J Clin Pathol 1983;79(4):426–30.
18. Sharma S, Narayan S, Kaur M. Acute lymphoblastic leukaemia with giant intra-cytoplasmic inclusions–a case report. Indian J Pathol Microbiol 2000;43(4): 485–7.
19. Yanagihara ET, Naeim F, Gale RP, et al. Acute lymphoblastic leukemia with giant intracytoplasmic inclusions. Am J Clin Pathol 1980;74(3):345–9.
20. Schumacher HR, Champion JE, et al. Acute lymphoblastic leukemia–hand mirror variant. An analysis of a large group of patients. Am J Hematol 1979;7(1):11–7.
21. Horigome H, Sumazaki R, Iwasaki N, et al. Fatal eosinophilic heart disease in a child with neurofibromatosis-1 complicated by acute lymphoblastic leukemia. Heart Vessels 2005;20(3):120–2.
22. Brunning RD, McKenna RW. Acute leukemias. Tumors of the bone marrow. Washington, DC: Armed Forces Institute of Pathology; 1994. p. 100–36.

23. Cantu-Rajnoldi A, Invernizzi R, Biondi A, et al. Biological and clinical features of acute lymphoblastic leukaemia with cytoplasmic granules or inclusions: description of eight cases. Br J Haematol 1989;73(3):309–14.

24. Li S, Lew G. Is B-lineage acute lymphoblastic leukemia with a mature phenotype and I1 morphology a precursor B-lymphoblastic leukemia/lymphoma or Burkitt leukemia/lymphoma? Arch Pathol Lab Med 2003;127(10):1340–4.

25. Nelson BP, Treaba D, Goolsby C, et al. Surface immunoglobulin positive lymphoblastic leukemia in adults; a genetic spectrum. Leuk Lymphoma 2006;47(7):1352–9.

26. Bene MC, Castoldi G, Knapp W, et al. Proposals for the immunological classification of acute leukemias. European Group for the Immunological Characterization of Leukemias (EGIL). Leukemia 1995;9(10):1783–6.

27. Pilozzi E, Pulford K, Jones M, et al. Co-expression of CD79a (JCB117) and CD3 by lymphoblastic lymphoma. J Pathol 1998;186(2):140–3.

28. Faber J, Kantarjian H, Roberts MW, et al. Terminal deoxynucleotidyl transferase-negative acute lymphoblastic leukemia. Arch Pathol Lab Med 2000;124(1):92–7.

29. Coustan-Smith E, Mullighan CG, Onciu M, et al. Early T-cell precursor leukaemia: a subtype of very high-risk acute lymphoblastic leukaemia. Lancet Oncol 2009; 10:147–56.

30. Faderl S, Jeha S, Kantarjian HM. The biology and therapy of adult acute lymphoblastic leukemia. Cancer 2003;98(7):1337–54.

31. Mancini M, Scappaticci D, Cimino G, et al. A comprehensive genetic classification of adult acute lymphoblastic leukemia (ALL): analysis of the GIMEMA 0496 protocol. Blood 2005;105(9):3434–41.

32. Ross ME, Zhou X, Song G, et al. Classification of pediatric acute lymphoblastic leukemia by gene expression profiling. Blood 2003;102(8):2951–9.

33. Yeoh EJ, Ross ME, Shurtleff SA, et al. Classification, subtype discovery, and prediction of outcome in pediatric acute lymphoblastic leukemia by gene expression profiling. Cancer Cell 2002;1(2):133–43.

34. Pui CH, Campana D, Evans WE. Childhood acute lymphoblastic leukaemia–current status and future perspectives. Lancet Oncol 2001;2(10):597–607.

35. Ramakers-van Woerden NL, Pieters R, Loonen AH, et al. TEL/AML1 gene fusion is related to in vitro drug sensitivity for L-asparaginase in childhood acute lymphoblastic leukemia. Blood 2000;96(3):1094–9.

36. Stam RW, den Boer ML, Meijerink JP, et al. Differential mRNA expression of Ara-C-metabolizing enzymes explains Ara-C sensitivity in MLL gene-rearranged infant acute lymphoblastic leukemia. Blood 2003;101(4):1270–6.

37. Kager L, Cheok M, Yang W, et al. Folate pathway gene expression differs in subtypes of acute lymphoblastic leukemia and influences methotrexate pharmacodynamics. J Clin Invest 2005;115(1):110–7.

38. Mullighan CG, Goorha S, Radtke I, et al. Genome-wide analysis of genetic alterations in acute lymphoblastic leukaemia. Nature 2007;446(7137):758–64.

39. Armstrong SA, Staunton JE, Silverman LB, et al. MLL translocations specify a distinct gene expression profile that distinguishes a unique leukemia. Nat Genet 2002;30(1):41–7.

40. Armstrong SA, Mabon ME, Silverman LB, et al. FLT3 mutations in childhood acute lymphoblastic leukemia. Blood 2004;103(9):3544–6.

41. Mullighan CG, Miller CB, Radtke I, et al. BCR-ABL1 lymphoblastic leukaemia is characterized by the deletion of Ikaros. Nature 2008;453(7191):110–4.

42. Taketani T, Taki T, Sugita K, et al. FLT3 mutations in the activation loop of tyrosine kinase domain are frequently found in infant ALL with MLL rearrangements and pediatric ALL with hyperdiploidy. Blood 2004;103(3):1085–8.

43. Hatano M, Roberts CW, Minden M, et al. Deregulation of a homeobox gene, HOX11, by the t(10;14) in T cell leukemia. Science 1991;253(5015):79–82.

44. Kennedy MA, Gonzalez-Sarmiento R, Kees UR, et al. HOX11, a homeobox-containing T-cell oncogene on human chromosome 10q24. Proc Natl Acad Sci U S A 1991;88(20):8900–4.

45. Ballerini P, Blaise A, Busson-Le Coniat M, et al. HOX11L2 expression defines a clinical subtype of pediatric T-ALL associated with poor prognosis. Blood 2002;100(3):991–7.

46. Bernard OA, Busson-LeConiat M, Ballerini P, et al. A new recurrent and specific cryptic translocation, t(5;14) (q35;q32), is associated with expression of the Hox11L2 gene in T acute lymphoblastic leukemia. Leukemia 2001;15(10): 1495–504.

47. Valge-Archer V, Forster A, Rabbitts TH. The LMO1 and LDB1 proteins interact in human T cell acute leukaemia with the chromosomal translocation t(11;14) (p15;q11). Oncogene 1998;17(24):3199–202.

48. Carlson KM, Vignon C, Bohlander S, et al. Identification and molecular characterization of CALM/AF10 fusion products in T cell acute lymphoblastic leukemia and acute myeloid leukemia. Leukemia 2000;14(1):100–4.

49. Narita M, Shimizu K, Hayashi Y, et al. Consistent detection of CALM-AF10 chimaeric transcripts in haematological malignancies with t(10;11) (p13;q14) and identification of novel transcripts. Br J Haematol 1999; 105(4):928–37.

50. Asnafi V, Radford-Weiss I, Dastugue N, et al. CALM-AF10 is a common fusion transcript in T-ALL and is specific to the TCRgammadelta lineage. Blood 2003;102(3):1000–6.

51. Caudell D, Aplan PD. The role of CALM-AF10 gene fusion in acute leukemia. Leukemia 2008;22(4):678–85.

52. Ferrando AA, Neuberg DS, Staunton J, et al. Gene expression signatures define novel oncogenic pathways in T cell acute lymphoblastic leukemia. Cancer Cell 2002;1(1):75–87.

53. Graux C, Cools J, Michaux L, et al. Cytogenetics and molecular genetics of T-cell acute lymphoblastic leukemia: from thymocyte to lymphoblast. Leukemia 2006;20(9):1496–510.

54. Kees UR, Heerema NA, Kumar R, et al. Expression of HOX11 in childhood T-lineage acute lymphoblastic leukaemia can occur in the absence of cytogenetic aberration at 10q24: a study from the Children's Cancer Group (CCG). Leukemia 2003;17(5):887–93.

55. Weng AP, Ferrando AA, Lee W, et al. Activating mutations of NOTCH1 in human T cell acute lymphoblastic leukemia. Science 2004;306(5694):269–71.

56. Asnafi V, Beldjord K, Libura M, et al. Age-related phenotypic and oncogenic differences in T-cell acute lymphoblastic leukemias may reflect thymic atrophy. Blood 2004;104(13):4173–80.

57. Szczepanski T, Beishuizen A, Pongers-Willemse MJ, et al. Cross-lineage T cell receptor gene rearrangements occur in more than ninety percent of childhood precursor-B acute lymphoblastic leukemias: alternative PCR targets for detection of minimal residual disease. Leukemia 1999;13(2): 196–205.

58. van der Velden V, Bruggemann M, Hoogeveen PG, et al. TCRB gene rearrangements in childhood and adult precursor-B-ALL: frequency, applicability as MRD-PCR target, and stability between diagnosis and relapse. Leukemia 2004; 18(12):1971–80.

59. van Dongen JJ, Langerak AW. Immunoglobulin and T-cell receptor gene rearrangements. In: Pui CH, editor. Childhood leukemias. New York: Cambridge University Press; 2006. p. 210–34.

60. Breit TM, Verschuren MC, Wolvers-Tettero IL, et al. Human T cell leukemias with continuous V(D)J recombinase activity for TCR-delta gene deletion. J Immunol 1997;159(9):4341–9.

61. Beishuizen A, Hahlen K, Hagemeijer A, et al. Multiple rearranged immunoglobulin genes in childhood acute lymphoblastic leukemia of precursor B-cell origin. Leukemia 1991;5(8):657–67.

62. Szczepanski T, Willemse MJ, Brinkhof B, et al. Comparative analysis of Ig and TCR gene rearrangements at diagnosis and at relapse of childhood precursor-B-ALL provides improved strategies for selection of stable PCR targets for monitoring of minimal residual disease. Blood 2002;99(7): 2315–23.

63. Brady KA, Atwater SK, Lowell CA. Flow cytometric detection of CD10 (cALLA) on peripheral blood B lymphocytes of neonates. Br J Haematol 1999;107(4): 712–5.

64. Froehlich TW, Buchanan GR, Cornet JA, et al. Terminal deoxynucleotidyl transferase-containing cells in peripheral blood: implications for the surveillance of patients with lymphoblastic leukemia or lymphoma in remission. Blood 1981; 58(2):214–20.

65. Meru N, Jung A, Baumann I, et al. Expression of the recombination-activating genes in extrafollicular lymphocytes but no apparent reinduction in germinal center reactions in human tonsils. Blood 2002;99(2):531–7.

66. Onciu M, Lorsbach RB, Henry EC, et al. Terminal deoxynucleotidyl transferase-positive lymphoid cells in reactive lymph nodes from children with malignant tumors: incidence, distribution pattern, and immunophenotype in 26 patients. Am J Clin Pathol 2002;118(2):248–54.

67. McKenna RW, Washington LT, Aquino DB, et al. Immunophenotypic analysis of hematogones (B-lymphocyte precursors) in 662 consecutive bone marrow specimens by 4-color flow cytometry. Blood 2001;98(8):2498–507.

68. Kroft SH. Role of flow cytometry in pediatric hematopathology. Am J Clin Pathol 2004;122(Suppl):S19–32.

69. van Lochem EG, van der Velden V, Wind HK, et al. Immunophenotypic differentiation patterns of normal hematopoiesis in human bone marrow: reference patterns for age-related changes and disease-induced shifts. Cytometry B Clin Cytom 2004;60(1):1–13.

70. Dworzak MN, Fritsch G, Fleischer C, et al. Multiparameter phenotype mapping of normal and post-chemotherapy B lymphopoiesis in pediatric bone marrow. Leukemia 1997;11(8):1266–73.

71. Tiacci E, Pileri S, Orleth A, et al. PAX5 expression in acute leukemias: higher B-lineage specificity than CD79a and selective association with t(8;21)-acute myelogenous leukemia. Cancer Res 2004;64(20):7399–404.

72. Huh YO, Smith TL, Collins P, et al. Terminal deoxynucleotidyl transferase expression in acute myelogenous leukemia and myelodysplasia as determined by flow cytometry. Leuk Lymphoma 2000;37(3-4):319–31.

73. Rossi JG, Felice MS, Bernasconi AR, et al. Acute leukemia of dendritic cell lineage in childhood: incidence, biological characteristics and outcome. Leuk Lymphoma 2006;47(4):715–25.

74. Feuillard J, Jacob MC, Valensi F, et al. Clinical and biologic features of CD4(+)CD56(+) malignancies. Blood 2002;99(5):1556–63.

75. Chan NP, Ma ES, Wan TS, et al. The spectrum of acute lymphoblastic leukemia with mature B-cell phenotype. Leuk Res 2003;27(3):231–4.

76. Komrokji R, Lancet J, Felgar R, et al. Burkitt's leukemia with precursor B-cell immunophenotype and atypical morphology (atypical Burkitt's leukemia/lymphoma): case report and review of literature. Leuk Res 2003;27(6):561–6.

77. Navid F, Mosijczuk AD, Head DR, et al. Acute lymphoblastic leukemia with the (8;14) (q24;q32) translocation and FAB L3 morphology associated with a B-precursor immunophenotype: the Pediatric Oncology Group experience. Leukemia 1999;13(1):135–41.

78. Onciu M, Behm FG, Raimondi SC, et al. ALK-positive anaplastic large cell lymphoma with leukemic peripheral blood involvement is a clinicopathologic entity with an unfavorable prognosis. Report of three cases and review of the literature. Am J Clin Pathol 2003;120(4):617–25.

79. Juco J, Holden JT, Mann KP, et al. Immunophenotypic analysis of anaplastic large cell lymphoma by flow cytometry. Am J Clin Pathol 2003;119(2):205–12.

80. Ozdemirli M, Fanburg-Smith JC, Hartmann DP, et al. Differentiating lymphoblastic lymphoma and Ewing's sarcoma: lymphocyte markers and gene rearrangement. Mod Pathol 2001;14(11):1175–82.

81. Buresh CJ, Oliai BR, Miller RT. Reactivity with TdT in Merkel cell carcinoma: a potential diagnostic pitfall. Am J Clin Pathol 2008;129(6):894–8.

82. Dong HY, Liu W, Cohen P, et al. B-cell specific activation protein encoded by the PAX-5 gene is commonly expressed in merkel cell carcinoma and small cell carcinomas. Am J Surg Pathol 2005;29(5):687–92.

83. Denzinger S, Burger M, Hammerschmied CG, et al. Pax-5 protein expression in bladder cancer: a preliminary study that shows no correlation to grade, stage or clinical outcome. Pathology 2008;40(5):465–9.

84. Mhawech-Fauceglia P, Saxena R, Zhang S, et al. Pax-5 immunoexpression in various types of benign and malignant tumours: a high-throughput tissue microarray analysis. J Clin Pathol 2007;60(6):709–14.

85. Torlakovic E, Slipicevic A, Robinson C, et al. Pax-5 expression in nonhematopoietic tissues. Am J Clin Pathol 2006;126(5):798–804.

86. Gokbuget N, Hoelzer D. Treatment of adult acute lymphoblastic leukemia. Semin Hematol 2009;46(1):64–75.

87. Kantarjian H, Thomas D, O'Brien S, et al. Long-term follow-up results of hyperfractionated cyclophosphamide, vincristine, doxorubicin, and dexamethasone (Hyper-CVAD), a dose-intensive regimen, in adult acute lymphocytic leukemia. Cancer 2004;101(12):2788–801.

88. Pui CH, Relling MV, Evans WE. Role of pharmacogenomics and pharmacodynamics in the treatment of acute lymphoblastic leukaemia. Best Pract Res Clin Haematol 2002;15(4):741–56.

89. Yang JJ, Cheng C, Yang W, et al. Genome-wide interrogation of germline genetic variation associated with treatment response in childhood acute lymphoblastic leukemia. JAMA 2009;301(4):393–403.

90. Cheng Q, Yang W, Raimondi SC, et al. Karyotypic abnormalities create discordance of germline genotype and cancer cell phenotypes. Nat Genet 2005; 37(8):878–82.

91. Szczepanski T. Why and how to quantify minimal residual disease in acute lymphoblastic leukemia? Leukemia 2007;21(4):622–6.

92. Bruggemann M, Raff T, Flohr T, et al. Clinical significance of minimal residual disease quantification in adult patients with standard-risk acute lymphoblastic leukemia. Blood 2006;107(3):1116–23.

93. van Wering ER, Beishuizen A, Roeffen ET, et al. Immunophenotypic changes between diagnosis and relapse in childhood acute lymphoblastic leukemia. Leukemia 1995;9(9):1523–33.

94. Campana D. Determination of minimal residual disease in leukaemia patients. Br J Haematol 2003;121(6):823–38.

95. Campana D. Minimal residual disease in acute lymphoblastic leukemia. Semin Hematol 2009;46(1):100–6.

96. Campana D, Coustan-Smith E. Minimal residual disease studies by flow cytometry in acute leukemia. Acta Haematol 2004;112(1–2):8–15.

97. Coustan-Smith E, Sancho J, Hancock ML, et al. Use of peripheral blood instead of bone marrow to monitor residual disease in children with acute lymphoblastic leukemia. Blood 2002;100(7):2399–402.

98. Bruggemann M, van der Velden V, Raff T, et al. Rearranged T-cell receptor beta genes represent powerful targets for quantification of minimal residual disease in childhood and adult T-cell acute lymphoblastic leukemia. Leukemia 2004; 18(4):709–19.

99. Szczepanski T, van der Velden V, Raff T, et al. Comparative analysis of T-cell receptor gene rearrangements at diagnosis and relapse of T-cell acute lymphoblastic leukemia (T-ALL) shows high stability of clonal markers for monitoring of minimal residual disease and reveals the occurrence of second T-ALL. Leukemia 2003;17(11):2149–56.

100. Thorn I, Botling J, Hermansson M, et al. Monitoring minimal residual disease with flow cytometry, antigen-receptor gene rearrangements and fusion transcript quantification in Philadelphia-positive childhood acute lymphoblastic leukemia. Leuk Res 2009 Jan 19 [Epub ahead of print].

101. Mullighan CG, Su X, Zhang J, et al. Deletion of IKZF1 and Prognosis in Acute Lymphoblastic Leukemia. N Engl J Med 2009.

102. Lo NL, Cazzaniga G, Di Cataldo A, et al. Clonal stability in children with acute lymphoblastic leukemia (ALL) who relapsed five or more years after diagnosis. Leukemia 1999;13(2):190–5.

103. Chen W, Karandikar NJ, McKenna RW, et al. Stability of leukemia-associated immunophenotypes in precursor B-lymphoblastic leukemia/lymphoma: a single institution experience. Am J Clin Pathol 2007;127(1):39–46.

104. Zuna J, Cave H, Eckert C, et al. Childhood secondary ALL after ALL treatment. Leukemia 2007;21(7):1431–5.

105. Mullighan CG, Phillips LA, Su X, et al. Genomic analysis of the clonal origins of relapsed acute lymphoblastic leukemia. Science 2008;322(5906):1377–80.

The Myelodysplastic Syndromes

Phuong L. Nguyen, MD

KEYWORDS

- Myelodysplastic syndromes • Refractory anemia
- Refractory cytopenia • Ineffective hematopoiesis
- Bone marrow failure

The myelodysplastic syndromes (MDS) encompass a group of neoplastic hemato-poietic disorders that affect predominantly the elderly, typically manifest paradoxi-cally as peripheral blood cytopenia(s) despite bone marrow hypercellularity, and carry a variable probability of transformation into acute leukemia. There have been several attempts to classify MDS, with investigative efforts focused on prognostica-tion, delineation of molecular genetic aberrations, and identification of new thera-peutic options.

EPIDEMIOLOGY

The precise incidence of de novo MDS is not known, but among North American and western European populations, it is estimated to be approximately 3.3 to 4.5 per 100,000 individuals before adjustments for age.[1–3] In 2003, there were approximately 10,500 incident cases of MDS diagnosed in the United States.[4] MDS affect predom-inantly the elderly, with the median age at diagnosis in the seventh to eighth decade. They are uncommon in individuals younger than 50 years, among whom the annual incidence is estimated to be 0.5 per 100,000. This contrasts with the estimated annual incidences of 7.1 to 15 and greater than 20 for individuals between the age of 60 to 69 years and above 70 years, respectively.[1,5] With or without adjustments for age, MDS are diagnosed two to three times more frequently than acute myeloid leukemia (AML),[1–3] and the diagnosis of MDS among men is approximately two to three times more frequent than among women.[1,2] MDS are rare in the pediatric population; a discussion of childhood MDS is at the end of this article.

It is important to distinguish between de novo MDS, in which there are no known predisposing risk factors or exposures, and therapy-related MDS, which are associ-ated with well-documented earlier exposure to certain chemotherapeutic agents and/or ionizing radiation. A discussion of therapy-associated MDS is given at the end of this article.

Division of Hematopathology, Department of Laboratory Medicine and Pathology, Hilton 8-00C, Mayo Clinic, 200 First Street SW, Rochester, MN 55905, USA
E-mail address: nguyen.phuong@mayo.edu

Hematol Oncol Clin N Am 23 (2009) 675–691
doi:10.1016/j.hoc.2009.04.008
0889-8588/09/$ – see front matter © 2009 Elsevier Inc. All rights reserved.

CLINICAL PRESENTATION

The clinical manifestation of MDS is somewhat nonspecific and varies according to the MDS subtype. Thus, for the lowest-grade MDS, in which there are no increased blasts, patients may be asymptomatic, and the diagnosis of MDS is made during the course of an evaluation for other comorbid conditions, or the patient may present with symptoms related to anemia, such as fatigue and a decline of living activities. Patients with higher-grade MDS with increased blasts may present more acutely. Other symptoms related to neutropenia and thrombocytopenia may include frequent and unexplained infections and easy bruisability, respectively. Organomegaly in the form of hepatomegaly, splenomegaly, and lymphadenopathy is uncommon in MDS.

LABORATORY FINDINGS

Complete blood counts: Laboratory evaluation reveals in nearly all adult MDS patients a hypoproliferative anemia with an inadequate reticulocyte response. The anemia may be macro- or normocytic; less commonly, it may be microcytic. A neutropenia and/or a thrombocytopenia may accompany the anemia, with pancytopenia seen in approximately half of MDS patients.[6] An isolated neutropenia or thrombocytopenia is uncommon and is reported in less than 5% of adult MDS patients.

The presence of a neutrophilia, monocytosis, or thrombocytosis should introduce either the possibility of a hybrid myelodysplastic/myeloproliferative neoplasm or other possibilities such as infections or inflammations. There is, however, one exception: patients with MDS associated with isolated del(5q) may present with a normal or elevated platelet count.

Morphologic findings: Because morphologic assessment of cellular atypia is still an inexact art subject to interobserver variability, because preservation of cellular morphologic features is predicated on proper specimen handling and processing, including staining, and because some of the morphologic features of dysmyelopoiesis overlap with those seen in certain metabolic and nonmalignant hematologic disorders, the reader is cautioned to weigh carefully the qualitative abnormalities against the patient's clinical history and other laboratory results including cytogenetics, and to consider other possibilities in the differential diagnosis (**Box 1**), especially when the morphologic features are equivocal to minimal.

Red cell series: In some patients with MDS, especially those with ring sideroblasts, a dimorphic pattern may be seen in the blood smear where both a normochromic and a hypochromic population of erythrocytes may be observed. There is no poikilocytosis specific to MDS; the presence of schistocytes, spherocytes, or acanthocytes should thus raise a concern of other concomitant comorbidities. Similarly, because marked myelofibrosis is not characteristic of MDS, the presence of marked dacryocytes should at least introduce other diagnostic considerations.

In the bone marrow, morphologic features of dyserythropoiesis include nuclear/cytoplasmic asynchrony (so-called "megaloblastoid" changes), cytoplasmic vacuolization, bizarre multinucleation, irregular nuclear lobulations, and increased karyorrhexis (**Fig. 1**A). Ring sideroblasts, where five or more iron granules encircle at least one-third of the nuclear circumference,[7] may be present (see **Fig. 1**B). Maturation of the erythroid series may be left-shifted, but a complete maturational arrest is uncommon.

Granulocytic series: The blood may show circulating blasts, but the proportion does not reach 20%, in which case the diagnosis of acute leukemia is warranted. The presence of Auer rods does not preclude the diagnosis of MDS as long as there are fewer than 20% blasts in the blood and in the bone marrow.

Box 1
Differential diagnosis of MDS

Cytopenia(s)

Pancytopenia: Bone marrow failure syndromes; medication or toxic exposure (especially if onset is acute or subacute); hemophagocytic syndromes

Isolated anemia: MDS must be a diagnosis of exclusion

Isolated neutropenia: T-cell large granular lymphocytic leukemia; medication (eg, trimethoprim-sulfamethoxazole; ganciclovir; the cephalosporins) or toxic exposure; hypersplenism; autoimmune disorders; familial or cyclic neutropenia; ethnic variations; in the pediatric population, congenital neutropenia due to ELA2-, HAX1-, or G-CSF-receptor mutations

Isolated thrombocytopenia in adults: pseudothrombocytopenia; idiopathic thrombocytopenic purpura; hypersplenism

Combined neutropenia and thrombocytopenia with a relatively preserved hemoglobin level: hypersplenism

Dyseythropoiesis

Ring sideroblasts: alcohol; arsenic poisoning; zinc toxicity; copper deficiency; pyridoxine deficiency; hereditary sideroblastic anemia; antituberculosis medications; in the pediatric population, Pearson syndrome, and other mitochondrial cytopathies

Other morphologic features of dyserythropoiesis:

Severe hemolysis with brisk erythropoietic compensation

Congenital dyserythropoietic anemia

Deficiency of vitamin B12 and/or the covitamin folate

Medications: antimetabolites; valproic acid; azathioprine

Dysgranulopoiesis

Medications: trimethoprim-sulfamethoxazole; granulocyte- or granulocyte-macrophage colony-stimulating factor

Dysmegakaryopoiesis

Sectioning artifacts, if the abnormalities are seen only in biopsy

Megakaryocyte immaturity

Morphologic features of dysgranulopoiesis can be seen in either a blood or bone marrow aspirate smear and include cytoplasmic hypogranularity (**Fig. 2**A) and nuclear hyposegmentation (so-called "pseudo-Pelger-Huet" or "Pelgeroid" anomaly) (see **Fig. 2**C). Nuclear hypersegmentation is less common and should necessitate first and foremost a consideration of a deficiency of vitamin B12 or folate; when seen in MDS, the hypersegmented neutrophil is usually bizarre with abnormal chromatin bridging. In patients with MDS related to abnormalities involving 17p/p53, the neutrophils may be abnormally small with abnormally condensed and unilobed/unsegmented nuclei.[8] Chédiak-Higashi-type granulation abnormalities may also be seen.

The presence of cytologically abnormal monocytes or increased immature monocytic precursors,especially promonocytes, should prompt the consideration of a myelomonocytic neoplasm.

The proportions of circulating and medullary blasts form one of the cornerstones in the classification of MDS. In the latest World Health Organization (WHO) classification,

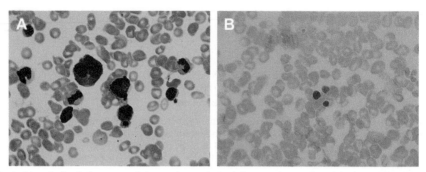

Fig. 1. Morphologic features of dyserythropoiesis. (*A*) Irregular nuclear lobulations in several erythroid precursors (Wright stain, original magnification ×1000). (*B*) Ring sideroblasts, where more than five iron granules encircle at least one-third of the nuclear circumference of two erythroid precursors (Dacie stain, original magnification ×1000).

besides the 20% cut-off that separates MDS from AML, the other critical separations lie at less than 1%, 1%, 2% to 4%, and 5% blasts in the blood, and 5% and 10% in the marrow (**Table 1**). Because of differences in prognoses and management decisions associated with these blast proportions, accurate manual differential counts of at least

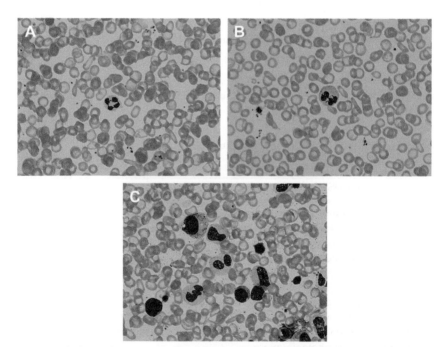

Fig. 2. Morphologic features of dysgranulopoiesis. (*A*) Cytoplasmic hypogranularity in a segmented neutrophil. (*B*) The normal content of cytoplasmic granulation in a segmented neutrophil seen elsewhere in the same blood smear excludes the possibility of poor staining as an explanation for the hypogranulation seen in *A*. (*C*) Nuclear hyposegmentation, so-called pseudo-Pelger-Huet or Pelgeroid anomaly in a mature neutrophil (Wright stain, original magnification ×1000).

200 cells and 500 cells in well-prepared and well-sampled blood and bone marrow aspirate smears, respectively, are crucial, with additional cells counted and/or additional sampling evaluated as necessary.[9] In particular, the International Working Group on Morphology of MDS recommends that a 500-cell manual differential count of a blood sample be performed in view of the reported differences in prognosis associated with such small differences in the proportion of circulating blasts.[7]

Platelets and megakaryocytic series: Dysplastic megakaryocytes may have hypolobated nuclei (**Fig. 3**A), or they may have abnormally disconnected nuclear lobes resembling those seen in osteoclasts (see **Fig. 3**B). The platelets themselves may be abnormally large and hypogranular. In MDS associated with isolated del(5q), the megakaryocytes are normal-sized, but the nuclei are characteristically hypolobated.

SPECIAL STUDIES

Iron stains are Prussian blue–based stains of bone marrow aspirate smears or of undecalcified clot sections that can be helpful in demonstrating ring sideroblasts.

Although mild reticulin fibrosis does not preclude the diagnosis of MDS, marked diffuse reticulin fibrosis is atypical and should introduce other diagnostic considerations, in addition to the MDS category of refractory anemia with excess blasts with fibrosis.

Immunohistochemical studies with antibodies directed against megakaryocytic lineage-associated antigens such as CD61 and factor VIII antigen can highlight abnormally small megakaryocytes that may be difficult to visualize otherwise on routine hematoxylin-and-eosin-stained biopsy sections. CD34 immunohistochemistry can be of help in enumerating CD34+ blasts when the bone marrow aspirate slide is hemodilute; it also enables one to determine the distribution of such CD34+ blasts, where a clustered distribution may portend focal/early blast proliferations.

Flow cytometry immunophenotyping is defined as abnormal gains or losses of lineage-specific antigenic expression or as altered (usually reduced) intensity of antigenic expression, flow cytometric immunophenotypic abnormalities affecting erythroid and myelomonocytic precursors have been detected in up to 90% to 95% of cases that are diagnosable as MDS by morphologic and/or cytogenetic criteria.[10–12] Such high degrees of correlation with morphology and cytogenetics have suggested a potential role for flow cytometric immunophenotyping analysis in the diagnosis of MDS. In particular, in situations where the morphologic findings are borderline and results of cytogenetic analysis are normal or noncontributory, it has been suggested that detection of three or more flow cytometric immunophenotypic abnormalities might be considered as "suggestive" of an MDS diagnosis.[13] Scoring systems advancing the diagnostic and prognostic value of flow cytometric immunophenotyping have also been put forth.[14] To date, however, the diagnosis of MDS remains one by morphology and/or cytogenetics, with contributions from flow cytometry immunophenotyping still under active investigation.

The role of flow cytometric immunophenotyping in enumerating blasts deserves a special note. The proportions of blood and marrow blasts as outlined in the various classification and prognostication systems are based upon manual differential counts derived during a morphologic/microscopic evaluation. In general, for blast enumeration, there are good agreements between flow cytometry immunophenotyping and the more traditional method of morphology-based manual differential counts. However, for a variety of legitimate reasons, discrepancies between the two methods are not uncommon and do occur. For example, the sample for flow cytometry is often collected after that for morphology and subject to hemodilution; further processing in

Table 1
Classifications of MDS

FAB	WHO-2001	WHO-2008	WHO-2008 Diagnostic Criteria
RA	RA	RCUD	
(n/a)	RA	RA	Anemia (Hb <10 g/dL); ± neutropenia or thrombocytopenia; <1% circulating blasts; <5% medullary blasts; unequivocal dyserythropoiesis in ≥10% erythroid precursors; dysgranulopoiesis and dysmegakaryopoiesis, if present, in <10% nucleated cells; <15% RS; no Auer rods
(n/a)	(n/a)	RN	Neutropenia (absolute neutrophil count <1.8 × 10⁹/L); ± anemia or thrombocytopenia; <1% circulating blasts; <5% medullary blasts; ≥10% dysplastic neutrophils; <10% dyserythropoiesis and dysmegakaryopoiesis; <15% RS; no Auer rods
(n/a)	(n/a)	RT	Thrombocytopenia (platelet count <100 × 10⁹/L); ± anemia or neutropenia; <1% circulating blasts; <5% medullary blasts; ≥10% dysplastic megakaryocytes of ≥30 megakaryocytes; <10% dyserythropoiesis and dysgranulopoiesis; <15% RS; no Auer rods
RARS	RARS	RARS	Anemia; no circulating blasts; <5% medullary blasts; dyserythropoiesis only, with RS among >15% of 100 erythroid precursors; no Auer rods
(n/a)	RCMD	RCMD	Cytopenia(s); <1 × 10⁹/L circulating monocytes; <1% circulating blasts; <5% medullary blasts; dysplasia among >10% cells of ≥2 lineages; no Auer rods
	and RS	(n/a)	(n/a)
RAEB	RAEB-1	RAEB-1	Cytopenia(s); <1 × 10⁹/L circulating monocytes ; <5% circulating blasts; 5%–9% medullary blasts; dysplasia involving ≥1 lineage(s); no Auer rods

(n/a)	RAEB-2	Cytopenia(s); <1 × 10⁹/L circulating monocytes; 5%–19% circulating blasts; 10%–19% medullary blasts; dysplasia involving ≥1 lineage(s); ± Auer rods
(n/a)	RAEB-F	Similar to RAEB-1 or RAEB-2, with at least bilineage dysplasia and with diffuse coarse reticulin fibrosis, with or without collagenous fibrosis
RAEB-T	(AML)	(n/a)
(n/a)	MDS, U	Pancytopenia; <1 × 10⁹/L circulating monocytes; ≤1% circulating blasts; <5% circulating blasts; dysplasia in <10% cells of ≥1 lineage(s); demonstration of MDS-associated chromosomal abnormality(ies), exclusive of +8, del(20q), and -Y
MDS, isolated del(5q)	MDS, isolated del(5q)	Anemia; platelet count may be normal or increased; <1% circulating blasts; <5% medullary blasts; megakaryocytes with characteristic nuclear hypolobulation; isolated del(5q) cytogenetic abnormality involving bands q31-q33
(MDS/MPN)	(MDS/MPN)	(n/a)
CMML	RCC	Thrombocytopenia, anemia, and/or neutropenia; <2% circulating blasts; <5% medullary blasts; unequivocal dysplasia in ≥2 lineages, or in >10% cells of one lineage; no RS
(n/a)	(n/a)	

Abbreviations: CMML, chronic myelomonocytic leukemia; MDS, U, myelodysplastic syndrome, unclassifiable; MPN, myeloproliferative neoplasm; n/a, not applicable; RAEB-F, refractory anemia with excess blasts with fibrosis; RAEB-T, refractory anemia with excess blasts in transformation; RCC, refractory cytopenia of childhood; RN, refractory neutropenia; RS, ring sideroblasts; RT, refractory thrombocytopenia.

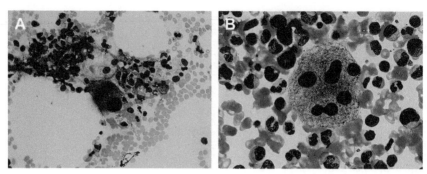

Fig. 3. Dysplastic megakaryocytes with (*A*) nuclear hypolobulation or (*B*) abnormally disconnected nuclear lobes, so-called "osteoclast-like" or "multinucleated" (Wright stain, original magnification ×1000).

the flow cytometry laboratory can selectively remove subpopulations of non-blast nucleated cells, thus lowering the denominator and elevating the final blast percentage. For these reasons, blast enumerations by flow cytometry may be used in the diagnosis and classification of MDS only exceptionally, when those obtained by manual differential counts are otherwise unavailable or unacceptable, and even then, only when there is no possibility of obtaining another blood and/or bone marrow sample for accurate diagnosis, subclassification, and prognostication.

Cytogenetics: Approximately 50% of patients with primary MDS have clonal chromosomal abnormalities, although this number varies according to the MDS subtypes, ranging from as low as none as detected by G-banded or fluorescence in situ hybridization (FISH) analysis in the very low-grade MDS subtype of refractory anemia to as high as 80% among MDS patients with increased blasts.[15–17]

Although the presence of a clonal chromosomal abnormality typically implies a neoplastic process and thus can aid in the diagnosis of MDS, it should be noted that certain abnormalities, such as trisomy 8, loss of chromosome Y, del(20q), and trisomy 15, when seen as sole abnormalities, do not necessarily or clinically indicate MDS, because patients with these particular abnormalities have shown no hematologic deficits on follow-up.[13,18] On the other hand, other abnormalities such as monosomy 7, del(7q), i(17q), and t(17p) are not only diagnostic of MDS, but they also portend poor prognosis. When present as an isolated abnormality, del(5)(q13q33) [and less commonly del(5)(q15q33) and del(5)(q22q33)] is associated with a good prognosis, with recent clinical trials demonstrating excellent clinical, hematologic, and cytogenetic responses to lenalidomide.[19] Cytogenetic analysis thus provides valuable diagnostic and prognostic information in the evaluation of patients with MDS, with cytogenetic results incorporated in virtually all recent prognostic scoring systems.

Molecular genetics: Advances in molecular genetics have uncovered genetic abnormalities previously undetectable by G-banded karyotypic analysis or by interphase FISH analysis. Thus, for example, by high-resolution single nucleotide polymorphism arrays, Gondek and colleagues[20,21] detected chromosomal defects in 78% of their MDS patients as compared with 59% by metaphase cytogenetics. Moreover, the additionally detected defects often involved a copy number-neutral loss of heterozygosity, consistent with the pattern of uniparental disomy described in other solid tumors.[22]

At an epigenetic level, DNA hypermethylation of genes involved in cell-cycle control and apoptosis, such as CDK1 p15INK4b and CDK1 p15INK4a, has been shown to be a common feature in high-risk MDS.[23,24] The reversibility of such silencing of transcriptional activity by DNA methylation is believed to account for the efficacy in MDS of demethylating agents such as 5-azacytidine and 5-aza-2'-deoxycytidine. Analogously, the role of acetylation and deacetylation of nucleosomal histones in the regulation of transcriptional activity may explain the efficacy of valproic acid, a histone deacetylase inhibitor, in subsets of MDS patients.[25]

In all, continued advances in the application of molecular genetic analysis to the study of MDS promise not only to shed further light on the pathogenesis of this family of disorders, but also to provide testable targets for future therapeutic strategies.

CLASSIFICATION

The earliest classification of MDS by the French-American-British (FAB) cooperative group recognized the importance of distinguishing those MDS with increased blasts versus those with fewer than 5% blasts (see **Table 1**).[26] However, in retrospect, there was insufficient distinction among those MDS without increased blasts, such that it was not possible in the FAB schema to separate a patient with only a refractory anemia and no other morphologic features of dysmyelopoiesis from another patient with bicytopenia and with morphologic features of dysgranulopoiesis, both patients with fewer than 5% blasts in the blood and bone marrow.

Building upon the FAB classification, the WHO published its classification of MDS in 2001 with 4 substantial changes. First, the category "refractory anemia with excess blasts in transformation" was removed, because the threshold of blasts required for the diagnosis of AML was lowered to 20%. Instead, the category "refractory anemia with excess blasts" ("RAEB") was subdivided into RAEB-1 (<5% circulating blasts and 5%–9% bone marrow blasts) and RAEB-2 (5%–19% circulating blasts, 10%–19% bone marrow blasts, or Auer rods). Second, the category "chronic myelomonocytic leukemia" was moved to "myelodysplastic/myeloproliferative diseases." Third, the categories "refractory cytopenia with multilineage dysplasia [without] or [with] ringed sideroblasts" were added to account for those patients without enough blasts to be under "RAEB," but with more dysmyelopoietic features than can be accommodated under "refractory anemia" ("RA"). Last, the entity of "MDS with associated del(5q)" was formally recognized as its own category (see **Table 1**).[27]

In the latest WHO classification, the most notable change involves the category "RA," which has been redefined as "refractory cytopenias with unilineage dysplasia," under which "refractory anemia" is still the most common subtype, followed by the rare instances of "refractory neutropenia" in which dysmyelopoiesis, if present, should be limited to the granulocytic lineage, and by the rare instances of "refractory thrombocytopenia" in which any dysmyelopoiesis is limited only to platelets and the megakaryocytic lineage.[28] Because of potential confusion between these subtypes and the category "MDS-unclassifiable," the latter is evoked when there is "unequivocal dysplasia in LESS (added emphasis) than 10% of cells in one or more myeloid cell lines," when there is pancytopenia but only unilineage dysplasia, or when there are 1% circulating blasts in what otherwise looks like refractory cytopenia with unilineage dysplasia (RCUD) or refractory cytopenia with multilineage dysplasia (RCMD).[29] The other change relates to the category "RCMD" where there is no longer any distinction between those with and those without ring sideroblasts.

PROGNOSTICATION

Although those MDS with "excess" blasts in the FAB classification system clearly had a worse outcome with a greater likelihood of and a shorter interval to acute leukemia evolution, the FAB classification system was primarily a codification of diagnostic subtypes that did not incorporate other prognostic parameters such as cytogenetics. The International Prognostic Scoring System (IPSS) published in 1997 (**Table 2**) was an attempt to provide a means to prognosticate using a combination of laboratory parameters that were easy to obtain. Thus, in their meta-analysis of data from nearly 1000 MDS patients, Greenberg and colleagues[30] demonstrated that patients with MDS could be stratified into four risk categories according to a sum of three scores, each score value reflecting the "severity" of marrow blasts, cytogenetic abnormality, and cytopenias. An MDS patient with a summed IPSS score of 2.5 to 3.5 would fall into the "high-risk" category and would have an estimated median survival of less than 1 year. Patients in the "intermediate-1" (summed IPSS score 0.5–1.0) or "intermediate-2" (summed IPSS score 1.5–2.0) risk category would have an estimated median survival of approximately 2.5 to 5 years and 1 to 2 years, respectively. In contrast, patients with an IPSS score of less than 0.5 are in the "low-risk" category and have an estimated median survival of more than 10 years if younger than 60 years, or approximately 4 to 5 years if older than 60 years.[30]

Subsequent to the publication of the WHO classification in 2001, other prognostication attempts have incorporated WHO categories and other promising prognostic variables, including characterizations of transfusion dependency (see **Table 2**).[31]

TREATMENT

The goals in the management of patients with MDS are to improve overall survival, decrease progression to acute leukemia, improve quality of life, and control symptoms related to cytopenias,[30] balanced with considerations of the patient's age, performance status, and prognostic risk category.[32]

Treatment options for patients with MDS have been expanded beyond the historical limitations of supportive care (including transfusion support) versus antileukemic therapy. A brief summary of some of these developments is given in the following paragraphs; a detailed discussion of therapeutics is beyond the scope of this article.

Red blood cell transfusion and iron chelation: Long a mainstay in the treatment of MDS patients to control symptoms related to anemia, repeated RBC transfusions carry with them the risk for iron overload and end-organ damage. However, unlike the situation with patients with β-thalassemia major, the benefits of iron chelation in MDS patients with iron overload (more than 20–30 transfusions, serum ferritin >1000 μg/L) have not been clearly established. Studies suggest that the worse prognosis of MDS patients with greater transfusion dependency may be independent of the effects of iron overload.[33]

Erythropoietin (EPO) and darbepoetin: Approximately 20% to 50% of MDS patients respond to EPO, although it may take as long as 6 months to see the benefits, and responses were more likely among those with suboptimally elevated serum EPO concentrations (<100 or <200 mU/mL) and with lower-grade MDS (eg, refractory anemia) and "good" cytogenetics.[34,35]

Hematopoietic growth factors: Even in the face of severe neutropenia with resultant infectious complications, the use of granulocyte- or granulocyte-macrophage colony-stimulating factor (G- or GM-CSF) as monotherapy has not been shown to be of benefit in the setting of MDS. The combined use of EPO and G-CSF (and to a lesser extent GM-CSF) seems to have a synergistic effect in improving the anemia.[36]

Immunosuppression: For subsets of patients with so-called "hypocellular MDS" who tend to be younger with marrow hypoplasia, normal cytogenetics, and HLA-DR15(DR2) haplotype, treatment with ATG and/or cyclosporine has resulted in normalization of hematologic parameters and transfusion independence.[37]

Table 2
Prognostic classifications of MDS

International Prognostic Scoring System (IPSS)[30]

Variable	Score value				
	0	0.5	1.0	1.5	2.0
Medullary blasts	<5%	5%–10%	—	11%–20%	21%–30%
Karyotype[a]	Good	Intermediate	Poor	—	—
Cytopenia[b]	0 or 1	2 or 3	—	—	—

Proposed WHO Classification-Based Prognostic Scoring System (WPSS)[31]

Variable	Score value			
	0	1	2	3
WHO-2001 category	RA, RARS, 5q-	RCMD, RCMD-RS	RAEB-1	RAEB-2
Karyotype[a]	Good	Intermediate	Poor	—
Transfusion Dependency[c]	None	Regular	—	—

IPSS risk groups: low, 0 summed score values; intermediate-1, 0.5–1.0 summed score values; intermediate-2, 1.5–2.0 summed score values; high, >2.5 summed score values.

WPSS risk groups: very low, 0 summed score values; low, 1 summed score values; intermediate, 2 summed score values; high, 3–4 summed score values; very high, 5–6 summed score values.

Abbreviation: 5q-, MDS with isolated del(5q).

[a] Karyotype: *good*, del(5q), del(20q), -Y; *poor*, abnormalities involving chromosome 7 and/or >3 abnormalities; *intermediate*, others.
[b] Cytopenia: hemoglobin <10 g/dL; absolute neutrophil count <1.5 × 10^9/L; platelets <100 × 10^9/L.
[c] Transfusion dependency: ≥1 RBC transfusion every 8 weeks for a period of 4 months.

Paroxysmal nocturnal hemoglobinuria-type cells were described in a small number of such patients who responded to immunosuppression.[38] It remains unclear whether this subset of responders may represent immune-mediated hematopoietic suppression apart from MDS.

Lenalidomide: One of the most exciting developments in the treatment of MDS has been the rediscovery of this thalidomide derivative as an effective and potentially curative therapeutic option for those patients with MDS associated with isolated 5q-, with a more variable efficacy in those with other chromosomal abnormalities. The reader is referred to several recent and definitive primary reports on this subject.[19,39]

Azacytidine and decitabine: A pyrimidine nucleoside analog of cytidine, 5-azacytidine is thought to achieve its antineoplastic effect by causing hypomethylation and direct cytotoxicity on abnormal hematopoietic cells. When compared against best supportive care alone or to conventional care plus best supportive care in prospective randomized phase III studies, 5-azacytidine has been shown to result in not only better complete and partial responses and quality of life measures, but also in improved overall survival.[40,41]

The use of decitabine, another pyrimidine nucleoside analog of cytidine, has been shown in phase II studies to be effective in MDS patients, including those previously treated with azacytidine and those in relapse. However, toxicity up to death appears appreciable.[42]

Antileukemic chemotherapy: Although in general it has disappointing results, aggressive antileukemic chemotherapy may have a role in the treatment of those MDS patients with more than 10% blasts who are younger than 60 years with a good performance status and good-risk cytogenetics.

Hematopoietic stem cell transplantation: Although it offers potentially the best chance of cure, allogeneic myeloablative hematopoietic stem cell transplant is an option for only approximately 25% of MDS patients, that is, those younger than 60 years with an HLA-matched sibling donor. Further, among those suitable for transplant, judicious timing appears predictive of best outcome, with the recommendation that transplant be delayed for those patients in the low to intermediate-1 IPSS risk groups until there are signs of significant disease progression. In contrast, for those patients in the intermediate-2 and high IPSS risk groups, transplant is recommended at the time of diagnosis.[43]

SPECIAL CONSIDERATIONS
Childhood Myelodysplastic Syndromes

Contrasts with adult MDS: De novo MDS is rare in the pediatric population and accounts for less than 5% of all malignant hematopoietic neoplasms among children under the age of 14 years.[44,45] Unlike adults with MDS, among whom anemia is a common finding at presentation, children with MDS present with anemia as an initial sign in only approximately half of the times, with thrombocytopenia seen more frequently, in approximately 75% of cases.[46] Whereas bone marrow hypocellularity is encountered in only approximately 10% of cases of adult MDS, it is reported in most cases of childhood MDS. Lastly, certain subtypes of adult MDS, such as refractory anemia with ring sideroblasts (RARS) and MDS associated with isolated del (5q), are exceedingly rare among the pediatric population. For these reasons, the WHO proposes a slightly different classification schema for childhood MDS.

Refractory cytopenia of childhood: For pediatric patients with MDS in whom there are fewer than 2% circulating blasts and fewer than 5% medullary blasts, the term "refractory cytopenia of childhood" is proposed, because anemia is not a common sign at presentation for this patient population.[47]

Because marrow hypocellularity is a common finding in childhood MDS, the differential diagnosis must include acquired aplastic anemia and other inherited bone marrow failure syndromes, such as Fanconi anemia, Shwachman-Diamond syndrome, and amegakaryocytic thrombocytopenia, among others. In addition, marrow hypoplasia due to infections and nutritional deficiencies must be ruled out. The presence of ring sideroblasts in a child should raise the question of Pearson syndrome or other mitochondrial cytopathies. To aid in the differential diagnosis of childhood MDS, it is recommended that unequivocal morphologic features of dysmyelopoiesis involving two or more hematopoietic lineages or affecting at least 10% of cells of a single lineage be present as a minimal diagnostic criterion.[47] Moreover, the need for adequate bone marrow biopsy samplings (at least 1–2 cm in length) cannot be overemphasized, to address the possibility of patchy hematopoiesis in some bone marrow failure syndromes, with a repeat bone marrow biopsy as necessary.

RAEB: For childhood MDS with 2% or more of circulating blasts or 5% or more of medullary blasts, the designation "refractory anemia with excess blasts" is retained. Although it is not clear whether or not the different natural history associated with RAEB-1 and RAEB-2 described in adults also applies to childhood MDS, it is recommended that this distinction be maintained until further data suggest otherwise.

Therapy-Related Myelodysplastic Syndromes

In the latest WHO classification, MDS and AML that arise in association with prior cytotoxic chemotherapy and/or ionizing radiation therapy are considered together as "therapy-related myeloid neoplasms," to reflect the shared unique clinical outcome.[48,49]

Clinical features: Regardless of the underlying primary disease for which the treatment was administered, patients with prior exposure to alkylating agents and/or ionizing radiation are at increased risk for developing a therapy-related myeloid neoplasm, generally at 5 to 10 years after such exposure. The reader is referred to standard texts of hematology and medical oncology for a complete list of such potentiating agents, but these classes of agents are typically encountered in the setting of treatments of lymphoma and multiple myeloma and include melphalan, cyclophosphamide, busulfan, chlorambucil, carboplatin, and cisplatin, among others. For those patients who have had previous exposure to inhibitors of topoisomerase II, such as etoposide, doxorubicin, daunorubicin, and so on, the latency period is shorter, at 1 to 5 years.[50]

Pathology

Pathology: The MDS seen after alkylating chemotherapy and/or ionizing radiation therapy typically show dysplasia involving two or more hematopoietic lineages, with or without increased blasts; it is uncommon for therapy-related MDS to present as RA or RARS. Cytogenetic abnormalities are seen in more than 90% of cases and typically involve chromosomes 5 and 7, among others. In contrast, patients whose myeloid neoplasms are caused by previous exposure to the topoisomerase II inhibitors typically present with acute leukemia, with cytogenetic analysis typically showing balanced translocations involving 11q23.

Prognosis: The prognosis of therapy-related myeloid neoplasms is poor.

REFERENCES

1. Rollison DE, Howlader N, Smith MT, et al. Epidemiology of myelodysplastic syndromes and chronic myeloproliferative disorders in the United States, 2001–2004: utilizing data from the NAACCR and SEER Programs. Blood 2008;112(1):45–52.
2. Aul C, Gatterman N, Schneider W. Age-related incidence and other epidemiological aspects of myelodysplastic syndromes. Br J Haematol 1992;82(2):358–67.
3. Germing U, Strupp C, Kundgen A, et al. No increase in age-specific incidence of myelodysplastic syndromes. Haematologica 2004;89(8):905–10.
4. Ma X, Does M, Raza A, et al. Myelodysplastic syndromes: incidence and survival in the United States. Cancer 2007;109(8):1536–42.
5. Williamson PJ, Kruger AR, Reynolds PJ, et al. Establishing the incidence of myelodysplastic syndrome. Br J Haematol 1997;87(4):743–5.
6. Groupe Français de Morphologie Hematologique. French registry of acute leukemia and myelodysplastic syndromes. Age distribution and hemogram analysis of the 4496 cases recorded during 1982–1983 and classified according to FAB criteria. Groupe Français de Morphologie Hematologique. Cancer 1987; 60(6):1385–94.
7. Mufti GJ, Bennett JM, Goasguen J, et al. Diagnosis and classification of myelodysplastic syndrome: International Working Group on Morphology of Myelodysplastic Syndrome (IWGM-MDS) consensus proposals for the definition and enumeration of myeloblasts and ring sideroblasts. Haematologica 2008;93(11):1712–7.
8. Lai JL, Preudhomme C, Zandecki M, et al. Myelodysplastic syndromes and acute myeloid leukemia with 17p deletion. An entity characterized by specific dysgranulopoiesis and a high incidence of P53 mutations. Leukemia 1995;9(3): 370–81.
9. Lee SH, Erber WN, Porwit A, et al. ICSH guidelines for the standardization of bone marrow specimens and reports. Int J Lab Hematol 2008;30(5):349–64.
10. Stetler-Stevenson M, Arthur DC, Jabbour N, et al. Diagnostic utility of flow cytometric immunophenotyping in myelodysplastic syndrome. Blood 2001;98(4):979–87.
11. Della Porta MG, Malcovati L, Invernizzi R, et al. Flow cytometry evaluation of erythroid dysplasia in patients with myelodysplastic syndrome. Leukemia 2006; 20(4):549–55.
12. Kussick SJ, Fromm JR, Rossini A, et al. Four-color flow cytometry shows strong concordance with bone marrow morphology and cytogenetics in the evaluation for myelodysplasia. Am J Clin Pathol 2005;124(2):170–81.
13. Brunning RD, Orazi A, Germing U, et al. "Myelodysplastic syndromes/neoplasms, overview". In: Swerdlow SH, Campo E, Harris NL, editors. World Health Organization classification of tumours of haematopoietic and lymphoid tissues. Lyon: IARC Press; 2008. p. 92–3.
14. van de Loosdrecht AA, Westers TM, Westra AH, et al. Identification of distinct prognostic subgroups in low- and intermediate-1-risk myelodysplastic syndromes by flow cytometry. Blood 2008;111(3):1067–77.
15. Third MIC Cooperative Study Group. Recommendations for a morphologic, immunologic, and cytogenetic (MIC) working classification of the primary and therapy-related myelodysplastic disorders. Report of the workshop held in Scottsdale, Arizona, USA, on February 23–25, 1987. Third MIC Cooperative Study Group. Cancer Genet Cytogenet 1988;32(1):1–10.
16. Toyama K, Ohyashiki K, Yoshida Y, et al. Clinical implications of chromosomal abnormalities in 401 patients with MDS: a multicentric study in Japan. Leukemia 1993;7(4):499–508.

17. Haase D, Germing U, Schanz J, et al. New insights into the prognostic impact of the karyotype in MDS and correlation with subtypes: evidence from a core data-set of 2124 patients. Blood 2007;110(13):4385–95.
18. Hanson CA, Steensma DP, Hodnefield JM, et al. Isolated trisomy 15: a clonal chromosome abnormality in bone marrow with doubtful hematologic significance. Am J Clin Pathol 2008;129(3):478–85.
19. List A, Dewald G, Bennett J, et al. Lenalidomide in the myelodysplastic syndrome with chromosome 5q deletion. N Engl J Med 2006;355(14):1456–65.
20. Gondek LP, Tiu R, O'Keefe CL, et al. Chromosomal lesions and uniparental dis-omy detected by SNP arrays in MDS, MDS/MPD, and MDS-derived AML. Blood 2008;111(3):1534–42.
21. Gondek LP, Haddad AS, O'Keefe CL, et al. Detection of cryptic chromosomal lesions including acquired segmental uniparental disomy in advanced and low-risk myelodysplastic syndromes. Exp Hematol 2007;35(11):1728–38.
22. Mohamedali A, Gaken J, Twine NA, et al. Prevalence and prognostic significance of allelic imbalance by single-nucleotide polymorphism analysis in low-risk mye-lodysplastic syndromes. Blood 2007;110(9):3365–73.
23. Quesnel B, Guillerm G, Vereecque R, et al. Methylation of the p15(INK4b) gene in myelodysplastic syndromes is frequent and acquired during disease progres-sion. Blood 1998;91(8):2985–90.
24. Aoki E, Uchida T, Ohashi H, et al. Methylation status of the p15INK4B gene in hematopoietic progenitors and peripheral blood cells in myelodysplastic syndromes. Leukemia 2000;14(4):586–93.
25. Kuendgen A, Knipp S, Fox F, et al. Results of a phase 2 study of valproic acid in 75 patients with myelodysplastic syndrome and relapsed or refractory acute myeloid leukemia. Ann Hematol 2005;84(Suppl 1):61–6.
26. Bennett JM, Catovsky D, Daniel MT, et al. Proposals for the classification of the myelodysplastic syndromes. Br J Haematol 1982;51(2):189–99.
27. Brunning RD, Bennett JM, Flandrin G, et al. Myelodysplastic syndromes. In: Jaffe ES, Harris NL, Stein H, editors. World Health Organization classification of tumours of haematopoietic and lymphoid tissues. Lyon: IARC Press; 2001. p. 63–73.
28. Brunning RD, Hasserjian RP, Porwit A, et al. Refractory cytopenia with unilineage dysplasia. In: Swerdlow SH, Campo E, Harris NL, editors. World Health Organi-zation classification of tumours of haematopoietic and lymphoid tissues. Lyon: IARC Press; 2008. p. 94–5.
29. Orazi A, Brunning RD, Baumann I, et al. Myelodysplastic syndrome, unclassifi-able. In: Swerdlow SH, Campo E, Harris NL, editors. World Health Organization classification of tumours of haematopoietic and lymphoid tissues. Lyon, France: IARC Press; 2008. p. 103.
30. Greenberg P, Cox C, LeBeau MM, et al. International scoring system for evalu-ating prognosis in myelodysplastic syndromes. Blood 1997;89(6):2079–88.
31. Malcovati L, Germing U, Kuendgen A, et al. Time-dependent prognostic scoring system for predicting survival and leukemic evolution in myelodysplastic syndromes. J Clin Oncol 2007;25(34):3503–10.
32. Myelodysplastic syndromes v.1, NCCN Clinical Practice Guidelines in Oncology™. Available at: www.nccn.org. Accessed January 10, 2009.
33. Chee CE, Steensma DP, Wu W, et al. Neither serum ferritin nor the number of red blood cell transfusions affect overall survival in refractory anemia with ringed sideroblasts. Am J Hematol 2008;83(8):611–3.

34. Gabrilove J, Paquette R, Lyons RM, et al. Phase 2, single-arm trial to evaluate the effectiveness of darbepoetin alfa for correcting anaemia in patients with myelodysplastic syndromes. Br J Haematol 2008;142(3):379–93.
35. Stasi R, Abruzzese E, Lanzetta G, et al. Darbepoetin alfa for the treatment of anemic patients with low- and intermediate-1-risk myelodysplastic syndromes. Ann Oncol 2005;16(12):1921–7.
36. Negrin RS, Stein R, Doherty K, et al. Maintenance treatment of the anemia of myelodysplastic syndromes with recombinant human G-CSF plus erythropoietin: evidence for in vivo synergy. Blood 1996;87(10):4076–81.
37. Saunthararajah Y, Nakamura R, Nam JM, et al. HLA-DR15(DR2) is overrepresented in myelodysplastic syndrome and aplastic anemia and predicts a response to immunosuppression in myelodysplastic syndrome. Blood 2002; 100(5):1570–4.
38. Wang H, Chuhjo T, Yasue S, et al. Clinical significance of a minor population of paroxysmal nocturnal hemoglobinuria-type cells in bone marrow failure syndrome. Blood 2002;100(12):3897–902.
39. Raza A, Reeves JA, Feldman EJ, et al. Phase 2 study of lenalidomide in transfusion-dependent, low-risk, and intermediate-1 risk myelodysplastic syndromes with karyotypes other than deletion 5q. Blood 2008;111(1):86–93.
40. Silverman LR, Demakos EP, Peterson BL, et al. Randomized controlled trial of azacitidine in patients with the myelodysplastic syndrome: a study of the cancer and leukemia group B. J Clin Oncol 2002;20(10):2429–40.
41. Fenaux P, Mufti GJ, Santini V, et al. Azacitidine (AZA) treatment prolongs overall survival (OS) in higher-risk MDS patients compared with conventional care regimens (CCR): results of the AZA-100 phase II study [abstract]. Blood 2007;110:250.
42. Lubbert M, Wijermans P, Kunzmann R, et al. Cytogenetic responses in high-risk myelodysplastic syndrome following low-dose treatment with the DNA methylation inhibitor 5-aza-2'-deoxycytidine. Br J Haematol 2001;114(2):349–57.
43. Cutler CS, Lee SJ, Greenberg P, et al. A decision analysis of allogeneic bone marrow transplantation for the myelodysplastic syndromes: delayed transplantation for low-risk myelodysplasia is associated with improved outcome. Blood 2004;104(2):579–85.
44. Hasle H, Wadsworth LD, Massing BG, et al. A population-based study of childhood myelodysplastic syndrome in British Columbia, Canada. Br J Haematol 1999;106(4):1027–32.
45. Stary J, Baumann I, Creutzig U, et al. Getting the numbers straight in pediatric MDS: distribution of subtypes after exclusion of Down syndrome. Pediatr Blood Cancer 2008;50(2):435–6.
46. Kardos G, Baumann I, Passmore SJ, et al. Refractory anemia in childhood: a retrospective analysis of 67 patients with particular reference to monosomy 7. Blood 2003;102(6):1997–2003.
47. Baumann I, Niemeyer CM, Bennett JM, et al. Childhood myelodysplastic syndrome. In: Swerdlow SH, Campo E, Harris NL, editors. World Health Organization classification of tumours of haematopoietic and lymphoid tissues. Lyon: IARC Press; 2008. p. 104–7.
48. Vardiman JW, Arber DA, Brunning RD, et al. Therapy-related myeloid neoplasms. In: Swerdlow SH, Campo E, Harris NL, editors. World Health Organization classification of tumours of haematopoietic and lymphoid tissues. Lyon: IARC Press; 2008. p. 127–9.

49. Singh ZN, Huo D, Anastasi J, et al. Therapy-related myelodysplastic syndrome: morphologic subclassification may not be clinically relevant. Am J Clin Pathol 2007;127(2):197–205.
50. Smith SM, LeBeau MM, Huo D, et al. Clinical-cytogenetic association in 306 patients with therapy-related myelodysplasia and myeloid leukemia: the University of Chicago series. Blood 2003;102(1):43–52.

The Myeloproliferative Neoplasms: Insights into Molecular Pathogenesis and Changes in WHO Classification and Criteria for Diagnosis

John Anastasi, MD

KEYWORDS

- Myeloproliferative neoplasms • Polycythemia vera
- Primary myelofibrosis • Essential thrombocytosis
- Tyrosine kinase

In the fourth edition of the World Health Organization (WHO)-sponsored classification of hematopoietic and lymphoid malignancies, published in 2008, changes were made in the classification and criteria for the diagnosis of some of the myeloproliferative disorders (MPD).[1] The group of entities was also given a new name by substituting "neoplasms" for "disorders." Although the name change and its abbreviation, "MPN," might tongue-tie those accustomed for so many years to "MPD," the other changes were appropriately related to insights into the pathogenesis of these malignancies gained after the third edition of the classification was published in 2001.[2] These new insights include the notable discoveries of associated mutations in the tyrosine kinases (TK) of signal transduction pathways in several entities, and in particular the Janus Kinase 2 (*JAK2*) mutation (*JAK2*V617F) in a substantial number of the more common types of these diseases.[3–5] In this review, the changes made to the MPN, and the basis of the new classification and altered diagnostic criteria, are summarized and discussed. The MPN and associated diseases include chronic myelogenous leukemia (CML); the common *BCR-ABL1*-negative MPN, including polycythemia vera (PV), primary myelofibrosis (PMF), and essential thrombocythemia (ET); the new group of myeloid and lymphoid neoplasms with eosinophilia associated

Department of Pathology, University of Chicago, 5841 South Maryland Avenue, MC 0008, Chicago, IL 60637, USA
E-mail address: john.anastasi@uchospitals.edu

Hematol Oncol Clin N Am 23 (2009) 693–708
doi:10.1016/j.hoc.2009.04.002
0889-8588/09/$ – see front matter © 2009 Elsevier Inc. All rights reserved.

with TK rearrangements (listed separately in the WHO scheme) and the related chronic eosinophilic leukemia (CEL), and hypereosinophilic syndrome (HES); and, lastly, the less common BCR-ABL1-negative diseases, including mast cell disease (MCD) and chronic neutrophilic leukemia (**Table 1**).

THE UNKNOWN GROWTH STIMULUS AND THE TYROSINE KINASE STORY

William Dameshek, a preeminent hematologist of his time and founding editor of the journal *Blood*, postulated in 1951 that the then-considered-unrelated entities of CML, PV, myelofibrosis with myeloid metaplasia (now PMF), and what he referred to as "megakaryocytic leukemia" (now ET) should all be considered together as a single disease type, which he proposed to call the "myeloproliferative syndromes."[6] He further went on to speculate that the different entities were closely related disorders caused by a proliferative activity of marrow cells because of some type of an "unknown growth stimulus." Despite the addition of a number of other diseases to the list that Dameshek initially generated, and despite habitual changes in the names and terminology used to identify them, it is now accepted that these entities are closely related myeloid progenitor-cell malignancies, and that many are indeed the result of an "abnormal growth stimulus." This growth stimulus has been identified to be an uncontrolled signal from a constitutively activated TK that is part of the normal signal transduction pathway for the regulation of growth and differentiation of normal myeloid cells (**Table 1**).[7] The unrelenting signaling leads to unchecked proliferation of erythroid, megakaryocytic, or granulocytic myeloid cells, or a combination thereof, and then to the characteristic clinical and laboratory features associated with the different diseases.[8]

These new insights into the molecular pathogenesis of the MPN constitute what can be referred to as the "TK story." This story began with CML, and has made CML a tremendously useful model for the other chronic myeloid neoplasms. The

Table 1 The myeloproliferative neoplasms	
Disease	**TK Involved (% of cases)**
CML	ABL (100%)
PV	JAK2V617F (~95%), JAK2 (exon 12 mutations)(~4%)
PMF	JAK2V617F(~50%), MPLW515K/L (5%–9%)
ET	JAK2V617F(~50%), MPLW515K/L (~1%)
The myeloid neoplasms with eosinophilia and TK mutations	
- with PDGFRA rearrangement	PDGFRA (100%)
- with PDGFRB rearrangement	PDGFRB (100%)
- 8p11 MPN	FGFR1 (100%)
CEL	None identified, (clonal or associated with increased blasts)
HES	None identified (nonclonal, no increased blasts)
MCD	KIT (D816V) (95% of SM)
CNL	JAK2 mutation ("occasional")
MPN, unclassified	Unknown

subsequent successful development of a rationally designed drug to inhibit the excessive TK signaling in CML has further elevated the role model status of CML. It is now a much-emphasized model for how scientific inquiry into the pathogenesis of a disorder can lead to the logical development of a successful targeted therapy.

CHRONIC MYELOID LEUKEMIA

CML has been a model disease from the onset when it was the disease for which the name "leukemia" was coined. Reported with only weeks between publications, the disease was first described in 1845 by Virchow in Germany and by Bennett in England.[9,10] Both of them reported autopsy cases with marked hepatosplenomegaly and blood that oozed out of the cut surface of organs that had the look of purulent material or pus (**Fig. 1**). The two differed about what to call the entity, with Bennett suggesting the somewhat more accurate term, "leukocythemia," or, white cell blood (**Fig. 1**), and Virchow suggesting "weisses Blut," (white blood) or leukemia. Virchow, who was far more established than Bennett, apparently won out.

The first advance into the inquiry of the molecular basis of the disease came in 1960 when Nowell and Hungerford[11] identified a small G-group chromosome that they believed had some missing genetic material at its tip compared with its normal counterpart. It was not until 10 years later, with the use of chromosomal banding, that Rowley[12] identified that the small G-group chromosome resulted from a reciprocal translocation between the long arm of chromosome 9 and the long arm of

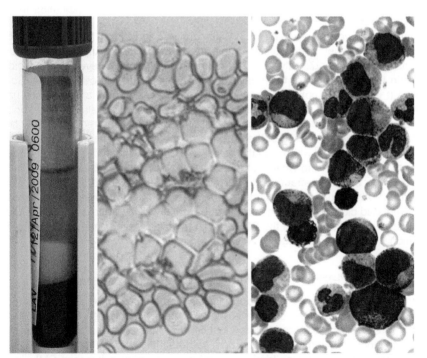

Fig. 1. A modern day approximation of the purulent blood of CML initially described by Virchow and Bennett (*left;* CML blood with WBC = 350 × 10^9/L) with its microscopic appearance (*unstained*) showing leukocythemia (*middle*); this is compared with a typical Wright-stained smear of CML (*right*). (Image on left is *courtesy of* Bakul Dalal, MD, Vancouver, British Columbia.)

chromosome 22. The genes involved in the translocation were identified within another 10 years when various investigators recognized a homolog to a murine oncogene, ABL1, on chromosome 9 and a newly identified gene denoted BCR, for breakpoint cluster region, on chromosome 22.[13] The fusion gene, BCR-ABL1, on the derivative chromosome 22 was shown to be the cause of the disease through the constitutive activation of the ABL1 TK with the excessive signaling apparently driving the myeloid proliferation.[14,15] The idea to inhibit the overactive ABL1 TK as a possible treatment occurred early on, but the first-attempted naturally occurring TK inhibitors were weak, and the synthetic compounds tried next were nonspecific. In the late 1990s a specifically tailored or designed drug named imatinib was developed.[16] This exceeded all expectations, and has proven to be a tremendous success in specifically inhibiting the ABL TK activity. The drug reverses the myeloid and megakaryocytic proliferation and greatly increases disease-free survival by markedly reducing disease progression.[17,18] Once a uniformly fatal disease, CML is now manageable, and some patients can achieve a complete remission even at the molecular level.

In the 2008 edition of the WHO publication, there are essentially no changes in the classification or diagnostic criteria for CML. The identification of a marked leukocytosis due to a neutrophilia of all stages of maturation with a myelocyte "bulge," lack of significant circulating blasts, absolute basophilia, frequent thrombocytosis, and mild anemia are still the key factors in the initial diagnosis (**Fig. 1**). Review of a bone marrow biopsy with its marked granulocytic and "dwarf" megakaryocytic proliferations, and the correlation of these findings with cytogenetic or molecular studies that show the t(9;22) and/or BCR-ABL1 is typically done to confirm the morphologic diagnosis of the chronic phase.

There was some discussion by the WHO committee and clinical advisors involved in the project as to whether the concept of the accelerated phase of the disease had outlived its usefulness, especially in the age of imatinib therapy. However, it was decided to retain the recognition of this phase of CML, at least for the current time. Some believe it is probably not synonymous with imatinib resistance, and may still have usefulness as a herald of blast crisis. Further discussion and evaluation is ongoing. Some other issues under discussion in CML include questions regarding how best to standardize the monitoring of therapy with quantitative polymerase chain reaction (PCR) for BCR-ABL1,[19] when, and the best way to identify mutation-associated resistance to imatinib,[20,21] and what strategies to use to develop new treatments for those patients who become refractory to imatinib and the subsequent second tier of TK inhibitors.[22] Additionally, the findings of rare cases of CML with an apparent previous JAK2 mutated clone has resurrected the question of whether there is a clonal expansion before the acquisition of the BCR-ABL in the initial development of CML.[23] This question was raised years ago by Raskind and colleagues.[24]

THE MYELOID NEOPLASMS WITH EOSINOPHILIA AND TYROSINE KINASE MUTATIONS

The myeloid neoplasms with eosinophilia and TK mutations are rare, but historically were the focus of the next chapter in the "TK story." Compared to the hard-won inquiry in CML with its decades-long, logical, scientific progression of knowledge, the discovery in the eosinophilic disorders came somewhat indirectly. After imatinib was approved for use, it was tried in a number of disorders other than CML. In the trials, the eosinophilic disorders were found to be exquisitely sensitive.[25–27] This implied that the diseases were the result of an overactivity of an inhibitable TK, which was later realized to be the receptor TK, PDGFRB, or PDGFRA. These had previously been shown to be altered in rare chromosomal translocations involving 5q12 and deletions of 4q, respectively.[28,29] In the initial publications, the eosinophilic diseases were referred to as chronic myelomonocytic leukemia with eosinophilia or MCD with eosinophilia, but in the latest classification they are simply denoted as "myeloid neoplasms associated with eosinophilia" and abnormalities of PDGFRA or PDGFRB.

Another disease added to this group was the 8p11 myeloproliferative syndrome.[30,31] Although quite rare, this disorder presents with neutrophilia, frequently with eosinophilia, and is associated with rearrangement of the fibroblast growth factor receptor (FGFR1), another TK receptor. Uniquely, the 8p11 disease may present as a myeloid proliferation, but subsequently can develop into a precursor T-cell acute lymphoblastic leukemia (although the reverse progression can also happen). As such, it resembles CML in chronic phase transforming to a lymphoid blast crisis. Unfortunately and unlike CML or the other myeloid neoplasms associated with eosinophilia, the 8p11 MPN is not responsive to imatinib. Clinical trials of FGFR1 inhibitors are under way.

An approach to assessing a patient with marked eosinophilia and a possible MPN with eosinophilia is illustrated in **Box 1**.[7] One must first rule out reactive causes clinically and then through the evaluation of the peripheral blood (PB) and bone marrow (BM). The evaluation should consider infectious or immune-mediated (allergy) causes, causes related to an abnormal T-cell proliferation, and reactive causes due to diseases that stimulate normal eosinophils, such as Hodgkin lymphoma, T-cell lymphoma (including Sézary syndrome and mycosis fungoides), and acute lymphoblastic leukemia (ALL) with t(5;14)(q31;q32). Bone marrow assessment for disorders that have clonal eosinophilia should be considered next, and this includes ruling out CML, acute myeloid leukemia (AML), and other MPN associated with a substantial eosinophilic component. If these are all negative, one would assess for alterations of PDGFRA, PDGFRB, or FGFR1 by cytogenetic, molecular, or fluorescent in situ

---

Box 1
An approach to the assessment of a possible myeloid neoplasm with eosinophilia

1. Document prolonged eosinophilia greater than 1.5×10^9/L for 6 months, then

2. Rule out reactive causes (infections, allergy, etc) by clinical history and other clinical information, then

3. Evaluate peripheral blood and bone marrow (biopsy and aspirate)

   a. Rule out abnormal T-cell clone

   b. Rule out another malignancy associated with eosinophilia (eg, Hodgkin lymphoma, T-cell lymphoma/leukemia, acute lymphoblastic leukemia with t[5;14])

   c. Rule out clonal eosinophilia due to another malignancy (eg, CML, AML), then

4. Assess for TK translocations/mutations by cytogenetics, molecular or FISH. If positive, diagnose MPN with eosinophilia with mutations of PDGFRA, PDGFB or FGFR1. If negative, then

5. Assess for clonality of the process, or for blasts in blood (>1%), BM (>5%), if positive, diagnosis CEL; if negative, then

6. Diagnose HES

Data from Tefferi A, Vardiman JW. Classification and diagnosis of myeloproliferative neoplasms: the 2008 World Health Organization criteria and point-of-care diagnostic algorithms. Leukemia 2008;22:14.

hybridization (FISH) analysis; if these are positive, the disease may be diagnosed and subclassified by the particular molecular abnormality found. If negative, evaluate for clonality or for increased blasts, and diagnose CEL if clonality is identified or if the PB or BM blasts are greater than1% and 5% respectively. One would revert to a diagnosis of HES if a reactive condition is excluded, if a specific myeloid disorder with eosinophilia is ruled out, if a TK abnormality (*PDGFRA, PDGFRB* or *FGFR1*) is not detected, if there is no identifiable clonality, and if there is no increase in blasts.

JAK2

Just as Bennet and Virchow were within weeks of one another in their publication of the first cases of CML, so too were four different laboratories that reported another major discovery regarding most cases of the more common MPN, that is, a mutation in the TK called JAK2.[32–35] Given the precedents of CML and the myeloid neoplasms with eosinophilia, the four different laboratories were clearly in a race to identify dysregulation of a TK-associated signaling pathway. There had been some earlier work suggesting that there was a gene of interest on chromosome 9p.[36] However, the laboratories took different approaches, including a candidate gene approach, a high-throughput specimen-sequencing approach, a loss of heterozygosity satellite mapping approach, and an inhibition approach using siRNA. Notwithstanding some intrigue and the question of which laboratory was first with the discovery, the four laboratories identified a mutation in the negative regulatory domain of *JAK2* and recognized that it was present in the majority of cases of PV, PMF, and ET. Each laboratory published its discovery between March and April of 2005.

The hallmark discovery and the initial data regarding the incidence of the *JAK2*V617F in the myeloid neoplasms have been confirmed and expanded in numerous subsequent reports. It is now accepted that the mutation is present in ~95% of cases of PV, in about 50% of cases of PMF and ET, but only rarely <1%–5% in cases of AML, myelodysplastic syndrome (MDS), CML, MCD, and chronic myelomonocytic leukemia. It is reported in about ~20% of cases of "atypical CML" and juvenile myelomonocytic leukemia[4] and in a slightly higher percentage of cases of refractory anemia with ring sideroblasts and thrombocytosis.[37–39]

There are numerous approaches to assay for *JAK2*V617F, including direct DNA sequencing, allele-specific PCR, DNA-melting curve analysis, and pyrosequencing,[4] and they can be easily performed on cells from the peripheral blood. Allele-specific oligonucleotide PCR with quantitative assay is sensitive and seems to be commonly used.[40] The sensitivity of this assay is on the range of 1% to 3%.

Although the association of *JAK2*V617F with PV, PMF, and ET continues the "TK story" for the more common *BCR-ABL1*-negative MPN, many questions still remain concerning the exact mechanism of disease, or, more importantly, whether a *JAK2*-specific TK inhibitor is clinically useful.[41] Whether the *JAK2*V617F is actually the cause of the disease or only a disease modifier is still not clear. Some data point to a pre-*JAK2*V617F clone as an initiation step followed by the development of a subclone with the mutation.[42,43] This multistep process with the mutation developing later may even occur in familial cases of MPN with *JAK2*V617F.[44] How the mutation results in the different diseases or phenotypes is also an issue under investigation. It seems that dosage of the mutation and the level of progenitor cell affected are important factors.[45] It seems, for example, that in PV there is higher dosage with frequent homozygous mutations that probably occur in a more primitive progenitor. This is in contrast to ET, where the dosage is less, and the stem cell involved is believed to be more lineage-restricted. Whether inhibition of the *JAK2*V617F-associated constitutive activity benefits patients with these *BCR-ABL1*-negative MPN is a pressing question that, at the moment, is still unanswered. However, a rigorous inquiry is being undertaken in ongoing clinical trials of a large number of newly synthesized inhibitors.[41]

POLYCYTHEMIA VERA

The new discoveries regarding *JAK2*V617F in the MPN have had most impact on PV, particularly with regard to its diagnosis.[5] Before the recent discoveries, difficulties with the diagnosis stemmed mainly from problems with ruling out reactive causes of erythrocytosis. A somewhat complex set of five major and four minor criteria was established with an even more complex set of rules for accepting different combinations of the criteria deemed necessary for a diagnosis.[2] With the initial observations that *JAK2*V617F is seen in ~95% of cases of PV, the problem of ruling out a reactive cause has become largely alleviated. The *JAK2*V617F is only rarely seen in hematologically normal patients.[46] The discovery that 80% of the *JAK2*V617F-negative cases of PV have a mutation, but in a different exon of *JAK2*, exon 12,[47] makes the identification of a *JAK2* mutation an even more important measure for helping to correctly diagnose PV. Essentially, one of the two mutations is seen in about 99% of cases.

The new and much simplified WHO criteria for diagnosing PV are listed in **Box 2**.[1]

For most cases, one essentially needs to first identify sufficiently elevated hemoglobin levels, hematocrit, or red cell mass above a set threshold, then demonstrate a normal or low erythropoietin (EPO) level to show that the erythroid proliferation is not related to physiologic causes. One would then attempt to demonstrate the *JAK2*V617F or, if not found, evaluate for a mutation in *JAK2* exon12. A bone marrow evaluation is usually obtained as a baseline for comparison to future evaluations, or it might be necessary as a diagnostic criterion to illustrate a myeloproliferation if the EPO is not reduced. The criterion of illustrating exogenous erythroid colony formation is entirely appropriate, as this is a direct manifestation of the abnormal TK signaling. However, it seems less relevant, as it is not a test that most laboratories have

---

Box 2

WHO 2008 diagnostic criteria for PV

The diagnosis of PV requires (1) both major and one minor criterion or (2) the first major and two minor criteria.

Major criteria

1. Hemoglobin greater than 18.5 g/dL in men

Hemoglobin greater than 16.5 g/dL in woman or

Other evidence of increased red cell volume

2. Presence of *JAK2*V617F or other functionally similar mutation, such as *JAK2* exon 12 mutation

Minor criteria

1. Bone marrow biopsy showing hypercellularity for age with trilineage growth (panmyelosis) with prominent erythroid, granulocytic, and megakaryocytic proliferation.

2. Serum erythropoietin level below the reference range.

3. Endogenous erythroid colony formation.

Data from Swerdlow SH Campo E, Harris NL, et al, editors. WHO classification of tumours of haematopoietic and lymphoid tissues. Lyon: IARC; 2008. p. 40.

available. The *JAK2* mutation-negative cases can still be diagnosed as PV by meeting the first criterion and two of the minor criteria. However, such cases would be quite rare.

PRIMARY MYELOFIBROSIS, FIBROTIC STAGE

In addition to changing the name from "MPD" to "MPN," the WHO committee has once again changed the renamed "chronic idiopathic myelofibrosis" to PMF.[1,48] This seems to be in keeping with the long tradition for renaming this entity and the thought that it might as well be called the "syndrome of pseudonyms."[49] In contrast to PV, the *JAK2*V617F has not had much impact in the diagnosis of PMF, or at least not in the diagnosis of the fibrotic stage of the disease, which is considered first.

The WHO diagnostic criteria for PMF are noted in **Box 3**, and they apply to a prefibrotic and fibrotic stage. The diagnostic criteria are changed compared with those in the 2001, third edition.[2] They comprise three major and four minor criteria.[1] The major criteria include morphologic features, exclusionary features, and molecular features, or, in the absence of the latter, additional exclusions. The molecular features include the finding of *JAK2*V617F, a mutation in the thrombopoietin receptor *MPL*, *MPL*W515K/L,[50] or a clonal cytogenetic abnormality. The latter are seen in up to 35% of cases and include del(13q), del(20q), and 1q abnormalities, although none of these are specific to PMF.[51] The minor criteria include clinical features (splenomegaly), laboratory features (anemia and elevated lactate dehydrogenase), and morphologic features of the peripheral blood (leukoerythroblastosis). Although a diagnosis requires meeting all three major and two of the four minor criteria, it is worth pointing out that a firm diagnosis of the fibrotic stage of PMF can usually be made

---

Box 3
Diagnostic criteria for PMF

Major criteria

1. Presence of megakaryocytic proliferation and atypia, usually accompanied with either reticulin or collagen fibrosis, or in the absence of fibrosis, the megakaryocytic proliferation must be accompanied by an increase in marrow cellularity characterized by granulocytic proliferation and often decreased erythroid elements.

2. Not meeting the WHO criteria for PV, CML, MDS, or other myeloid neoplasms

3. Demonstration of *JAK2*V617F or other clonal marker, such as *MPL*W515K/L or in the absence of a clonal marker, no evidence that the bone marrow fibrosis or other changes are secondary to infection, autoimmune disorder or other chronic inflammatory condition, hairy cell leukemia, or other lymphoid neoplasm, metastatic malignancy, or toxic (chronic) myelopathies.

Minor criteria

1. Leukoerythroblastosis

2. Increase in serum lactate dehydrogenase

3. Anemia

4. Splenomegaly.

The diagnosis of PMF requires satisfying each of the three major and two of the minor criteria.
Data from Swerdlow SH, Campo E, Harris NL, et al, editors. WHO classification of tumours of haematopoietic and lymphoid tissues. Lyon: IARC; 2008. p. 44.

morphologically, coupled with the knowledge that the patient has splenomegaly. Exclusion of postpolycythemic myelofibrosis or the postessential thrombocythemic myelofibrosis must be made with appropriate history.

PMF most commonly presents in a fibrotic stage, reportedly in close to two-thirds of cases. In this presentation, patients have splenomegaly and characteristic blood and marrow findings, which are a result of the extramedullary hematopoiesis that is subsequent to the marrow fibrosis. The characteristic findings include a peripheral blood smear with mild anemia, the classic leukoerythroblastosis composed of circulating immature granulocytes, and nucleated red blood cells. This is typically associated with tear-drop–shaped red cells (dacrocytes). The bone marrow is also characteristic with a highly abnormal megakaryocytic proliferation with bizarre, various-sized cytoplasm, and bulbous nuclei, associated with reticulin or collagen fibrosis, granulocytic proliferation, and sinusoidal hematopoiesis (**Fig. 2**).[8] In the fibrotic stage, the morphologic features are usually quite straightforward and are similar to what have been used for decades in identifying patients with this disease. The diagnosis can usually be made without knowledge of the JAK2V617F or MPLW515K/L, which are seen in only one-half or in 5% to 9% of cases, respectively. The morphologic findings in the fibrotic stage satisfy the first criterion and can be used to rule out the exclusionary diseases in the second and third criteria. For the latter, this includes ruling out other causes of marrow fibrosis.

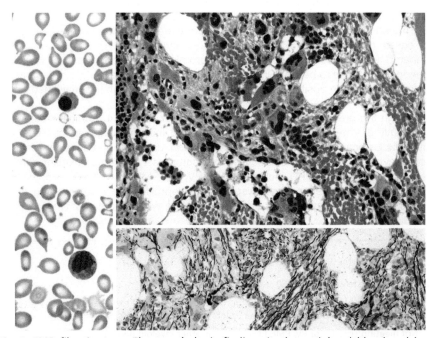

Fig. 2. PMF, fibrotic stage. The morphologic findings in the peripheral blood and bone marrow biopsy can be diagnostic. In the peripheral blood, there is a leukoerythroblastic picture with nucleated red blood cells (*top left*) and immature granulocytes (*bottom left*) associated with tear-drop forms. In the bone marrow, there is a marked, highly atypical megakaryocytic proliferation in a background of granulocytic proliferation, and sinusoidal hematopoiesis (*top right*), and this is associated with sever fibrosis as illustrated on a reticulin stain (*bottom right*).

Significant marrow fibrosis can be seen in other MPN, AML, myelodysplastic syndromes, lymphoma, hairy cell leukemia, ALL, myeloma, metastatic carcinoma, and nonneoplastic causes, such as collagen vascular disease (autoimmune myelofibrosis), toxicity, hyperthyroidism, osteopetrosis, and storage disease.[52] Although this is a long list, the disorders in the differential have associated morphologic features (dysplasia, metastatic tumor cells, a lymphomatous infiltrate, etc) that make them less problematic to rule out histologically. For future treatment purposes and possibly for prognostic implications, it may be critical to identify whether the *JAK2V617F* is present. However, for the vast majority of cases, the diagnosis of the fibrotic stage of PMF can be made mainly at the microscope.

ESSENTIAL THROMBOCYTHEMIA AND THE PREFIBROTIC STAGE OF PMF

The diagnostic criteria for ET have changed in two major ways after the previous WHO publication (**Box 4**). First, the threshold for the platelet elevation has been lowered. In the earlier criteria, it was required that the platelet count be 600×10^9/L or more,[2] whereas in the revised criteria, it was lowered to 450×10^9/L or more.[1] This change was made in hopes of identifying cases earlier in their course for better intervention. The second change was the inclusion of the finding of the *JAK2V617F* or other clonal markers, or in their absence, no cause for a reactive thrombocytosis. The *JAK2* mutation is seen in ~50% of cases of ET and can be a tremendous help in ruling out a reactive thrombocytosis. The *MPL* mutation, present in only 1% of cases, and cytogenetic clones, which are also rare, make these less useful in this regard. The presence of the *JAK2* mutation in ET may have a morphologic correlate as well. It is believed that positive cases may resemble PV with increased erythropoiesis and granulopoiesis compared with negative cases with more prominent thrombopoiesis.[53] However, there does not seem to be any clinical associations. There apparently is no increased risk for thrombosis in positive versus negative cases,[54] although this may need additional study.

Although the presence of *JAK2V617F* is useful for ruling out a reactive cause of significantly elevated platelets, it must be realized that the diagnosis of ET is still mostly exclusionary. In the absence of the mutation, one must first consider reactive thrombocytosis and then other diseases that can present with high platelet counts. These include the other MPN, including CML, PV, and PMF, as well as myelodysplastic syndromes, the overlap myelodysplastic/myeloproliferative disorders and AML, and particularly the myeloid disorders associated with del(5q), t(3;3)(q21;q26.2)/

Box 4
2008 WHO criteria for the diagnosis of ET

1. Sustained platelet count of 450×10^9/L or more

2. Bone marrow biopsy specimen showing proliferation mainly of megakaryocytes that are large and mature. There is no increase or left shift in granulocytes or erythroid elements.

3. Not meeting criteria for PV, PMF, CML, MDS, or other myeloid neoplasm

4. Demonstration of *JAK2V617F* or other clonal marker, or in the absence of *JAK2V617F*, no evidence of reactive thrombocytosis.

All four criteria must be met.
Data from Swerdlow SH, Campo E, Harris NL, et al, editors. WHO classification of tumours of haematopoietic and lymphoid tissues. Lyon: IARC; 2008. p. 48.

inv(3)(q21q26.2).[52] In the presence of the *JAK2* mutation one still has to exclude PV, PMF, and some of the other disorders that can occasionally have the mutation.

Most of the entities to be considered in the differential of ET can be excluded by fairly straightforward means, including clinical history, careful morphologic evaluation of blood and bone marrow, cytogenetic study, and molecular analysis. ET should not show dysplasia in the erythroid or granulocytic lines, should not have elevated blasts, the small "dwarf" megakaryocytes of CML, or the *BCR-ABL1*. It should also not show the cytogenetic abnormalities seen in AML or MDS with increased platelets, that is, t(3;3)(q21;q26.2)/inv(3)(q21q26.2) or those related to del(5q). Despite the reasonable ability to exclude most entities in the differential, the distinction between ET and an early prefibrotic phase of PMF can be difficult. It is entirely independent of the presence or absence of *JAK2V617F* or *MPL* mutations, because these can be seen in both entities.

It is believed that about one-third of patients with PMF present with a prefibrotic phase. This is obviously an early phase of the disease in which fibrosis has not yet developed. In the absence of fibrosis and the subsequent extramedullary hematopoiesis that it typically causes, there is no extramedullary hematopoiesis, no splenomegaly, no leukoerythroblastosis, and no circulating tear-drop forms. Without fibrosis, morphologic and clinical features of prefibrotic PMF overlaps significantly with ET, and the diagnostician is sometimes left undecided in distinguishing between the two. One must ask whether distinguishing one from the other is important regarding immediate therapy, and it may be that there is no immediate consequence for not being able to do so. However, some investigators would argue that distinguishing ET from the prefibrotic stage of PMF has great significance regarding prognosis. According to carefully performed studies from Germany, correctly classifying a case as prefibrotic PMF versus ET improves the ability to predict outcome. Correctly identifying a case as ET versus PMF leads to an ability to predict improved life expectancy. This is opposed to correctly identifying prefibrotic PMF from a suspected ET, which leads to an accurate prediction of worsened life expectancy.[55]

The histologic features that are believed to separate prefibrotic PMF from ET are listed in **Table 2** and are illustrated in **Fig. 3**. They are somewhat subtle and, in some cases, might not be as easily recognized as hoped. These include a less prominent cellularity in ET compared with a more densely cellular marrow in prefibrotic PMF; loose clusters of hyperlobated megakaryocytes with a large to giant size and a staghorn appearance in ET versus dense clusters of more atypical, often

Table 2
Morphologic differences between prefibrotic PMF and ET

	ET	Prefibrotic PMF
Cellularity	Less cellular	More cellular
Megakaryocytes	Less clustered	More clustered
	Large and giant	Various sized, small to large
	Lobulated (staghorn)	Bulbus (cloudlike)
	Less atypical	Maturation defects, hyperchromatic
	Mature cytoplasm	Varied cytoplasm, naked nuclei
Granulopoiesis	Less proliferation	More proliferation
	Less left-shifted	More frequently left-shifted

Data from Thiele J, Kvasnicka HM, Schmitt-Graeff A, et al. Follow-up examinations including sequential bone marrow biopsies in essential thrombocythemia (ET): a retrospective clinicopathological study of 120 patients. Am J Hematol 2002;70:283–91.

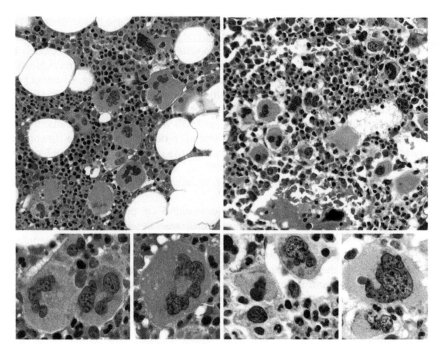

Fig. 3. ET versus prefibrotic PMF. In ET (*left*), the marrow is less cellular, and the megakaryocytes are less clustered. The megakaryocytes are large and larger. The background hematopoiesis is normal with erythroid and granulocytic maturation. The megakaryocytes (*bottom left*) have abundant cytoplasm and lobulated nuclei, sometimes with a staghorn appearance. In prefibrotic PMF, the cellularity is usually higher, and the megakaryocytes are in tighter clusters. The background hematopoietic activity is predominantly granulocytic. The megakaryocytes (*bottom right*) are atypical and small to large, sometimes with less cytoplasm and sometimes with hyperchromic nuclei. Some large forms (*bottom, far right*) have a cloud like appearance to the nucleus.

hyperchromatic megakaryocytes with maturational defects and naked nuclei in prefibrotic PMF; and the absence of erythroid, particularly of neutrophilic proliferation in ET, compared with the presence of a predominant background granulocytic proliferation with a left shift in prefibrotic PMF.[56] However, whether these can be used consistently or even reproducibly, and whether they can accurately predict the progress of a patient to a fibrotic stage (PMF) or otherwise (ET) has been questioned.[57,58] It seems reasonable to accept that in some instances a diagnosis of one or the other disease cannot be firmly established early on.

MAST CELL DISEASE AND CNL

In the revised WHO classification of hematological tumors, the MCD entities have been appropriately moved to the MPN section; however, the list of major entities has remained the same.[1] These include cutaneous mastocytosis, indolent systemic mastocytosis, systemic mastocytosis (SM) with associated clonally hematological nonmast cell disease, aggressive systemic mastocytosis, mast cell sarcoma, and extracutaneous mastocytoma.

A more in-depth focus on MCD is beyond the scope of this review, but suffice it to say that the association of another TK abnormality, (a *KIT* mutation [D816V] in most cases of SM), allows it to fit nicely with the other MPN in the "TK story."[59] Abnormalities in the *KIT* gene in MCD may even be useful in the diagnosis if the cases are morphologically challenging. Because the disease is rare, there is less familiarity with its morphologic features, and many cases can be overlooked or can be difficult to recognize. This is especially the case when they are associated concurrently with other myeloid or even lymphoid neoplasms, as they commonly are. Despite the association of MCD with a TK mutation, the disease is generally not responsive to imatinib, although other TK inhibitors are being tried.

CNL is a rare entity, and only about 150 cases have been published.[1] It is also a disease that has yet to be understood fully. The presence of myeloma in at least one-third of cases and the knowledge that the plasma cell–derived cytokines might constitute a reactive stimulus for neutrophils in such cases, raises the question of whether some of the cases are reactive or even malignant. A firm diagnosis is made when the white blood cell (WBC) count is $25 \times 10^9/L$ or more, when segmented neutrophils are 80% or more of the leukocytes, when there are less than 1% blasts in the peripheral blood, when the marrow is hypercellular with less than 5% blasts, when there is hepatosplenomegaly, and when other diseases such as CML, myeloid neoplasms with eosinophilia, PV, ET, PMF, and MDS are ruled out. The identification of clonality in the neutrophils can greatly facilitate the diagnosis, but this is not easy to show in most cases.[60] *JAK2*V617F mutation has been described in occasional cases of CNL.

SUMMARY

Starting with CML and progressing to the myeloid neoplasms with eosinophilia, and subsequently to the common MPN, PV, ET, and PMF and to MCD, the "TK story" unifies the MPN and fulfills the insightful speculations of Dameshek[6] in his 1951 musings. The recent insights into the molecular pathogenesis of the disorders have initiated a significant change in the classification of the different entities and in the criteria for diagnosis of many of the diseases. Although the insights and the changes have been remarkable, it is prudent to remember that the significance of the TK mutations is not entirely clear. Many unanswered questions remain. Nevertheless, the new insights into the molecular pathogenesis of this group of disease are exciting and could have great potential with regard to the development of future therapies. Near the end of his 1951 commentary, Dameshek[6] speculated that "putting these disorders together ... may prove useful and even productive." Given the tremendous success of imatinib in CML and the hopes for other TK inhibitors for the other diseases, the remark in retrospect seems quite prophetic.

REFERENCES

1. Swerdlow SH, Campo E, Harris NL, et al, editors. WHO classification of tumours of haematopoietic and lymphoid tissues. Lyon: IARC; 2008.
2. Jaffe ES, Harris NL, Stein H, et al, editors. WHO classification of tumours. Pathology and genetics of tumours of haematopoietic and lymphoid tissues. Lyon: IARC Press; 2001.
3. Levine RL, Gilliland DG. Myeloproliferative disorders. Blood 2008;112:2190–8.
4. Smith CA, Fan G. The saga of JAK2 mutations and translocations in hematologic disorders: pathogenesis, diagnostic and therapeutic prospects, and revised World Health Organization diagnostic criteria for myeloproliferative neoplasms. Hum Pathol 2008;39:795–810.

5. Tefferi A, Gilliland DG. Oncogenes in myeloproliferative disorders. Cell Cycle 2007;6:550–66.
6. Dameshek W. Some speculations on the myeloproliferative syndromes. Blood 1951;6:372–5.
7. Tefferi A, Vardiman JW. Classification and diagnosis of myeloproliferative neoplasms: the 2008 World Health Organization criteria and point-of-care diagnostic algorithms. Leukemia 2008;22:14–22.
8. Anastasi J. The myeloproliferative and overlap myelodysplastic/myeloproliferative disorders. In: Hsi ED, editor. Hematopathology. Philadelphia: Elsevier; 2007. p. 455–92.
9. Bennett JH. Two cases of disease and enlargement of the spleen in which death took place from the presence of purulent matter in the blood. Edinburgh Med Surg J 1845;64:413.
10. Virchow P. Weisses blut. Froriep's Notizen 1845;36:151.
11. Nowell PC, Hungerford DA. Chromosome studies on normal and leukemic human leukocytes. J Natl Cancer Inst 1960;25:85–109.
12. Rowley JD. Letter: a new consistent chromosomal abnormality in chronic myelogenous leukaemia identified by quinacrine fluorescence and Giemsa staining. Nature 1973;243:290–3.
13. Bartram CR, de Klein A, Hagemeijer A, et al. Translocation of c-ab1 oncogene correlates with the presence of a Philadelphia chromosome in chronic myelocytic leukaemia. Nature 1983;306:277–80.
14. Konopka JB, Witte ON. Detection of c-abl tyrosine kinase activity in vitro permits direct comparison of normal and altered abl gene products. Mol Cell Biol 1985;5:3116–23.
15. Shtivelman E, Lifshitz B, Gale RP, et al. Fused transcript of abl and bcr genes in chronic myelogenous leukaemia. Nature 1985;315:550–4.
16. Druker BJ, Tamura S, Buchdunger E, et al. Effects of a selective inhibitor of the Abl tyrosine kinase on the growth of Bcr-Abl positive cells. Nat Med 1996;2:561–6.
17. Deininger MW. Management of early stage disease. Hematology Am Soc Hematol Educ Program 2005;174–82.
18. Druker BJ, Sawyers CL, Kantarjian H, et al. Activity of a specific inhibitor of the BCR-ABL tyrosine kinase in the blast crisis of chronic myeloid leukemia and acute lymphoblastic leukemia with the Philadelphia chromosome. N Engl J Med 2001;344:1038–42.
19. Hughes T, Deininger M, Hochhaus A, et al. Monitoring CML patients responding to treatment with tyrosine kinase inhibitors: review and recommendations for harmonizing current methodology for detecting BCR-ABL transcripts and kinase domain mutations and for expressing results. Blood 2006;108:28–37.
20. Gorre ME, Mohammed M, Ellwood K, et al. Clinical resistance to STI-571 cancer therapy caused by BCR-ABL gene mutation or amplification. Science 2001;293:876–80.
21. Irving JA, O'Brien S, Lennard AL, et al. Use of denaturing HPLC for detection of mutations in the BCR-ABL kinase domain in patients resistant to imatinib. Clin Chem 2004;50:1233–7.
22. Walz C, Sattler M. Novel targeted therapies to overcome imatinib mesylate resistance in chronic myeloid leukemia (CML). Crit Rev Oncol Hematol 2006;57:145–64.
23. Kramer A. JAK2-V617F and BCR-ABL–double jeopardy? Leuk Res 2008;32:1489.

24. Raskind WH, Tirumali N, Jacobson R, et al. Evidence for a multistep pathogenesis of a myelodysplastic syndrome. Blood 1984;63:1318–23.
25. Apperley JF, Gardembas M, Melo JV, et al. Response to imatinib mesylate in patients with chronic myeloproliferative diseases with rearrangements of the platelet-derived growth factor receptor beta. N Engl J Med 2002;347:481–7.
26. Cools J, DeAngelo DJ, Gotlib J, et al. A tyrosine kinase created by fusion of the PDGFRA and FIP1L1 genes as a therapeutic target of imatinib in idiopathic hypereosinophilic syndrome. N Engl J Med 2003;348:1201–14.
27. Pardanani A, Reeder T, Porrata LF, et al. Imatinib therapy for hypereosinophilic syndrome and other eosinophilic disorders. Blood 2003;101:3391–7.
28. Golub TR, Barker GF, Lovett M, et al. Fusion of PDGF receptor beta to a novel ets-like gene, tel, in chronic myelomonocytic leukemia with t(5;12) chromosomal translocation. Cell 1994;77:307–16.
29. Pardanani A, Ketterling RP, Brockman SR, et al. CHIC2 deletion, a surrogate for FIP1L1-PDGFRA fusion, occurs in systemic mastocytosis associated with eosinophilia and predicts response to imatinib mesylate therapy. Blood 2003;102:3093–6.
30. Macdonald D, Aguiar RC, Mason PJ, et al. A new myeloproliferative disorder associated with chromosomal translocations involving 8p11: a review. Leukemia 1995;9:1628–30.
31. Macdonald D, Reiter A, Cross NC. The 8p11 myeloproliferative syndrome: a distinct clinical entity caused by constitutive activation of FGFR1. Acta Haematol 2002;107:101–7.
32. Baxter EJ, Scott LM, Campbell PJ, et al. Acquired mutation of the tyrosine kinase JAK2 in human myeloproliferative disorders. Lancet 2005;365:1054–61.
33. James C, Ugo V, Le Couedic JP, et al. A unique clonal JAK2 mutation leading to constitutive signalling causes polycythaemia vera. Nature 2005;434:1144–8.
34. Kralovics R, Passamonti F, Buser AS, et al. A gain-of-function mutation of JAK2 in myeloproliferative disorders. N Engl J Med 2005;352:1779–90.
35. Levine RL, Loriaux M, Huntly BJ, et al. The JAK2V617F activating mutation occurs in chronic myelomonocytic leukemia and acute myeloid leukemia, but not in acute lymphoblastic leukemia or chronic lymphocytic leukemia. Blood 2005;106:3377–9.
36. Kralovics R, Guan Y, Prchal JT. Acquired uniparental disomy of chromosome 9p is a frequent stem cell defect in polycythemia vera. Exp Hematol 2002;30:229–36.
37. Ceesay MM, Lea NC, Ingram W, et al. The JAK2 V617F mutation is rare in RARS but common in RARS-T. Leukemia 2006;20:2060–1.
38. Remacha AF, Nomdedeu JF, Puget G, et al. Occurrence of the JAK2 V617F mutation in the WHO provisional entity: myelodysplastic/myeloproliferative disease, unclassifiable-refractory anemia with ringed sideroblasts associated with marked thrombocytosis. Haematologica 2006;91:719–20.
39. Szpurka H, Tiu R, Murugesan G, et al. Refractory anemia with ringed sideroblasts associated with marked thrombocytosis (RARS-T), another myeloproliferative condition characterized by JAK2 V617F mutation. Blood 2006;108:2173–81.
40. Greiner TC. Diagnostic assays for the JAK2 V617F mutation in chronic myeloproliferative disorders. Am J Clin Pathol 2006;125:651–3.
41. James C. The JAK2V617F mutation in polycythemia vera and other myeloproliferative disorders: one mutation for three diseases? Hematology Am Soc Hematol Educ Program 2008;69–75.
42. Campbell PJ, Baxter EJ, Beer PA, et al. Mutation of JAK2 in the myeloproliferative disorders: timing, clonality studies, cytogenetic associations, and role in leukemic transformation. Blood 2006;108:3548–55.

43. Kralovics R, Teo SS, Li S, et al. Acquisition of the V617F mutation of JAK2 is a late genetic event in a subset of patients with myeloproliferative disorders. Blood 2006;108:1377–80.

44. Bellanne-Chantelot C, Chaumarel I, Labopin M, et al. Genetic and clinical implications of the Val617Phe JAK2 mutation in 72 families with myeloproliferative disorders. Blood 2006;108:346–52.

45. James C, Mazurier F, Dupont S, et al. The hematopoietic stem cell compartment of JAK2V617F-positive myeloproliferative disorders is a reflection of disease heterogeneity. Blood 2008;112:2429–38.

46. Xu X, Zhang Q, Luo J, et al. JAK2(V617F): prevalence in a large Chinese hospital population. Blood 2007;109:339–42.

47. Scott LM, Tong W, Levine RL, et al. JAK2 exon 12 mutations in polycythemia vera and idiopathic erythrocytosis. N Engl J Med 2007;356:459–68.

48. Mesa RA, Verstovsek S, Cervantes F, et al. Primary myelofibrosis (PMF), post polycythemia vera myelofibrosis (post-PV MF), post essential thrombocythemia myelofibrosis (post-ET MF), blast phase PMF (PMF-BP): consensus on terminology by the international working group for myelofibrosis research and treatment (IWG-MRT). Leuk Res 2007;31:737–40.

49. Silverstein MN. Agnogenic myeloid metaplasia. Acton (MA): Publishing Science Group; 1975.

50. Pardanani AD, Levine RL, Lasho T, et al. MPL515 mutations in myeloproliferative and other myeloid disorders: a study of 1182 patients. Blood 2006;108:3472–6.

51. Reilly JT, Snowden JA, Spearing RL, et al. Cytogenetic abnormalities and their prognostic significance in idiopathic myelofibrosis: a study of 106 cases. Br J Haematol 1997;98:96–102.

52. Foucar K. Bone marrow pathology. 2nd edition. Chicago: ASCP Press; 2001.

53. Campbell PJ, Scott LM, Buck G, et al. Definition of subtypes of essential thrombocythaemia and relation to polycythaemia vera based on JAK2 V617F mutation status: a prospective study. Lancet 2005;366:1945–53.

54. Carobbio A, Antonioli E, Guglielmelli P, et al. Leukocytosis and risk stratification assessment in essential thrombocythemia. J Clin Oncol 2008;26:2732–6.

55. Thiele J, Kvasnicka HM, Schmitt-Graeff A, et al. Follow-up examinations including sequential bone marrow biopsies in essential thrombocythemia (ET): a retrospective clinicopathological study of 120 patients. Am J Hematol 2002;70:283–91.

56. Thiele J, Kvasnicka HM, Zankovich R, et al. Relevance of bone marrow features in the differential diagnosis between essential thrombocythemia and early stage idiopathic myelofibrosis. Haematologica 2000;85:1126–34.

57. Spivak JL, Silver RT. The revised World Health Organization diagnostic criteria for polycythemia vera, essential thrombocytosis, and primary myelofibrosis: an alternative proposal. Blood 2008;112:231–9.

58. Wilkins BS, Erber WN, Bareford D, et al. Bone marrow pathology in essential thrombocythemia: interobserver reliability and utility for identifying disease subtypes. Blood 2008;111:60–70.

59. Tefferi A, Pardanani A. Clinical, genetic, and therapeutic insights into systemic mast cell disease. Curr Opin Hematol 2004;11:58–64.

60. Standen GR, Steers FJ, Jones L. Clonality of chronic neutrophilic leukaemia associated with myeloma: analysis using the X-linked probe M27 beta. J Clin Pathol 1993;46:297–8.

Plasma Cell Myeloma

Pei Lin, MD

KEYWORDS
- Myeloma • MGUS • Plasmacytoma • Amyloid
- Immunophenotype • Cytogenetics • Prognosis

Plasma cell myeloma is a B-cell neoplasm characterized by clonal expansion of plasma cells in the bone marrow, which produces lytic bone lesions and monoclonal protein. It is one of the most common hematological malignancies in the United States. Plasma cell myeloma is a rather heterogeneous disease with variable clinical presentation and outcome determined largely by the tumor biology as well as the host response. In recent years, approaches to identify different risk groups and strategies to improve clinical outcome have focused on the molecular genetics of the neoplastic cells as well as the bone marrow microenvironment that sustains the neoplastic cells. Although conventional cytogenetics remains a powerful tool in clinical assessment, new techniques such as array comparative genomic hybridization, gene expression profiling, and single nucleotide polymorphism (SNP) mapping allow genome-wide investigation of myeloma genetics and molecular classification of myeloma. The emergence of novel therapeutic agents such as immune modulators thalidomide, its derivative lenolidomide, and proteasome inhibitors such as bortezomib are rapidly changing the long-term outlook of myeloma patients, making "personalized medicine" in myeloma patient care highly achievable. We review here the current knowledge of plasma cell myeloma and briefly describe other related diseases such as monoclonal gammopathy of unknown significance, solitary plasmacytoma of bone or soft tissue, and monoclonal immunoglobulin deposition diseases.

EPIDEMIOLOGY

Multiple myeloma, or plasma cell myeloma, accounts for approximately 10% of all hematological malignances in the United States. The annual incidence has steadily increased to 19,920 new cases in 2008 according to the estimates of American Cancer Society. It is largely an incurable disease with an annual death rate of 10,690. Plasma cell myeloma affects mainly older people with a median age of 70 years. Only 1% to 2% of cases are diagnosed in people younger than 40 years. It is twice as common among black as white populations, and men are affected slightly more than women.[1] Previously described risk factors include family history, obesity, and exposure to petroleum, pesticides, or radiation, but many are controversial.

Department of Hematopathology, Box 72, University of Texas-MD Anderson Cancer Center, 1515 Holcombe Boulevard, Houston, TX 77070, USA
E-mail address: peilin@mdanderson.org

Hematol Oncol Clin N Am 23 (2009) 709–727
doi:10.1016/j.hoc.2009.04.012
0889-8588/09/$ – see front matter © 2009 Elsevier Inc. All rights reserved.

CLINICAL FEATURES

Presenting symptoms are variable and depend on the extent of tumor burden and activity. Most patients present with bone pain due to tumor infiltration and pathologic fractures. Fatigue and weakness secondary to anemia as well as renal failure and recurrent infection are also common. Less frequent symptoms include hyperviscosity syndrome, hypercalcemia, and spinal cord compression as a result of vertebral body fracture or epidural tumor mass. Some patients may be asymptomatic and the disease diagnosed incidentally.

Historically, the diagnosis of myeloma is established using major and minor criteria, defined largely by the extent of marrow plasmacytosis, lytic lesions, and levels of M protein. A minimum of 10% or more of monoclonal plasma cells and presence of M protein in the serum or urine are generally required. Those who meet the minimal criteria but are asymptomatic or with low tumor burdens are considered to have smoldering or indolent myeloma, which may require no immediate therapeutic intervention. Symptomatic patients with the clinical manifestations described here usually have monoclonal plasma cells 30% or more and serum M protein 30 g/L or more or Bence Jones protein 1 g/d or more.

The International Myeloma Working Group (IMWG) introduced a simplified diagnostic scheme in 2003, which no longer relies on the major or minor criteria.[2] Although the minimal diagnostic criteria remain the same in the IMWG scheme, cases with monoclonal plasma cells and M protein that are below the minimal criteria can still be diagnosed as long as evidence of related end organ or tissue impairment (RETI) is confirmed. RETI is defined as hypercalcemia, renal insufficiency, and anemia or bone lesions (**Box 1**). This modification is supported by the clinical observation that a small number of symptomatic patients have plasmacytosis less than 10% and M protein less than 3 g/dL. The diagnosis of smoldering myeloma is still reserved for patients who meet the minimal criteria but are asymptomatic clinically, and the category of indolent myeloma is discontinued.[2] The IMWG scheme is adopted by the new World Health Organization (WHO) classification published in 2008.[3]

RADIOGRAPHIC IMAGING

Imaging studies are essential for assessment of the extent and activity of the disease. Standard skeletal survey detects bone changes that may range from osteolysis in most cases to osteopenia or rarely osteosclerosis. The characteristic findings on bone survey are multiple "punched-out" lytic lesions within the axial skeleton, such as skull, vertebral bodies, pelvis, or upper part of the extremities (**Fig. 1**). Identification of lytic lesions excludes the diagnosis of monoclonal gammopathy of unknown significance (MGUS). Computerized tomography is usually unnecessary except in cases with a negative skeletal survey. MRI is useful in assessing for spinal cord compression and for extramedullary diseases, and PET scan may detect small lytic lesions not detected by skeletal survey. They are increasingly used in clinical staging.

MORPHOLOGY

Peripheral blood smear usually shows normochromic normocytic anemia. Rouleaux formation is a striking feature that results from high level of serum M protein. Circulating plasma cells are increased in plasma cell leukemia (PCL) and may resemble lymphocytes. Leukopenia and thrombocytopenia are usually features of an advanced stage of disease.

Box 1
World Health Organization diagnostic criteria of myeloma and MGUS

Symptomatic plasma cell myeloma:

M protein in serum and/or urine

Bone marrow (clonal) plasma cells or plasmacytoma

Related organ or tissue impairment (end organ damage, including bone lesions) (see later text)

Myeloma-Related Organ or Tissue Impairment (End organ damage):

Serum calcium >0.25 mmol/L (1 mg/dL) above the upper limit of normal or >2.75 mmol/L (11 mg/dL)

Renal insufficiency: creatinine >173 mmol/L (1.96 mg/dL)

Anemia: hemoglobin 2 g/dL below the lower limit of normal or hemoglobin <10 g/dL

Bone lesions: lytic lesions or osteopenia with compression fractures

Other: symptomatic hyperviscosity, amyloidosis, recurrent bacterial infections (>2 episodes in 12 mo)

Asymptomatic (smoldering) myeloma

M protein in serum >30 g/L and/or

Bone marrow clonal plasma cells >10%

No related organ or tissue impairment (including bone lesions) or symptoms

Monoclonal gammopathy of undetermined significance

M protein in serum <30 g/L

Bone marrow clonal plasma cells <10%, and low level of plasma cell infiltration in a trephine biopsy

No evidence of other B-cell proliferative disorders

No related organ or tissue impairment (including bone lesions)

Enumeration of plasma cells is routinely performed on Wright-Giemsa–stained bone marrow aspirate smears using a differential count of 200-500 cells. Since tumor infiltration can be patchy or associated with fibrosis resulting in a dry tap, trephine biopsy should be performed at least initially to allow more reliable assessment of tumor load

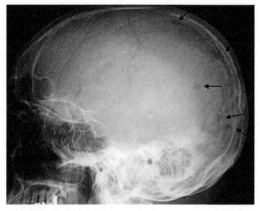

Fig. 1. "Punched-out" osteolytic lesions (*arrows*) characteristic of plasma cell myeloma on skull survey.

as well as detection of amyloid deposition and bone changes. In symptomatic myeloma, there are usually increased osteoclastic activity and microvascular density.[4]

Normal plasma cells are of "Marschalko" type with "spoke-wheel" nuclear chromatin pattern and perinuclear hof, comprising less than 4% of nucleated cells. Plasmacytosis, sometimes up to 30% to 40% and with binucleated or even trinucleated forms, can be observed in reactive conditions such as autoimmune diseases or viral infections. Reactive plasma cells, however, do not show immature or anaplastic features typical of neoplastic plasma cells. These features include immature chromatin and prominent nucleoli, bizarre nuclear shapes, and marked variation in nuclear size. They are strong evidence of myeloma even when the plasma cells are less than 10% or lack light chain restriction, as in cases of nonsecretory myeloma. Cytoplasmic inclusions such as Russell bodies or crystalline rods are immunoglobulin accumulations. Cells containing multiple immunoglobulin inclusions are described as flame cells, Mott cells, and Gaucher-like cells. Nuclear inclusions such as Dutcher bodies are usually an indication of neoplastic plasma cells, whereas cytoplasmic inclusions are nonspecific.

Two major grading systems, Greipp and the Bartl, are designed to capture the morphologic spectrum of myeloma cells.[5] The Greipp system consists of mature, intermediate, immature, and plasmablastic subtypes. The Bartl system consists of 3 tiers with 7 subtypes. The low grade consists of small-cell variant and Marschalko type. The intermediate grade consists of polymorphous, asynchronous type, and cleaved cell type; the high grade consists of blastic and sarcomatous types. (Fig. 2A–G) Bartl also described 6 patterns of infiltration as interstitial, interstitial with paratrabecular sheets, interstitial/nodular, nodular, packed, and sarcomatous.

Recognition of different subtypes helps to distinguish myeloma from mimics. For example, the asynchronous or blastic subtype may resemble acute monoblastic leukemia. Polymorphous type of myeloma with multinucleated neoplastic cells and fibrosis can be mistaken for primary myelofibrosis or acute panmyelosis with myelofibrosis. The small-cell variant closely resembles low-grade B-cell lymphoma or leukemia with plasmacytic differentiation, such as lymphoplasmacytic lymphoma or marginal zone B-cell lymphoma.

LABORATORY TESTS

M protein can be detected in most patients by serum or urine protein electrophoresis (SPEP/UPEP) as a narrow peak in the densitometer tracing or a distinct band on agarose gel (Fig. 3). The most common type of M protein is IgG (55%), followed by IgA (22%), light chain only (18%), IgD or IgE (2%), biclonal (2%), and IgM (<1%). About 1% of myeloma is nonsecretory type. The presence of M protein is usually accompanied by suppression of normal gamma globulin and sometimes albumin. In light chain only myeloma, hypogammaglobulinemia may be the only finding. Bence Jones protein can be detected in up to 80% of patients.

Immunofixation (IFE) determines the type of M protein and will detect serum M-protein of 0.2 g/L or greater and a urine M-protein of 0.04 g/L or greater. IFE is the gold standard for detection of M protein. Serum immunoglobulin quantification shows suppression of nonmyeloma immunoglobulin. Serial quantification of M protein allows easy assessment of tumor load reduction as indication of response to treatment.[6]

Serum or urine free immunoglobulin light chain (FLC) ratio (κ/λ) is considered to be most useful in MGUS, AL amyloidosis, light chain deposition disease (LCDD), and oligosecretory or nonsecretory myeloma when the M protein levels are low. It is also used to assess treatment response six. Recently, it has been shown that FLC ratio

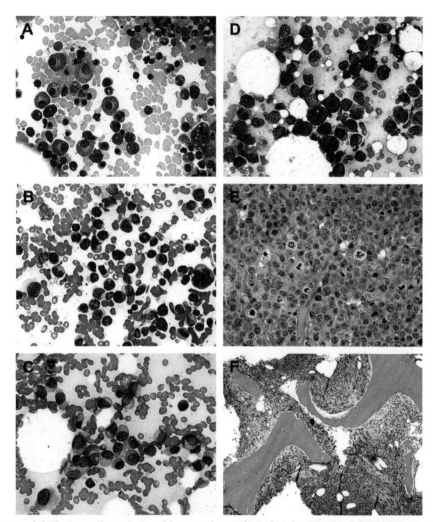

Fig. 2. (*A*) Plasma cell myeloma of low-grade cytology (Wight-Giemsa, x500); (*B*) intermediate-grade cytology, polymorphous type (Wight-Giemsa, x500); (*C*) intermediate-grade, asynchronous type (Wight-Giemsa, x500); (*D*) high-grade cytology, plasmablastic subtype (Wright-Giemsa, x500); (*E*) Sheets of immature plasma cells and increased mitotic figures (Hematoxylin and eosin, 400x); (*F*) myeloma infiltrate associated with fibrosis (Hematoxylin and eosin, 100x).

of <0.03 or >32 at initial diagnosis predicts greater risk for asymptomatic myeloma to evolve to a symptomatic one.[7,8] However, the sensitivity and specificity of FLC analysis in comparison to SPEP and IFE are still controversial. In many instances, FLC analysis cannot replace SPEP and IFE.

Serum level of β2 microglobulin (β2M) reflects tumor turnover and renal function. C-reactive protein (CRP) regulated by interleukin-6 (IL-6) can be a surrogate marker for myeloma activity. Serum carboxy-terminal telopeptide of type-1 collagen is a specific and sensitive marker for bone resorption.[9] LDH is usually elevated in patients with extensive lymph node involvement and is associated with a poor

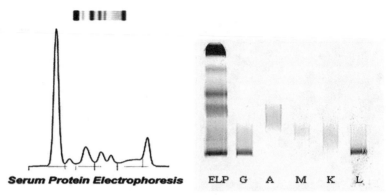

Serum Protein Electrophoresis   ELP G A M K L

Fig. 3. Serum protein electrophoresis demonstrates a spike, and immune fixation electrophoresis confirms IgG λ M protein.

prognosis. The plasma cell labeling index (PCLI) measures synthesis of DNA by using a monoclonal antibody (BU-1). BU-1 reacts with bromodeoxyuridine that is incorporated into DNA by cells in S phase. PCLI is usually greater than 1% in symptomatic myeloma or greater than 5% in advanced disease.[2]

IMMUNOPHENOTYPE

Flow cytometry (FCM) immunophenotyping helps identifying neoplastic plasma cells in morphologically challenging or nonsecretory cases. Aberrant markers identified may serve as potential therapeutic targets or facilitate detection of minimal residual disease.[10] Myeloma cells typically express CD138 (syndecan-1), CD38, and monotypic cytoplasmic immunoglobulin light chain. Expression of other markers is variable, and the frequency of those commonly assessed in clinical laboratory is summarized in **Table 1**. CD56 expression is usually indicative of malignancy and is more common in myeloma than in primary PCL or extramedullary disease. CD117 expression is associated with favorable clinical features, whereas CD28 expression is associated with aggressive clinical features.[11] Unlike plasma cells in B-cell lymphomas with plasmacytic differentiation or reactive conditions, myeloma cells rarely express CD19. Most cases also lack other B-cell–associated antigens such as CD20, CD22, and CD24. The myeloma cells are also usually negative or weakly positive for CD45. However, CD20 and CD45 can be positive in a subset of myeloma cases at moderate or greater intensity. It is also common that a subpopulation within a tumor expresses markers different from the remaining population. Using a 2-step acquisition procedure with a live gate for plasma cells (gate drawn on the CD138++ CD38++ population) **(Fig. 4)**, FCM can detect minimal residual disease in 1 in 10^4 to 10^5 cells, and the

Table 1								
Expression frequency of commonly assessed markers in plasma cell myeloma								
Marker	CD138	CD38	CD56	CD117	CD28	CD45	CD20	CD19
Frequency (%)	98–100	100	65	25–30	15–45	10–20	20–30	<5
Pattern	Bright	Bright	Bright	Moderate-bright	Moderate-bright	Moderate-bright	Moderate-bright	Dim-moderate

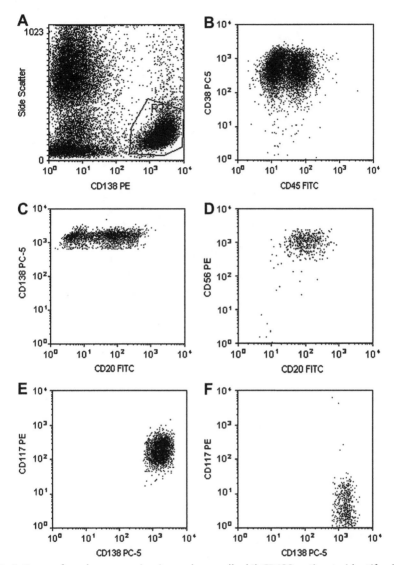

Fig. 4. Patterns of marker expression in myeloma cells. (*A*) CD138 gating to identify plasma cells. (*B*) Subsets of CD138-positive myeloma cells show different patterns of CD45 expression, one negative and another positive. (*C*) CD20 is expressed in a subset of myeloma cells. (*D*) The myeloma cells are positive for CD56 and CD20. (*E*) The myeloma cells express CD117. (*F*) CD117 is negative.

detection sensitivity is enhanced in cases with aberrant marker expression or aneuploidy.[10] A small number of monotypic B cells expressing identical isotype of surface light chain as the myeloma cells can be detected concurrently in the peripheral blood and bone marrow.[12,13]

Immunohistochemical stain for CD138 readily identifies plasma cells in the biopsy sections, allowing assessment of the extent and pattern of infiltration (**Fig. 5**A). In contrast to reactive conditions or MGUS, myeloma cells infiltrate in sheets or large

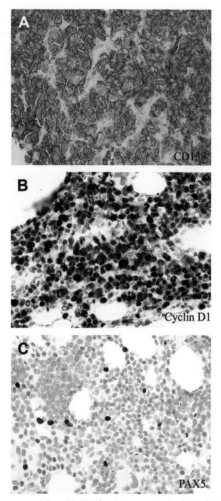

Fig. 5. The plasma cells are positive CD138 by immunostain (400x), A case of IgM myeloma positive for cyclin D1 (nuclear and cytoplasmic staining) and t(11;14) (400x). They are negative for PAX5/BSAP (immunohistochemistry, 400x).

clusters. A caveat to keep in mind is that CD138 also stains the neoplastic cells of immunoblastic or plasmablastic lymphomas and epithelial tumors. Rarely, cases of myeloma may be negative or weakly positive for CD138. Myeloma cells also frequently expressed MUM1 and CD79a. Approximately 30% to 45% of cases are immunoreactive for cyclin D1 in a cytoplasmic and nuclear pattern (see **Fig. 5**B), a feature helpful to distinguish CD20-positive or IgM-secreting myeloma from mantle cell lymphoma, which typically stains positive in a nuclear pattern.[14,15] Expression of cyclin D1 can be seen in myeloma cases without t(11;14). PAX5/BSAP, a B-cell transcription factor downregulated in the terminally differentiated B cells and plasma cells, is usually negative, or weak and variable in myeloma (see **Fig. 5**C). EBV-encoded RNA in situ hybridization is usually positive in plasmablastic lymphoma but negative in myeloma or plasmacytoma.

GENETICS AND MOLECULAR GENETICS

Conventional cytogenetic analysis detects numerical or structural aberrations in only about 30% to 40% of newly diagnosed myeloma cases due to low metaphase yield. However, interphase fluorescence in situ hybridization (FISH) can detect abnormalities in nearly all cases. FISH also allows for comparison of genetic aberrations across different stages of disease, thereby providing insight into tumor biology.

Translocations involving immunoglobulin heavy-chain gene, usually the switch region on chromosome 14q32, are the most common cytogenetic aberrations, occurring in about 50% to 70% myeloma more than 50 partner genes have been described; the 5 most common ones, representing 40% of all cases with IgH translocation, are located at 11q, 4p, 16q, 6p, and 20q. The genes and their functions are mostly related to expression of cyclin D family protein and cell cycle regulation (**Table 2**).[16] These 5 IgH translocations are also detectable in MGUS and are considered therefore primary and possibly initiating events.

Apart from structural aberrations, numerical aberrations are also common. Trisomy most frequently involves chromosomes 3, 5, 7, 9, 11, 15, 19, and 21, whereas monosomy and partial deletions affect mainly chromosomes 6, 13, 16, and 22. Gains of 1q are the most common structure aberrations in myeloma, detectable in up to 40% of those with an abnormal karyotype.

Monosomy 13 or interstitial deletion of 13 (q14) is detectable in 15% to 20% of newly diagnosed MM by conventional cytogenetics and 50% of cases by interphase FISH. Deletion 13 can also be found in MGUS.

Based on the number of chromosomes, myeloma cases can be broadly divided into 2 groups: the hyperdiploid (HRD; 48–75 chromosomes) and nonhyperdiploid myeloma (NHRD; <48 or >75 chromosomes). HRD represents about half of cases and frequently carries trisomies. The 5 recurrent translocations described here and del13 are by far more common in NHRD than HRD, suggesting that different molecular genetic pathways are involved in pathogenesis of the 2 subgroups.[17] The precise underlying mechanisms are still under investigation.

Other genetic aberrations described in myeloma include *MYC* rearrangement, usually variant involving non-IgH, occurring in 10% to 15% of cases, amplification of 1q21 (putative [cyclin-dependent kinase subunit 1] *CKS1B* gene amplification) in 30% to 40%, *N or K-RAS* mutations in 30-40% % of cases, *p16* methylation in 20%–30%, and P53 mutations in 10% of cases.[17] Recent studies found that mutations of the nuclear factor-kappa B (NF-kB) pathway components, such as TRAF3, cIAP1/2, CYLD, and NIK, also contribute to pathogenesis of myeloma.[17] Unlike the 5 primary translocations and 13q deletions, *MYC* rearrangement or *RAS* mutations

Table 2
Most common partner genes involved in translocation of immunoglobulin heavy chain gene in plasma cell myeloma

Chromosome	Gene	Frequency (%)	Functions
11q13	CCND1	15–20	Cell cycle regulator
4p16	FGFR-3 & MMSET	15	Growth factor receptor tyrosine kinase Transcription factor
16q23	C-MAF	5	Transcription factor
6p21	CCND3	3	Cell cycle regulator
20q11	MAFB	2	Transcription factor

are usually absent or rare in MGUS, suggesting that they are unlikely to be early initiating events.

The advent of new genomic technology allows global investigation of genes altered in myeloma.[18] Biologic subgroups identified by DNA microarray are represented in the TC (translocation/cyclin D) classification scheme, which proposes 8 molecular subgroups—6q21, 11q13, D1, D1+D2, D2, non, 4p16, and maf—based on the predominant activation pattern of cyclin D protein and the pattern of IgH translocations.[19–21] Array has discovered novel biomarkers such as *CKS1B* and Dickkopf-1, predicting high risk and bone disease, respectively.[19,20,22–24] The 17-gene model proposed by the Arkansas group emphasizes the predicting power of a limited number of genes and the potential of array as a guide to clinical practice.[18] Other technologies such as array comparative genomic hybridization (aCGH) and single nucleotide polymorphism based mapping array also allow investigation of key candidate genes in the context of complex chromosomal gain and loss.[25] Similarly, proteinomics has shown promise in delineating pathways controlling myeloma growth and disease progression.

PATHOGENESIS

Myeloma cells are thought to arise from antigen-exposed post–germinal center B cells with IgH gene rearrangement, somatic hypermutation of the V regions, and isotype switching. Differentiation of B cells to plasma cells requires upregulation of XBP-1, BLIMP1, and MUM1/IRF4 and downregulation of transcription factor BCL6.[26]

Growth and expansion of the neoplastic clone requires support of the bone marrow microenvironment. Adhesion molecules on extracellular matrix proteins and bone marrow stromal cells regulate the homing of myeloma cells. The adherence of myeloma cells to stromal cells leads to the overproduction of several cytokines and growth factors, such as IL-6, insulin-like growth factor 1 (IGF-1), tumor necrosis factor-α (TNF-a), stromal-cell-derived factor-1α (SCF-1), and vascular endothelial growth factor (VEGF) through autocrine and paracrine loops. These then activate multiple signaling pathways including JAK/STAT, PI3k/Akt/NF-κB, and Wnt,[27] which in turn promote angiogenesis, survival, and drug resistance of myeloma cells. Conversely, myeloma bone lesions develop as a result of increased cytokines, such as macrophage inflammatory protein 1α (MIP-1 a), released by myeloma cells, causing overexpression of the receptor activator of nuclear factor-κB ligand (RANKL) by osteoblasts and reduction of its decoy receptor osteoprotegerin. The imbalance of the two molecules leads to increased bone resorption and decreased bone formation, which then releases a range of cytokines further promoting myeloma growth.

In support of the new myeloma disease model, novel therapeutic agents targeting myeloma cells and their microenvironment have been shown to be effective in treating myeloma cases that are refractory to the conventional cytotoxic chemoagents.[28,29] The antimyeloma effects of immune modulating agents such as thalidomide and lenalidomide derive from their ability to block myeloma cell binding to extracellular matrix proteins and stromal cells, modulate cytokine secretion, inhibit angiogenesis, and enhance host immunity.[30] Proteosome inhibitor bortezomib (Velcade) downregulates the MAPK cascade and NFκB pathway, thereby promoting myeloma cell apoptosis via cell cycle arrest.[31]

Although still controversial and much under investigation, the concept of myeloma stem cells is gaining increasing attention. Myeloma stem cells, like the normal stem cells, are chemoresistant and may be responsible for relapse after treatment.[32] Evidence suggests that pathways involved in embryonic stem cells such as Wnt, Notch, and Hedgehog are activated in myeloma stem cells.[32–38] Targeting these pathways may be effective in eradicating the neoplastic clones and prevent future relapse.

PROGNOSIS

The median survival of myeloma patients averages approximately 3 years with standard therapy and 5 years with dose-intensive therapy and stem cell transplantation. Myeloma, however, is a heterogeneous disease with a survival duration ranging from less than 1 year to more than 10 years.

Besides age and performance status, disease stage is one of most useful prognostic indicators. The Durie-Salmon system (**Box 2**) was widely used before the International Staging System (ISS) was introduced in 2003. Both staging systems essentially measure tumor burdens and disease activities. The Durie-Salmon system stratifies patients into 3 risk subgroups (see **Box 2**), and the medium survival for stage I, II, and III myeloma is approximately 6.5, 5, and 2 years, respectively. The ISS proposes a simplified approach based on serum levels of β2M and albumin (**Table 3**).[39] The median survival for ISS stage I, II, and III diseases is approximately 62, 44, and 29 months, respectively. Besides elevated β2M and hypoalbuminemia, adverse prognostic factors described in the literature also include high PCLI, high LDH, CRP, and Ki67 labeling.[31]

Cytogenetic and molecular genetic profiles of the tumor cells are also major determinants of the disease behavior. For example, an abnormal karyotype identified by conventional cytogenetic analysis signifies a tumor capable of proliferating independent of the bone marrow microenvironment and therefore predicts an inferior survival. In the cytogenetic risk model proposed by the Mayo group (**Table 4**), patients with 13q deletions and hypodiploidy, identified by metaphase analysis or t(4;14), t(14;16), 17p deletions detected by FISH, belong to the high-risk group with a shorter median overall survival.[40] This risk model is now adopted by the WHO classification. The 1p21 deletion and 1q/CKS1B amplification are also described by some investigators to be associated with an inferior outcome.[16,40–43] The impact of genetic composition of a tumor is best interpreted in the context of the disease stage.[44] Moreau and colleagues have shown that the median overall survival of patients with t(4;14) treated

---

Box 2
Durie-salmon staging system

Stage 1 (All criteria need to be met)

Hgb >100 g/L

Normal serum calcium

Normal bone x-ray or single bone plasmacytoma

Low M protein levels: IgG <50 g/L, IgA <30 g/L, Urine light chain <4 g/24 h

Stage 2

Neither Stage 1 nor 3

Stage 3 (One or more criteria need to be met)

Hgb <85 g/L

Serum calcium >12 mg/dL

Multiple lytic bone lesions

High M protein levels: IgG >70 g/L, IgA >50 g/L, Urine light chain >12 g/24 h

Table 3
International staging system for plasma cell myeloma

Stage	Criteria	Median Survival (mo)
I	Serum β2M <3.5 mg/L, serum albumin ≥3.5 g/dL	62
II	Not stage I or III	44
III	Serum β2M ≥5.5 mg/L	29

There are 2 categories for stage II: Serum β2M <3.5 mg/L but serum albumin <3.5 g/dL; or serum β2M 3.5 to 5.5 mg/L, irrespective of the serum albumin level.

with high-dose therapy ranged from 19 months for those with an advanced stage of disease (B2M >4 and Hb <10) to 54.6 months for those with early stage of disease (B2M <4 and Hb >10).[44]

One also needs to keep in mind that many of the negative prognostic factors were identified through analyzing patients treated before the age of novel therapeutic agents. Data regarding the impact of certain genetic aberrations may be controversial depending on the treatment regimens the study cohort received.[45–47] Some investigators argue that the prognostic impact of del13 is largely related to its close correlation with t(4;14) and t(14;16); in fact, 90% of myeloma cases with t(4;14) or t(14;16) also carry del13.[46] Data from the Leukemia Research Fund, United Kingdom, Myeloma Forum Cytogenetic Database laboratory on the other hand suggest that the impact of t(4;14) is evident only in cases that exhibit an abnormal karyotype particularly del13.[47] A German study of more than 100 patients treated with allogeneic bone marrow transplantation found that only del(13)(q14) and del(17)(p13) significantly influenced the incidence of relapse, whereas only del(17)(p13) retained their negative prognostic value for event-free survival.[48] Recent data suggest that bortezimab may overcome the negative effect of t(4;14).[49] The novel agents will likely change the long-term survival of high-risk patients and redefine the prognostic model.

CLINICAL VARIANTS

PCL is an aggressive disease associated with a high tumor burden, extramedullary dissemination, and an adverse prognosis. It is defined as an absolute plasma cell count of more than 2×10^9/L or plasma cells comprising more than 20% of the total leukocytes in the peripheral blood. Primary PCL is diagnosed at initial presentation of disease, comprising less than 5% of newly diagnosed cases of myeloma. Secondary PCL is essentially peripheralized myeloma occurring at a terminal stage of disease due to excessive tumor growth, representing only 1% of myeloma cases. The neoplastic cells in primary PCL often have a small-cell morphology (**Fig. 6**).

Table 4
The cytogenetic risk model

Unfavorable	Favorable[a]
Deletion 13, aneuploidy, hypoploidy	Hyperdiploidy
t(4;14) or t(14;16) or t(14;20) by FISH	t(11;14) or t(6;14) by FISH
Del17p13 by FISH	—

[a] Requires absence of unfavorable cytogenetic aberrations.
Data from Stewart AK, Bergsagel PL, Greipp PR, et al. A practical guide to defining high-risk myeloma for clinical trials, patient counseling and choice of therapy. Leukemia 2007;21:529–34.

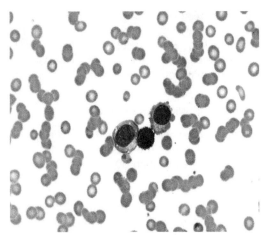

Fig. 6. Peripheral blood smear of a case of primary plasma cell leukemia. The circulating plasma cells are small, resembling plasmacytoid lymphocytes. The background red blood cells show rouleaux formation (Wight-Giemsa ×1000).

Immunophenotypically, the tumor cells are more likely positive for CD20 (50%), less likely positive for CD56 (45%) compared with myeloma, and are usually negative for CD117.[50] Of the five most common IgH translocations described here, 11q13 (cyclin D1) is almost exclusively and frequently seen in primary PCL, whereas all five can be observed in secondary PCL cases, indicating that primary PCL has distinct biology.[51] Del13 is more common in PCL (70%–85%) than myeloma (50%).

Solitary plasmacytoma of the bone (SPB), representing 3% of plasma cell neoplasms, is a tumor localized to a single bone at presentation.[52] It primarily affects the axial skeleton, mostly commonly thoracic or lumbosacral vertebrae, causing localized bone pain or neurologic symptoms secondary to spinal cord or root compression. The diagnosis requires extensive radiographic imaging to rule out occult systemic disease. Low levels of serum or urine M protein are detectable in 24% to 60% of patients by IFE. Most (70%) eventually develop systemic disease at a median of 2 to 4 years despite radiation treatment. The overall median survival is 7 to 12 years.

Solitary extramedullary plasmacytoma occurs most commonly in head and neck region, in 85% of all cases, followed by gastrointestinal tract.[52] Most of the tumors (>75%) do not produce detectable serum M protein. It is possible that those arising from the aerodigestive tract will represent extranodal marginal zone lymphomas with marked plasmacytic differentiation. The diagnosis again requires exclusion of occult systemic disease by extensive radiographic imaging. Local recurrence occurs in less than 10% of cases, and approximately 15% of patients subsequently develop myeloma. Risk for local recurrence and dissemination is high if serum monoclonal protein persists after local therapy. The 10-year survival rate is approximately 70% compared with 40% in SPB.

Osteosclerotic myeloma is a rare variant of myeloma (<1%) usually seen in POEMS (polyneuropathy, organomegaly, endocrinopathy, monoclonal gammopathy, and skin changes) syndrome. The bone changes are characterized by osteosclerotic rather than lytic lesions. The monoclonal protein is usually of IgA lambda type and is generally less than 3 g/dL.

Nonsecretory myeloma represents approximately 3% of cases of plasma cell neoplasms. Demonstration of the plasma cell origin (CD138+) and cytoplasmic immunoglobulin light chain restriction by flow cytometry immunophenotyping or immunohistochemistry is helpful in establishing the diagnosis. Exclusion of plasmablastic lymphoma or diffuse large B-cell lymphoma with plasmablastic differentiation may be difficult in some cases, and detection of myeloma-associated cytogenetic aberrations such as t(11;14) may confirm the diagnosis of myeloma.[51]

MONOCLONAL GAMMOPATHY OF UNKNOWN SIGNIFICANCE

MGUS is an asymptomatic plasma cell neoplasm that is usually diagnosed incidentally during routine laboratory evaluation. The incidence of MGUS increases with age, occurring in 1% of population older than 50 years, 5% older than 70 years, and 10% older than 80 years.[53] Patients are observed without therapy and monitored for progression.

MGUS is distinguished from smoldering myeloma by less than 10% monoclonal plasmacytosis and M protein less than 30 g/L. Bone marrow biopsy and aspirate show mild and interstitial plasmacytosis (median 3%–5%) without significant cytologic atypia. Immunoglobulin κ to λ ratio may fall within normal range when analyzed by immunohistochemistry, as polytypic plasma cells are frequently intermixed. The most common type of M protein is IgG (75%), followed by IgM (15%) and IgA (10%). Kappa is more common than lambda, 60% versus 40%. Urine Bence-Jones protein is usually absent or minimal.

Interphase FISH analysis reveals that aneuploidy is a constant finding in MGUS, and cytogenetic aberrations common in myeloma are also detectable in MGUS. For example, deletion 13q and 14q32 translocations are detectable in 40% to 50% and 50% of cases, respectively. Usually, deletion 13 is present in a subset of the clonal population. Microarray analysis reveals significant overlap between the gene expression patterns of MGUS and myeloma, further support that MGUS is part of the spectrum of plasma cell neoplasms.[54]

MGUS can evolve to myeloma or other related diseases.[53,55,56] The incidence of progression is about 1% each year. The cumulative incidence of progression is approximately 10% in 5 years, 15% in 10 years, and 20% in 15 years. The risk of progression is higher in patients with an abnormal serum κ to λ FLC ratio, a serum M protein 15 g/L or more, and IgM or IgA subtype.[53] The progress of MGUS to

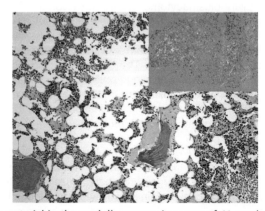

Fig. 7. Amorphous material in the medullary space in a case of AL amyloidosis hematoxylin and eosin stain, 400x, inset: Congo red stain shows apple green birefringent material under polarized light (400x).

myeloma is associated with the accumulation of additional genetic events such as *RAS* mutation and increased microvascular density (MVD) in the bone marrow. About 30% to 50% of myeloma patients have a preceding history of MGUS, and the onset of transformation may be sudden. The latency period may range from 2 to more than 20 years (median, 10 years). By contrast, patients with smoldering myeloma have a much shorter latency period, with 10% converting to overt myeloma in the first 5 years of diagnosis.

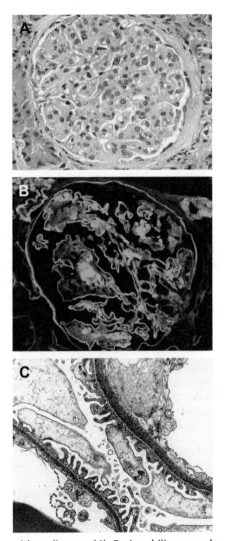

Fig. 8. Light chain deposition disease. (*A*) Eosinophilic amorphous material and base membrane thickening (Hematoxylin-eosin, original magnification x200. (*B*) Abnormal immunoglobulin appears as a linear ribbon-like deposition along the renal glomerular and tubular basement membrane (immunofluorescence stain). (*C*) Electrondense deposit (electronic microcopy). (*B and C courtesy of* Neriman Gokden, MD, Little Rock, AK.)

MONOCLONAL IMMUNOGLOBULIN DEPOSITION DISEASES

Primary amyloidosis (AL), light chain and/or heavy chain deposition diseases (LCDD and/or HCDD) are other plasma cell neoplasms that may occur as complications of myeloma or primary entities. Approximately 15% to 20% of patients with overt myeloma develop amyloidosis, and about 10% of overt myeloma patients develop LCDD or LHCDD. In most cases, monoclonal immunoglobulin deposition disease (MIDD) presents as primary disease with minimal monoclonal plasmacytosis and low levels of serum or urine M protein.

Deposition of monoclonal proteins in the vital organs, cause tissue damage and organ dysfunction. In AL, the amyloid fibers with monoclonal λ (75%) or κ (25%) light chains form insoluble proteins with a β-pleated sheet configuration. In LCDD or LHCDD, the monoclonal light chains, more often κ (75%), lack a β sheet structure. Symptoms of AL or LCDD and LHCDD are similar.[57] Kidney, heart, soft tissue, gastrointestinal tract, and nerve are commonly involved, and patients may suffer nephritic syndrome, cardiomyopathy, polyneuropathy, and coagulation disorders.

Rectal biopsy may detect amyloid in 80% of cases. Abdominal subcutaneous fat-pad aspiration detects amyloid in 70% of cases, whereas bone marrow biopsy may reveal amyloid in approximately 50% to 60% of cases; the combined methods allow detection in 90% to 95% cases.[35] The bone marrow vasculature and periosteum are the common sites as are the medullary cavities. Amyloid fibers have an amorphous, eosinophilic appearance, often associated with cracking artifact and multinucleated giant cell reaction (**Fig. 7**). They appear "apple-green" birefringent when stained with Congo red and viewed under polarized light. Immunohistochemical staining using monoclonal antibody against κ and λ may confirm monoclonality and identify the associated clonal plasma cells. The amyloid fibers appear as a mass of non-branching linear fibrils of 7 to 10 nm diameter and of variable length by electromicroscopy. Mass spectrometry may also identify amyloid components.

LCDD or/and HCDD are usually diagnosed by renal biopsy with appropriate ancillary studies. Light microscopic findings typically include nodular glomerulosclerosis resembling diabetic nephropathy, with the abnormal protein appearing as amorphous eosinophilic material resembling amyloid but negative by Congo red stain (**Fig. 8**). Other findings include basement membrane thickening, increased mesangial matrix, and proliferative vasculopathy.[58] By immunofluorescence, the abnormal immunoglobulin appears as a linear ribbon-like deposition along the renal glomerular and tubular basement membrane. The abnormal immunoglobulin typically appears as discrete, electron-dense, punctate deposits on electron microscopy.

Patients with MIDD are treated with chemotherapy with or without stem cell transplantation to control the monoclonal proteins. The overall survival of these patients is poor.

REFERENCES

1. Kyle RA, Rajkumar SV. Multiple myeloma. Blood 2008;111:2962–72.
2. International Myeloma Working Group. Criteria for the classification of monoclonal gammopathies, multiple myeloma and related disorders: a report of the International Myeloma Working Group. Br J Haematol 2003;121:749–57.
3. McKenna R, Kyle R, Kuehl W, et al. Plasma cell neoplasms. In: Swerdlow SH, Elias C, Harris NL, et al, editors. WHO classification of tumours of haematopoietic and lymphoid tissues. Lyon, France: IARC; 2008. p. 200–13.
4. Rajkumar SV, Greipp PR. Angiogenesis in multiple myeloma. Br J Haematol 2001; 113:565.

5. Bartl R, Frisch B, Fateh-Moghadam A, et al. Histologic classification and staging of multiple myeloma. A retrospective and prospective study of 674 cases. Am J Clin Pathol 1987;87:342–55.
6. Durie BG, Harousseau JL, Miguel JS, et al. International uniform response criteria for multiple myeloma. Leukemia 2006;20:1467–73.
7. Snozek CL, Katzmann JA, Kyle RA, et al. Prognostic value of the serum free light chain ratio in newly diagnosed myeloma: proposed incorporation into the international staging system. Leukemia 2008;22:1933–7.
8. Dispenzieri A, Kyle RA, Katzmann JA, et al. Immunoglobulin free light chain ratio is an independent risk factor for progression of smoldering (asymptomatic) multiple myeloma. Blood 2008;111:785–9.
9. Jakob C, Sterz J, Liebisch P, et al. Incorporation of the bone marker carboxy-terminal telopeptide of type-1 collagen improves prognostic information of the International Staging System in newly diagnosed symptomatic multiple myeloma. Leukemia 2008;22:1767–72.
10. Lin P, Owens R, Tricot G, et al. Flow cytometric immunophenotypic analysis of 306 cases of multiple myeloma. Am J Clin Pathol 2004;121:482–8.
11. Mateo G, Montalban MA, Vidriales MB, et al. Prognostic value of immunophenotyping in multiple myeloma: a study by the PETHEMA/GEM cooperative study groups on patients uniformly treated with high-dose therapy. J Clin Oncol 2008; 26:2737–44.
12. Bergsagel PL, Smith AM, Szczepek A, et al. In multiple myeloma, clonotypic B lymphocytes are detectable among CD19+ peripheral blood cells expressing CD38, CD56, and monotypic Ig light chain. Blood 1995;85:436–47.
13. Szczepek AJ, Seeberger K, Wizniak J, et al. A high frequency of circulating B cells share clonotypic Ig heavy-chain VDJ rearrangements with autologous bone marrow plasma cells in multiple myeloma, as measured by single-cell and in situ reverse transcriptase-polymerase chain reaction. Blood 1998;92: 2844–55.
14. Wilson CS, Butch AW, Lai R, et al. Cyclin D1 and E2F-1 immunoreactivity in bone marrow biopsy specimens of multiple myeloma: relationship to proliferative activity, cytogenetic abnormalities and DNA ploidy. Br J Haematol 2001;112: 776–82.
15. Hoyer JD, Hanson CA, Fonseca R, et al. The (11;14)(q13;q32) translocation in multiple myeloma. A morphologic and immunohistochemical study. Am J Clin Pathol 2000;113:831–7.
16. Stewart AK, Bergsagel PL, Greipp PR, et al. A practical guide to defining high-risk myeloma for clinical trials, patient counseling and choice of therapy. Leukemia 2007;21:529–34.
17. Chng WJ, Glebov O, Bergsagel PL, et al. Genetic events in the pathogenesis of multiple myeloma. Best Pract Res Clin Haematol 2007;20:571–96.
18. Shaughnessy JD Jr, Zhan F, Burington BE, et al. A validated gene expression model of high-risk multiple myeloma is defined by deregulated expression of genes mapping to chromosome 1. Blood 2007;109:2276–84.
19. Qian J, Xie J, Hong S, et al. Dickkopf-1 (DKK1) is a widely expressed and potent tumor-associated antigen in multiple myeloma. Blood 2007;110:1587–94.
20. Zhan F, Colla S, Wu X, et al. CKS1B, overexpressed in aggressive disease, regulates multiple myeloma growth and survival through SKP2- and p27Kip1-dependent and -independent mechanisms. Blood 2007;109:4995–5001.
21. Bergsagel PL, Kuehl WM. Molecular pathogenesis and a consequent classification of multiple myeloma. J Clin Oncol 2005;23:6333–8.

22. Pinzone JJ, Hall BM, Thudi NK, et al. The role of Dickkopf-1 in bone development, homeostasis and disease. Blood 2009;113:517–25.

23. Zhan F, Barlogie B, Mulligan G, et al. High-risk myeloma: a gene expression based risk-stratification model for newly diagnosed multiple myeloma treated with high-dose therapy is predictive of outcome in relapsed disease treated with single-agent bortezomib or high-dose dexamethasone. Blood 2008;111:968–9.

24. Qiang YW, Chen Y, Stephens O, et al. Myeloma-derived Dickkopf-1 disrupts Wnt-regulated osteoprotegerin and RANKL production by osteoblasts: a potential mechanism underlying osteolytic bone lesions in multiple myeloma. Blood 2008;112:196–207.

25. Walker BA, Leone PE, Jenner MW, et al. Integration of global SNP-based mapping and expression arrays reveals key regions, mechanisms, and genes important in the pathogenesis of multiple myeloma. Blood 2006;108:1733–43.

26. Schmidlin H, Diehl SA, Nagasawa M, et al. Spi-B inhibits human plasma cell differentiation by repressing BLIMP1 and XBP-1 expression. Blood 2008;112:1804–12.

27. Li ZW, Chen H, Campbell RA, et al. NF-kappaB in the pathogenesis and treatment of multiple myeloma. Curr Opin Hematol 2008;15:391–9.

28. Yasui H, Hideshima T, Richardson PG, et al. Recent advances in the treatment of multiple myeloma. Curr Pharm Biotechnol 2006;7:381–93.

29. Anargyrou K, Dimopoulos MA, Sezer O, et al. Novel anti-myeloma agents and angiogenesis. Leuk Lymphoma 2008;49:677–89.

30. Hideshima T, Raje N, Richardson PG, et al. A review of lenalidomide in combination with dexamethasone for the treatment of multiple myeloma. Ther Clin Risk Manag 2008;4:129–36.

31. Mateos MV, San Miguel JF. Bortezomib in multiple myeloma. Best Pract Res Clin Haematol 2007;20:701–15.

32. Ghosh N, Matsui W. Cancer stem cells in multiple myeloma. Cancer Lett 2009; 277:1–7.

33. Huff CA, Matsui W. Multiple myeloma cancer stem cells. J Clin Oncol 2008;26: 2895–900.

34. Huff CA, Matsui W, Smith BD, et al. The paradox of response and survival in cancer therapeutics. Blood 2006;107:431–4.

35. Matsui W, Huff CA, Wang Q, et al. Characterization of clonogenic multiple myeloma cells. Blood 2004;103:2332–6.

36. Matsui W, Wang Q, Barber JP, et al. Clonogenic multiple myeloma progenitors, stem cell properties, and drug resistance. Cancer Res 2008;68:190–7.

37. Noonan K, Matsui W, Serafini P, et al. Activated marrow-infiltrating lymphocytes effectively target plasma cells and their clonogenic precursors. Cancer Res 2005;65:2026–34.

38. Peacock CD, Wang Q, Gesell GS, et al. Hedgehog signaling maintains a tumor stem cell compartment in multiple myeloma. Proc Natl Acad Sci U S A 2007; 104:4048–53.

39. Greipp PR, San Miguel J, Durie BG, et al. International staging system for multiple myeloma. J Clin Oncol 2005;23:3412–20.

40. Chng WJ, Kuehl WM, Bergsagel PL, et al. Translocation t(4;14) retains prognostic significance even in the setting of high-risk molecular signature. Leukemia 2008; 22:459–61.

41. Wu KL, Beverloo B, Lokhorst HM, et al. Abnormalities of chromosome 1p/q are highly associated with chromosome 13/13q deletions and are an adverse prognostic factor for the outcome of high-dose chemotherapy in patients with multiple myeloma. Br J Haematol 2007;136:615–23.

42. Chang H, Ning Y, Qi X, et al. Chromosome 1p21 deletion is a novel prognostic marker in patients with multiple myeloma. Br J Haematol 2007;139:51–4.
43. Chang H, Qi C, Yi QL, et al. p53 gene deletion detected by fluorescence in situ hybridization is an adverse prognostic factor for patients with multiple myeloma following autologous stem cell transplantation. Blood 2005;105:358–60.
44. Moreau P, Attal M, Garban F, et al. Heterogeneity of t(4;14) in multiple myeloma. Long-term follow-up of 100 cases treated with tandem transplantation in IFM99 trials. Leukemia 2007;21:2020–4.
45. Avet-Loiseau H. Role of genetics in prognostication in myeloma. Best Pract Res Clin Haematol 2007;20:625–35.
46. Avet-Loiseau H, Attal M, Moreau P, et al. Genetic abnormalities and survival in multiple myeloma: the experience of the Intergroupe Francophone du Myelome. Blood 2007;109:3489–95.
47. Chiecchio L, Protheroe RK, Ibrahim AH, et al. Deletion of chromosome 13 detected by conventional cytogenetics is a critical prognostic factor in myeloma. Leukemia 2006;20:1610–7.
48. Schilling G, Hansen T, Shimoni A, et al. Impact of genetic abnormalities on survival after allogeneic hematopoietic stem cell transplantation in multiple myeloma. Leukemia 2008;22:1250–5.
49. Chng WJ, Gonzalez-Paz N, Price-Troska T, et al. Clinical and biological significance of RAS mutations in multiple myeloma. Leukemia 2008;22:2280–4.
50. Pellat-Deceunynck C, Barille S, Jego G, et al. The absence of CD56 (NCAM) on malignant plasma cells is a hallmark of plasma cell leukemia and of a special subset of multiple myeloma. Leukemia 1998;12:1977–82.
51. Tiedemann RE, Gonzalez-Paz N, Kyle RA, et al. Genetic aberrations and survival in plasma cell leukemia. Leukemia 2008;22:1044–52.
52. Soutar R, Lucraft H, Jackson G, et al. Guidelines on the diagnosis and management of solitary plasmacytoma of bone and solitary extramedullary plasmacytoma. Br J Haematol 2004;124:717–26.
53. Rajkumar SV, Lacy MQ, Kyle RA. Monoclonal gammopathy of undetermined significance and smoldering multiple myeloma. Blood Rev 2007;21:255–65.
54. Zhan F, Barlogie B, Arzoumanian V, et al. Gene-expression signature of benign monoclonal gammopathy evident in multiple myeloma is linked to good prognosis. Blood 2007;109:1692–700.
55. Kyle RA, Rajkumar SV. Monoclonal gammopathy of undetermined significance and smoldering multiple myeloma. Hematol Oncol Clin North Am 2007;21:1093–113, ix.
56. Kyle RA, Rajkumar SV. Epidemiology of the plasma-cell disorders. Best Pract Res Clin Haematol 2007;20:637–64.
57. Buxbaum J, Gallo G. Nonamyloidotic monoclonal immunoglobulin deposition disease. Light-chain, heavy-chain, and light- and heavy-chain deposition diseases. Hematol Oncol Clin North Am 1999;13:1235–48.
58. Gokden N, Barlogie B, Liapis H. Morphologic heterogeneity of renal light-chain deposition disease. Ultrastruct Pathol 2008;32:17–24.

Atypical Lymphoid Hyperplasia Mimicking Lymphoma

David J. Good, MD[a], Randy D. Gascoyne, MD[b],*

KEYWORDS

- Atypical lymphoid hyperplasia • Lymphoma • Pathology
- Immunophenotype • Reactive follicular hyperplasia

Much has been written and studied with regard to lymphoma and its presentation and diagnosis in lymph nodes. However, in routine pathology practice, many more lymph nodes are seen with reactive changes as opposed to malignant features. Many of these reactive changes can have atypical features and may often mimic lymphoma, making it difficult to differentiate these benign changes from malignant ones. This article discusses some of the more common atypical lymphoid proliferations found in lymph nodes that can mimic lymphoma and an approach to distinguish them from their malignant counterparts (**Table 1**).

REACTIVE FOLLICULAR HYPERPLASIA

One of the most common forms of benign lymphoid hyperplasia seen in excised lymph nodes is reactive follicular hyperplasia (RFH). The follicular pattern is typically a result of a humoral immune reaction, with antigenic stimulation and subsequent proliferation of B cells. Therefore, it is the most common type of reactive lymphoid hyperplasia in children and young adults, as they are exposed to a variety of new antigens. The differential diagnosis for RFH is broad, including many viral infections and autoimmune disorders such as rheumatoid arthritis. More commonly, florid RFH remains unexplained, particularly in younger patients.

Histologically, the lymph node follicles become enlarged and more numerous and may no longer be confined strictly to the cortex but can often be present throughout the entire node. There is considerable variation in the size and shape of the follicles. Most retain a round to oval structure, but, occasionally, they will coalesce and form irregular-shaped structures. The germinal centers are hyperplastic and comprise

[a] Department of Pathology and Laboratory Medicine, British Columbia Cancer Agency, 600 W 10th Avenue, Vancouver, BC V5Z 4E6, Canada
[b] Department of Pathology and Advanced Therapeutics, British Columbia Cancer Agency, British Columbia Cancer Research Centre, 675 W. 10th Avenue, Room 5-113, Vancouver, BC V5Z 4E6, Canada
* Corresponding author.
E-mail address: rgascoyn@bccancer.bc.ca (R.D. Gascoyne).

Hematol Oncol Clin N Am 23 (2009) 729–745
doi:10.1016/j.hoc.2009.04.005
0889-8588/09/$ – see front matter © 2009 Elsevier Inc. All rights reserved.

Table 1
Key features to distinguish between atypical proliferations and neoplastic mimics

Atypical Lymphoid Process	Neoplastic Mimics	Key Histologic Features	Key Immunophenotypic Features
Florid reactive follicular hyperplasia	Follicular lymphoma	Lower density of follicles than FL Well-defined mantle zones Polarity with admixed tingible body macrophages	Reactive follicles negative for BCL2 CD10 and BCL6 confined to the follicles
Florid progressive transformation of germinal centers	NLPHL Small B-cell lymphoma	Lack of LP cells May have large immunoblasts in PTGC areas	Lack of CD3+, CD57+, PD-1+ collarettes Immunoblasts epithelial membrane antigen negative
Infectious mononucleosis	Classical Hodgkin lymphoma Peripheral T-cell lymphoma Diffuse large B-cell lymphoma	Immunoblasts slightly smaller than RS cells, smaller but centrally located nucleoli Mottled appearance in paracortex, reactive germinal centers with intact sinuses	Immunoblasts CD20+, CD30±, EBV±, CD15-
Plasmablastic variant of multicentric Castleman Disease	HHV-8-positive plasmablastic lymphoma	Variable involution and hyalinization of germinal centers Scattered to small clusters of plasmablasts (should not be sheeting out)	Plasmablasts typically positive for HHV8, IgM, lambda light chain CD20±, CD138- Plasmablasts polyclonal by molecular analysis
Kikuchi-Fujimoto lymphadenopathy	Peripheral T-cell lymphoma	Patchy necrotic areas devoid of neutrophils Crescentic-shaped histiocytes admixed with plasmacytoid monocytes and small lymphocytes	Histiocytes positive for CD68, lysozyme, and myeloperoxidase T cell component predominantly cytotoxic (CD8, TIA-1, granzyme B, perforin +)
Dermatopathic lymphadenitis	Mycosis fungoides/Sézary syndrome	Paracortical expansion with large pale staining cells Histiocytes and antigen presenting cells ±pigment	Immunohistochemistry not overly useful to distinguish from MF/SS Molecular analysis to exclude clonality may be helpful

a mixture of centroblasts and centrocytes with numerous admixed mitotic figures and tingible body macrophages. In the majority of cases, a well-developed mantle zone is present surrounding the enlarged follicles. For the most part, the reactive follicles do not extend outside the capsule into the perinodal fat, even when highly stimulated. In a subset of cases, focal, progressively transformed germinal centers will be identified (discussed in a later section).

Most cases of RFH are quite apparent on hematoxylin and eosin examination, with little need for further ancillary studies. However, one of the major diagnostic difficulties occurs when there is prolonged antigenic stimulation and the RFH becomes florid with numerous enlarged follicles. Some of these cases are difficult to distinguish from follicular lymphoma (FL) on histologic grounds alone (**Fig. 1**A). Studies have attempted to define histologic criteria to reliably differentiate between florid RFH and FL.[1,2] The most significant feature is the density of the follicles, with them being less numerous and not as closely packed in RFH. They are also less uniform and more irregularly shaped in RFH than in FL. Additional histologic features that are important are polarity (light and dark zones in the follicles caused by areas of centrocytes and centroblasts), the relative persistence of mantle zones, and the presences of tingible body macrophages and mitoses in RFH. However, both tingible body macrophages and mitotic figures can be seen in higher-grade FL.

In these cases, immunohistochemical staining is invaluable to distinguish between these 2 entities. RFH will show CD20-positive B cells mainly confined to the germinal centers with little spread into the interfollicular areas. These germinal center B cells express the follicle center markers CD10 and BCL6. Reactive follicles will be negative for the antiapoptotic protein BCL2 (**Fig. 1**B). In cases of FL, the B cells tend to be no longer confined to the follicles. Therefore, it is common to find B cells positive for CD10 and BCL6 in the interfollicular areas. The majority of FL cases will be positive for BCL2, although approximately 10% to 15% of cases will be negative by immunohistochemistry.[3,4] In these cases, PCR analysis may help to provide evidence of a monoclonal B-cell population. Immunohistochemical staining for light chains can be useful in RFH, as there will typically be polytypic expression in the mantle zone B cells as well as in admixed plasma cells in the interfollicular areas. However, there have been rare cases reported in which there is apparent light chain restriction in otherwise reactive-appearing germinal centers.[5]

Although common in younger patients, florid RFH is unusual in patients older than 60 years, as the ability to mount a prominent humoral response is relatively subdued.

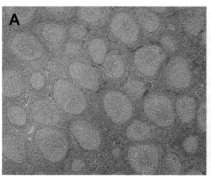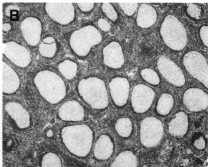

Fig. 1. (*A*) Florid reactive follicular hyperplasia mimicking follicular lymphoma. Note the very high overall density of lymphoid follicles. (*B*) The same case as that in *A*, stained with anti-BCL2 (Dako, clone 124), showing a virtual absence of staining within the follicles.

It appears that florid RFH in this age group may represent an immune system imbalance, often related to autoimmune conditions such as rheumatoid arthritis.[6,7] However, one study found a higher association with non-Hodgkin lymphoma (NHL), either concurrently present or subsequently developing.[8] Therefore, careful examination of the excised lymph node is necessary in these patients to exclude occult lymphoma. Lymphoma staging is also indicated in an attempt to identify other sites of lymphadenopathy that may be harboring lymphoma.

Rare cases have been reported in which the histologic appearance of the lymph node is consistent with RFH, but focal germinal centers are strongly positive for BCL2 protein, whereas most of the remaining GCs within the same lymph node are BCL2 negative.[9] In this study by Cong and colleagues, laser capture microdissection was performed followed by molecular clonality analysis, proving a monoclonal B-cell population in the majority of cases. The term "in situ FL" has been applied to these cases, as only a few follicles within the lymph node were involved, with the architectural and cytologic features otherwise being benign. It is recommended that clinical examination and lymphoma staging including a bone marrow biopsy be performed to identify if other sites of FL are present. If no FL is found, close clinical follow-up without therapy is advised. The opposite finding to these in situ cases has also been reported with the presence of usually single preserved germinal centers in a lymph node otherwise infiltrated by FL.[10] This finding appears to be strongly associated with limited stage disease. This process contrasts with the in situ localization of FL, as these cases have obvious involvement by FL with rare areas of preserved GC remnants, whereas the in situ cases by definition are devoid of identifiable lymphoma infiltrations.

Another issue when assessing the follicles in reactive lymph nodes is the differentiation between primary and secondary follicles. Primary follicles are present in nonstimulated lymphoid tissue and are composed of naïve small B cells and an underlying follicular dendritic cell (FDC) meshwork. Secondary B follicles develop on antigen exposure, forming the germinal center with a surrounding mantle zone. The histologic appearance of primary follicles characteristically shows small lymphocytes that have a monomorphic appearance, making it easy to mistake them for malignant follicles. Moreover, they are positive for BCL2 protein. However, they are not as densely packed, have reactive-appearing interfollicular areas, lack admixed large centroblasts, and are negative for the germinal center markers CD10 and BCL6, reflecting their lack of germinal center formation.

PROGRESSIVE TRANSFORMATION OF GERMINAL CENTERS

Progressive transformation of germinal centers (PTGC) is an atypical feature seen in lymph nodes, of which the pathogenesis is unknown. It is most commonly found in association with RFH.[11–13] In most cases, PTGC is localized, self-limited, and involves less than 5% of hyperplastic follicles. These cases have minimal clinical relevance and should not cause difficulties in being confused with lymphoma. However, in rare cases, PTGC is generalized or florid (**Fig. 2**) and can easily be mistaken for lymphoma, especially nodular lymphocyte predominant Hodgkin lymphoma (NLPHL).[11] These florid cases mostly occur in young men and manifest as an asymptomatic, solitary, enlarged lymph node frequently in the cervical region and less commonly in inguinal and axillary regions.

Histologically, florid PTGC shows very large transformed follicles involving numerous germinal centers.[12,14] In both focal and florid cases of PTGC, a similar process occurs, destroying the follicular microarchitecture and terminating the germinal-center reaction.[15] It is characterized by inward migration of numerous foci of perifollicular small

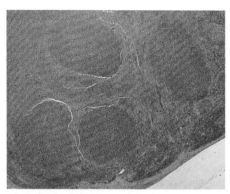

Fig. 2. Characteristic macronodular infiltrate seen in progressive transformation of germinal centers (PTGC). Occasional foci of PTGC in an otherwise reactive lymph node with secondary lymphoid follicles is common and not typically of concern. Florid PTGC must be carefully distinguished from nodular lymphocyte predominant Hodgkin lymphoma.

B cells with a mantle-zone phenotype into the follicle center.[16] This results in fragmentation of the germinal center into islands of centrocytes and centroblasts with obscuring of the mantle zone. Mitotic figures and tingible macrophages are still apparent in the transformed follicle, consistent with residual reactive germinal center remnants.

The differentiation of florid PTGC from lymphoma can be difficult as nodes with PTGC are more frequent in patients with a concurrent or prior diagnosis of NLPHL.[11,12,14,17,18] As well, patients with persistent PTGC appear at slightly increased risk of developing NLPHL.[13,19] Less commonly, PTGC changes can be associated with classic Hodgkin's lymphoma.[11,17]

The key to differentiating NLPHL from florid PTGC rests on identifying the malignant cells, now termed lymphocyte-predominant cells or LP cells in the 2008 WHO classification. However, in many cases the LP cells can be quite rare. In addition, in cases of PTGC, there may be cells within the effaced follicle that may mimic the malignant cells seen in NLPHL. Therefore, immunohistochemical staining is invaluable in highlighting the LP cells and distinguishing them from immunoblasts. LP cells express CD45, CD20, and epithelial membrane antigen (EMA). They are negative for CD15 and Epstein Barr virus (EBV) and only occasionally weakly positive for CD30, helping to differentiate them from classic Reed-Sternberg (RS) cells. Collarettes of CD3-positive, CD57-positive T cells surround the LP cells as well as a more recently described follicular T helper cell marker PD-1.[20] BCL6, a transcriptional repressor that regulates germinal center B-cell differentiation and inflammation, is present in a high proportion of LP cells. However, few cells in PTGC express this marker.[21]

The differential diagnosis of PTGC also includes follicular colonization by small cell B-cell lymphomas, usually marginal-zone lymphoma or rarely mantle cell lymphoma, leading to expansion of existing reactive germinal centers by small B cells. A helpful feature to distinguish between PTGC and B-cell lymphomas colonizing germinal centers is the clustering of T cells around the germinal center remnants in cases of PTGC. The floral variant of FL may also resemble PTGC in that there are often numerous reactive mantle-zone B cells and T cells intermixed with neoplastic B cells.[22,23] However, there are some key features to help distinguish between these entities. The presence of densely packed nodules of atypical follicular center cells with or without extranodal extension favors FL. PTGC is usually associated with a background of RFH. Immunohistochemical staining for CD10 can be useful, as only a few remnants of CD10+ follicle center B cells are present in PTGC, whereas numerous CD10+ cells are present in the follicles of FL. Additionally, the presence of CD10+ lymphocytic infiltrates outside of the follicles strongly supports the diagnosis of FL. In cases where the histologic features and immunohistochemical stains do not lead to a clear diagnosis, molecular studies to detect t(14;18) and clonal immunoglobulin gene rearrangement can be of utility to confirm the diagnosis of FL.

INFECTIOUS MONONUCLEOSIS AND OTHER IMMUNOBLASTIC PROLIFERATIONS

The histopathology of infectious mononucleosis (IM) and other morphologically related viral infections, including rubella, herpes zoster, and postvaccinal lymphadenitis, is important to recognize and to distinguish from malignant lymphoma. In most cases of IM, a combination of characteristic clinical, hematological, and serologic findings is used to make the diagnosis.[24] On occasion, establishing a diagnosis may be difficult due to an atypical clinical history or prolonged lymphadenopathy. In these cases, either lymph nodes or tonsils may be excised for evaluation.[25] However, as IM may often mimic lymphoma, a lymph node biopsy is not recommended if IM is suspected clinically, to prevent using many expensive and unnecessary ancillary tests to exclude a malignant diagnosis. More importantly, patients with IM run the risk of being labeled with a diagnosis of lymphoma, and, therefore, a biopsy is best avoided.

Histologically, lymph nodes with IM will show expansion of the paracortex with abundant immunoblasts and plasma cells and increased vascularity.[25,26] The extent of these changes varies considerably from case to case, with some cases having only mild paracortical expansion to others having an extensive and atypical cellular proliferation, severely altering the normal nodal architecture. Part of the reason for this variability is a result of the disease duration at the time the lymph node biopsy is performed. Early in the course of IM, reactive follicles may be present. As the process progresses, the follicles may become separated by the paracortical expansion, often pushing them toward the cortex of the node. In extreme cases, the follicles may be completely obliterated. The cellular composition of the paracortical expansion is also variable. It may be composed predominantly of immunoblasts or may contain a mixed cellular population in which immunoblasts are scattered among the small lymphocytes, imparting a mottled appearance (**Fig. 3**). Lymphocytes, plasma cells, plasmacytoid cells, and occasional histiocytes are present in varying numbers. Mitotic figures may be seen frequently among the proliferating immunoblasts, and focal areas of necrosis are often found. This paracortical expansion can often extend into the lymph node capsule. If the sinuses are not obliterated, they are often occupied by

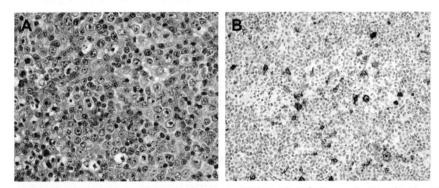

Fig. 3. (A) Immunoblastic reaction in a young patient with infectious mononucleosis. (B) Same case stained with anti-LMP (latent membrane protein) showing the presence of Epstein Barr virus (EBV).

immunoblasts with admixed monocytoid B cells and histiocytes. Similar immunoblastic proliferations are seen in tonsils of individuals with IM.

The difficulty with lymph nodes involved by IM is that the histologic changes are not specific and need to be differentiated from immunoblastic proliferations seen in other benign, atypical, and malignant lymphoproliferative disorders. A definitive diagnosis of IM cannot be made on histologic grounds alone. On the other hand, it can be easy to become focused on a malignant diagnosis, and, therefore, it is also important to keep IM and other similar viral infections in the differential when examining lymph nodes with interfollicular expansions of immunoblasts, especially in younger individuals.

The histologic changes and cellular composition in IM can be difficult to differentiate from both Hodgkin and NHL.[25,27,28] Frequently, the immunoblasts can be large and occasionally binuclear, mimicking RS cells. However, there are some cytologic features that may help to separate these two types of cells. Immunoblasts have large, open, round to oval nuclei with distinct nuclear borders and a single centrally located nucleolus surrounded by moderate basophilic cytoplasm. In contrast, diagnostic RS cells have two or more distinct nuclei, each containing a prominent single nucleolus that may occupy a considerable portion of the nucleus. The nucleoli are typically eosinophilic and surrounded by a perinucleolar halo in classical Hodgkin lymphoma (HL). In many cases of HL, diagnostic RS cells are relatively rare, and there may be considerable cytologic overlap between large immunoblasts and mononuclear Hodgkin cells. In these difficult cases, the cellular environment in which the large cells are found can be a key part in establishing the correct diagnosis. Generally, the mottled appearance in the paracortex due to immunoblasts scattered among the small lymphocytes is absent in HL. Additionally, the presence of intact sinuses with transformed lymphocytes and monocytoid B cells favors a benign diagnosis. Depending on the subtype of HL, the number of small lymphocytes may vary. However, there will often be a mixed inflammatory cellular infiltrate, including histiocytes and eosinophils with occasional plasma cells. Although the presence of reactive follicles would tend to favor a benign process, they do not exclude a diagnosis of HL, as partial involvement of lymph nodes is often confined to the paracortical areas, leaving intact follicles.

Immunohistochemical analysis may not be entirely helpful to distinguish between immunoblastic proliferations and HL. Immunoblasts may often be CD30 positive and be EBV positive (**Fig. 3**B), especially in cases of IM.[29,30] Although CD15 is usually negative in immunoblastic proliferations, it is not always expressed by RS cells. CD20 is usually positive in immunoblastic proliferations and typically shows weak and variable staining on RS cells. As well, immunoblasts usually lack the T-cell collarettes typically seen surrounding the RS cells. Therefore, the combination of histologic and cytologic appearances with possible addition of immunohistochemistry is needed to distinguish between these entities.

Differentiation of IM from the immunoblastic variant of diffuse large B-cell lymphoma (DLBCL) may be difficult when sheets of large immunoblasts partially efface the nodal architecture.[25,31] Therefore, it is especially important to examine the lymph node section under low magnification to appreciate the complete histologic picture. The presence of retained normal lymph node architecture, including follicles and sinuses, and the mottled appearance of the paracortex can be helpful features in differentiating benign, atypical lymphoid proliferations from lymphoma.

Nodal-based peripheral T-cell lymphomas such as angioimmunoblastic T-cell lymphoma (AILT) and peripheral T-cell lymphoma, not otherwise specified, with a T-zone pattern can also share certain features with IM. These features include RS-like cells, proliferation of immunoblasts, paracortical involvement with persistent or compressed follicles, prominent high endothelial venules, and a marked inflammatory background.[32–35] Although they are less common than HL and DLBCL, these entities should be considered in the differential diagnosis of viral lymphadenitis. Immunohistochemical studies can often help to distinguish between IM and peripheral T-cell lymphomas in histologically complex cases. In the nodal T-cell lymphomas, most of the interfollicular small lymphoid cells will be CD4+, whereas they are mainly CD8+ in IM.[36] In AILT specifically, the interfollicular T-cells will often characteristically co-express CD10, BCL6, and CXCL13.[35] DNA polymerase chain reaction (PCR) analysis can also be helpful to establish the presence of a T-cell clone in peripheral T-cell lymphomas. One's ability to distinguish between these overlapping entities is seriously hindered if a needle-core biopsy is used for evaluation, and, thus, an open excisional biopsy is strongly recommended.

CASTLEMAN DISEASE

The original description of Castleman disease (CD), also referred to as angiofollicular lymph node hyperplasia, was given in 1956 by Benjamin Castleman and colleagues. They described a series of patients with localized mediastinal masses resembling thymomas.[37] Today, these original cases constitute the hyaline vascular type of CD (HVCD). Although this type of CD is not usually mistaken for lymphoma, rarer types of CD have subsequently been described that have overlapping features with certain B-cell lymphomas and are further discussed.

Hyaline Vascular Castleman Disease

The typical clinical presentation of HVCD is the development of large solitary mediastinal masses or enlarged single peripheral lymph nodes in relatively younger patients.[38,39] Most of these patients lack constitutional symptoms. On histologic examination, it was found that most cases arise from lymph nodes although extranodal cases have been described.[39] The normal nodal architecture is partially effaced by an increased number of lymphoid follicles. These follicles are not restricted to the cortical areas but are often present throughout the entire node. They typically have regressed germinal centers with lymphocyte depletion, deposits of hyaline, and vascular proliferation with radially penetrating capillaries. The germinal centers also have prominent FDCs that sometimes appear dysplastic or have a disrupted pattern.[40] Surrounding these regressed germinal centers, the mantle zone is expanded and composed of concentric rings of small lymphocytes forming an "onion skin" appearance. The interfollicular areas can be mildly expanded and are composed of small lymphocytes, most of which are T cells, a prominent vascular proliferation including many high endothelial venules with variable hyalinization, and a variety of dendritic cells. Other inflammatory cells, including plasma cells, eosinophils, or histiocytes, are often present but are not numerous. The few interfollicular B cells and plasma cells are polyclonal. Areas of calcification and significant fibrosis may also be present. Caution needs to be exercised when making a diagnosis of HVCD, as various nonspecific reactive lymph nodes can have Castleman-like changes. These are particularly common in HIV-related lymphadenopathy. In addition, classical HL may have adjacent areas showing Castleman-like follicles.[41] Burnt out or regressively transformed germinal centers resembling those of HVCD may also be seen in AILT.[42]

Plasma Cell Type of Castleman Disease

Localized plasma cell type of Castleman disease (PCCD) is much less commonly observed than HVCD but occurs in a similar age group. A few clinical features are different from those of HVCD. Although it typically presents with a mass lesion in the mediastinum or abdomen, it is often an aggregate of lymph nodes as opposed to a single node.[38,39] Patients often have constitutional symptoms, including fever, night sweats, weight loss, and fatigue. Many patients will also have laboratory abnormalities, including anemia, leukocytosis, polyclonal hypergammaglobulinemia, and hypoalbuminemia. The histologic pattern is also different to that of HVCD. Instead of regressed follicles, many of the follicles are hyperplastic with reactive features and narrower mantle zones. The other key feature is the presence of sheets of plasma cells in the interfollicular areas and medulla of the lymph node. Virtually all of the plasma cells are mature and demonstrate polytypic light chain expression. Rare cases may show a marked predominance of one light chain over the other, making the distinction from a small B-cell lymphoma with plasmacytic differentiation difficult. PCR analysis for immunoglobulin gene rearrangements in these cases can be valuable, as the PCCD cases should not be clonal. However, rare cases may contain a detectable monoclonal lymphoid population, suggesting either the possible outgrowth of a neoplastic lymphoid clone that may eventually progress to lymphoma or the detection of an occult B-cell lymphoma being harbored by the patient but not histologically detectable in the lymph node sampled.[43,44]

As opposed to both HVCD and normal lymph nodes, there is elevated expression of interleukin (IL-6) by B cells in the germinal centers and immunoblasts in the mantle zones and interfollicular areas.[45,46] IL-6 mediates the differentiation of B-cells into plasma cells, is involved in the acute-phase inflammatory reaction, and may play a role in vascular proliferation. Therefore, the elevated IL-6 levels may help to explain many of the histologic findings, systemic symptoms, and laboratory abnormalities in PCCD.

Multicentric Castleman Disease

Multicentric Castleman disease (MCD) is a systemic lymphoproliferative disorder that can occur in children[47] but more typically occurs in older individuals with the median age between 50 and 60 years.[39,42,48] It occurs in more than one anatomic site with nodal involvement and frequent involvement of the liver and spleen. MCD also presents with similar constitutional symptoms and laboratory abnormalities as seen in PCCD.[49,50] Histologically, most cases of MCD closely resemble PCCD, although they may have intact and dilated sinuses in lymph nodes and there may be significant associated fibrosis. Splenic histology shows sheets of plasma cells in the white pulp often surrounded by a zone of fibrosis.[51] As with PCCD, most, but not all, cases are polyclonal. There is a significant association between MCD and infection with human herpes virus-8 (HHV-8) and human immunodeficiency virus (HIV) (**Fig. 4**). In one study of 31 patients with MCD, HHV-8 was detected in samples from all 14 HIV-positive patients, including 5 patients without Kaposi's sarcoma (KS), and in 41% of HIV-negative patients with MCD, including one case associated with cutaneous KS.[52] As MCD cases independent of HIV infection tend to occur in older patients, they may arise in a setting of immunoregulatory deficiency, such as immune senescence, that can occur with age.[42] The clinical course of MCD is variable, with some cases being aggressive and others that may wax and wane over long periods of time.

Plasmablastic Variant of Multicentric Castleman Disease

A variant of MCD has recently been recognized and is known as the plasmablastic variant of MCD (PBMCD).[51,53,54] Histologically, PBMCD contains HHV-8–positive plasmablasts, mainly in the mantle zones surrounding the follicles. IgM-positive immunoblasts have previously been described in the interfollicular region of MCD, but HHV-8–positive plasmablasts residing in the mantle zones are not present in

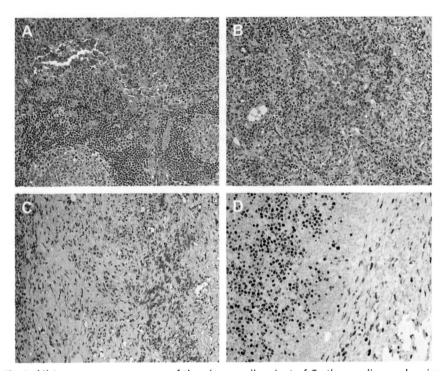

Fig. 4. (*A*) Low-power appearance of the plasma cell variant of Castleman disease showing reactive lymphoid follicles and sheets of mature plasma cells in the interfollicular zones. (*B*) A case of multicentric Castleman disease with an evolving plasmablastic lymphoma. Increased cells with plasmacytoid morphology are seen in and around lymphoid follicles). (*C*) Subcapsular area in the same case (*B*) showing a spindle cell neoplasm. (*D*) The same case stained with anti-HHV-8 showing the presence of the virus in both plasmablasts and the spindle cells of Kaposi's sarcoma.

HHV-8–negative MCD or in HVCD. Of particular importance, some cases contain small aggregates of plasmablasts that have been termed microlymphomas. These HHV-8–infected cells are naïve CD20-positive B cells that are usually monotypic by immunohistochemical staining (expressing IgMλ). However, in a study by Du and colleagues,[53] these cells were microdissected for PCR analysis. The majority of cases were found to be polyclonal. Two cases of microlymphomas revealed monoclonal HHV-8–positive plasmablasts as well as two cases of frank plasmablastic lymphoma. This indicates that HHV-8 infection invokes a phenotypically monoclonal but molecularly polyclonal B-cell proliferation in MCD patients and that in some cases, HHV-8–positive plasmablasts may form polyclonal or monoclonal microlymphomas or develop into frank monoclonal lymphomas.

KIKUCHI-FUJIMOTO LYMPHADENOPATHY

Kikuchi-Fujimoto lymphadenopathy (KFL) was initially independently described by two Japanese pathologists, Kikuchi[55] and Fujimoto, and colleagues[56] in 1972. Although this entity can affect patients of any age, gender, or ethnic background and can involve any anatomic site, including nodal and extranodal locations, most reports originate from Southeast Asia,[57–59] have a female:male ratio of approximately 3 to 4:1, and a mean age of 25 to 29 years for most larger series.

The typical presentation is cervical lymphadenopathy that is usually unilateral. However, it can be bilateral and may involve peripheral or abdominal lymph nodes, and in rare cases, patients may have systemic lymphadenopathy. The enlarged lymph nodes may be associated with pain, and some patients manifest systemic symptoms, including fever, myalgias, and skin rashes. The clinical course is typically benign, with resolution of the adenopathy in a few weeks to months.

Some key histologic features in lymph nodes involved by KFL allow for an accurate diagnosis. Importantly, KFL is typically the most common entity in the differential diagnosis of nongranulomatous necrotizing lymphadenitis. The lymph node architecture is partially maintained with patchy, mainly paracortical, involvement by irregularly shaped and occasionally confluent areas of fibrinoid necrosis. Abundant predominantly extracellular apoptotic debris is also present. Surrounding these necrotic areas, there is a mixture of benign histiocytes (so-called crescentic- or C-shaped forms), immunoblasts, plasmacytoid monocytes, and small lymphocytes. Granulocytes are noticeably absent, and plasma cells are rare or absent. Uninvolved areas of the lymph node may show paracortical hyperplasia with numerous immunoblasts. Reactive germinal centers may be present at the cortex of the node. The lymph node capsule may show partial thickening in the areas overlying necrotic lesions but is intact. Rare cases may be more florid and show extensive lymph node effacement with variable extension outside the capsule. These cases may be more difficult to differentiate from lymphoma with extensive necrosis.[60] In addition, there may be obliteration of the sinuses, and the large plasmacytoid monocytes may be mistaken for lymphoma cells (**Fig. 5**). However, the presence of reactive follicles and a mixture of lymphocytes and histiocytes can help in making the distinction between KFL and lymphoma.

Some authors have separated KFL into four different subtypes depending on which histologic features predominate: (1) early lymphoproliferative lesion, characterized by cellular proliferation of histiocytes; (2) phagocytic, with numerous histiocytes and single cell necrosis but lacking fibrinoid necrosis; (3) necrotic; and (4) xanthomatous (foamy cell), in which there are aggregates of vacuolated histiocytes surrounding foci of necrosis.[57] These morphologic variations are thought to correspond to different stages of an evolving process.

Immunohistochemical staining can be useful in the diagnosis of KFL. The histiocytes characteristically express CD68 (KP1), lysozyme, and myeloperoxidase, a feature unique to histiocytes in KFL and in lymph nodes involved by systemic lupus erythematosus.[61] The lymphoid component consists predominantly of mature T cells, the majority of which are CD8 positive and have a cytotoxic phenotype (TIA-1, granzyme B, perforin positive). A smaller number of CD4-positive cells are admixed.[57,61–63] Few B lymphocytes are present and are confined to the region of the germinal centers. The plasmacytoid monocytes will also express some myelomonocytic markers (CD4, CD68) and some endothelial markers (CD31), but they are negative for myeloperoxidase.[61,64,65]

DERMATOPATHIC LYMPHADENITIS

Dermatopathic lymphadenitis (DL) is a reactive lymphoid hyperplasia, usually associated with chronic dermatoses. It was initially called lipomelanocytic reticulosis due to the presence of lipid and melanin in large reticulum cells. The lymphoid reaction in DL is a result of the drainage of melanin and various skin antigens from affected skin lesions. DL can be seen in patients with chronic dermatosis, but the most florid

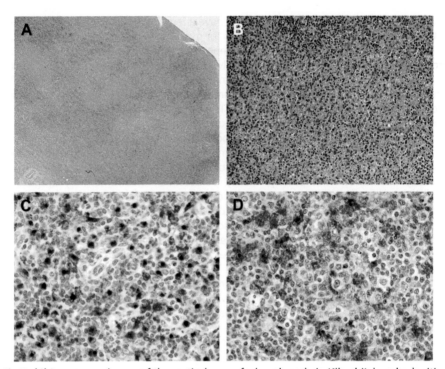

Fig. 5. (A) Low-power image of the cortical area of a lymph node in Kikuchi's lymphadenitis. (B) High-power image of the same case showing numerous histiocytic cells and abundant nuclear debris but no granulocytes. (C) The same case stained with anti-CD68, which highlights the macrophages. (D) The same case stained for myeloperoxidase, as the histiocytes/macrophages characteristically express this marker.

reaction is associated with cases of generalized exfoliative dermatitis. Occasionally, changes of DL are seen without evidence of significant skin disease.

This histologic changes associated with DL are best appreciated under low magnification (**Fig. 6**). There are varying degrees of nodular paracortical expansion as a result of the proliferation of large, pale, staining cells. As the paracortical areas further expand, the follicles can become compressed beneath the capsule or may be completely obliterated. In less florid DL, follicular hyperplasia may be present, often with associated sinus histiocytosis. The pale staining cells consist of a mixture of histiocytes, Langerhans cells, and interdigitating reticulum cells. The histiocytes may contain melanin and hemosiderin pigment. The Langerhans cells typically have complex, delicately folded nuclear membranes, fine chromatin, and inconspicuous nucleoli. Variable numbers of immunoblasts, plasma cells, and eosinophils may also be admixed among the numerous pale staining cells.

The difficulty in DL is distinguishing these reactive changes from early lymph node involvement by cutaneous T-cell lymphomas, specifically mycosis fungoides (MF) and Sézary syndrome (SS), as the histologic picture can be virtually identical. The malignant cells in MF and SS, characterized by convoluted or cerebriform nuclei, may be identified in the pale staining paracortical areas, but they are often hidden among the benign histiocytes. Later in the disease process, these atypical lymphocytes can completely replace the lymph node architecture, making it easier to identify.[66–68]

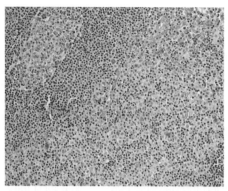

Fig. 6. Expanded paracortical area in a case of dermatopathic lymphadenopathy, showing a typical appearance with some melanin pigment–laden macrophages.

Various studies have looked at immunohistochemistry staining to help differentiate between DL and MF, but the results have not been conclusive.[67,69] Molecular analysis may be helpful in some cases to identify a clonal T-cell population in histologically indistinguishable cases of MF or SS.[70–74]

REFERENCES

1. Nathwani BN, Winberg CD, Diamond LW, et al. Morphologic criteria for the differentiation of follicular lymphoma from florid reactive follicular hyperplasia: a study of 80 cases. Cancer 1981;48(8):1794–806.
2. Crocker J, Jones EL, Curran RC. Study of nuclear sizes in the centres of malignant and benign lymphoid follicles. J Clin Pathol 1983;36(12):1332–4.
3. Horsman DE, Gascoyne RD, Coupland RW, et al. Comparison of cytogenetic analysis, southern analysis, and polymerase chain reaction for the detection of t(14;18) in follicular lymphoma. Am J Clin Pathol 1995;103(4):472–8.
4. Lai R, Arber DA, Chang KL, et al. Frequency of bcl-2 expression in non-Hodgkin's lymphoma: a study of 778 cases with comparison of marginal zone lymphoma and monocytoid B-cell hyperplasia. Mod Pathol 1998;11(9):864–9.
5. Nam-Cha SH, San-Millan B, Mollejo M, et al. Light-chain-restricted germinal centres in reactive lymphadenitis: report of eight cases. Histopathology 2008; 52(4):436–44.
6. Kojima M, Nakamura S, Shimizu K, et al. Florid reactive follicular hyperplasia in elderly patients. A clinicopathological study of 23 cases. Pathol Res Pract 1998;194(6):391–7.
7. Kojima M, Nakamura S, Itoh H, et al. Clinical implication of florid reactive follicular hyperplasia in Japanese patients 60 years or older: a study of 46 cases. Int J Surg Pathol 2005;13(2):175–80.
8. Osborne BM, Butler JJ. Clinical implications of nodal reactive follicular hyperplasia in the elderly patient with enlarged lymph nodes. Mod Pathol 1991;4(1): 24–30.
9. Cong P, Raffeld M, Teruya-Feldstein J, et al. In situ localization of follicular lymphoma: description and analysis by laser capture microdissection. Blood 2002;99(9):3376–82.
10. Adam P, Katzenberger T, Eifert M, et al. Presence of preserved reactive germinal centers in follicular lymphoma is a strong histopathologic indicator of limited disease stage. Am J Surg Pathol 2005;29(12):1661–4.

11. Osborne BM, Butler JJ, Gresik MV. Progressive transformation of germinal centers: comparison of 23 pediatric patients to the adult population. Mod Pathol 1992;5(2):135–40.
12. Ferry JA, Zukerberg LR, Harris NL. Florid progressive transformation of germinal centers. A syndrome affecting young men, without early progression to nodular lymphocyte predominance Hodgkin's disease. Am J Surg Pathol 1992;16(3):252–8.
13. Nguyen PL, Ferry JA, Harris NL. Progressive transformation of germinal centers and nodular lymphocyte predominance Hodgkin's disease: a comparative immunohistochemical study. Am J Surg Pathol 1999;23(1):27–33.
14. Burns BF, Colby TV, Dorfman RF. Differential diagnostic features of nodular L & H Hodgkin's disease, including progressive transformation of germinal centers. Am J Surg Pathol 1984;8(4):253–61.
15. Jones D. Dismantling the germinal center: comparing the processes of transformation, regression, and fragmentation of the lymphoid follicle. Adv Anat Pathol 2002;9(2):129–38.
16. Brauninger A, Yang W, Wacker HH, et al. B-cell development in progressively transformed germinal centers: similarities and differences compared with classical germinal centers and lymphocyte-predominant Hodgkin disease. Blood 2001;97(3):714–9.
17. Hansmann ML, Fellbaum C, Hui PK, et al. Progressive transformation of germinal centers with and without association to Hodgkin's disease. Am J Clin Pathol 1990; 93(2):219–26.
18. Hicks J, Flaitz C. Progressive transformation of germinal centers: review of histopathologic and clinical features. Int J Pediatr Otorhinolaryngol 2002;65(3):195–202.
19. Miettinen M, Franssila KO, Saxen E. Hodgkin's disease, lymphocytic predominance nodular. Increased risk for subsequent non-Hodgkin's lymphomas. Cancer 1983;51(12):2293–300.
20. Nam-Cha SH, Roncador G, Sanchez-Verde L, et al. PD-1, a follicular T-cell marker useful for recognizing nodular lymphocyte-predominant Hodgkin lymphoma. Am J Surg Pathol 2008;32(8):1252–7.
21. Kraus MD, Haley J. Lymphocyte predominance Hodgkin's disease: the use of bcl-6 and CD57 in diagnosis and differential diagnosis. Am J Surg Pathol 2000;24(8):1068–78.
22. Osborne BM, Butler JJ. Follicular lymphoma mimicking progressive transformation of germinal centers. Am J Clin Pathol 1987;88(3):264–9.
23. Goates JJ, Kamel OW, LeBrun DP, et al. Floral variant of follicular lymphoma. Immunological and molecular studies support a neoplastic process. Am J Surg Pathol 1994;18(1):37–47.
24. Hurt C, Tammaro D. Diagnostic evaluation of mononucleosis-like illnesses. Am J Med 2007;120(10):911.e1–8.
25. Childs CC, Parham DM, Berard CW. Infectious mononucleosis. The spectrum of morphologic changes simulating lymphoma in lymph nodes and tonsils. Am J Surg Pathol 1987;11(2):122–32.
26. Strickler JG, Fedeli F, Horwitz CA, et al. Infectious mononucleosis in lymphoid tissue. Histopathology, in situ hybridization, and differential diagnosis. Arch Pathol Lab Med 1993;117(3):269–78.
27. Lukes RJ, Tindle BH, Parker JW. Reed-Sternberg-like cells in infectious mononucleosis. Lancet 1969;2(7628):1003–4.
28. Tindle BH, Parker JW, Lukes RJ. "Reed-Sternberg cells" in infectious mononucleosis? Am J Clin Pathol 1972;58(6):607–17.

29. Segal GH, Kjeldsberg CR, Smith GP, et al. CD30 antigen expression in florid immunoblastic proliferations. A clinicopathologic study of 14 cases. Am J Clin Pathol 1994;102(3):292–8.
30. Reynolds DJ, Banks PM, Gulley ML. New characterization of infectious mononucleosis and a phenotypic comparison with Hodgkin's disease. Am J Pathol 1995; 146(2):379–88.
31. Otteman LA, Greipp PR, Ruiz-Arguelles GJ, et al. Infectious mononucleosis mimicking a B cell immunoblastic lymphoma associated with an abnormality in regulatory T cells. Am J Med 1985;78(5):885–90.
32. Nakamura S, Suchi T. A clinicopathologic study of node-based, low-grade, peripheral T-cell lymphoma. Angioimmunoblastic lymphoma, T-zone lymphoma, and lymphoepithelioid lymphoma. Cancer 1991;67(10):2566–78.
33. Ferry JA. Angioimmunoblastic T-cell lymphoma. Adv Anat Pathol 2002;9(5): 273–9.
34. Merchant SH, Amin MB, Viswanatha DS. Morphologic and immunophenotypic analysis of angioimmunoblastic T-cell lymphoma: emphasis on phenotypic aberrancies for early diagnosis. Am J Clin Pathol 2006;126(1):29–38.
35. Warnke RA, Jones D, Hsi ED. Morphologic and immunophenotypic variants of nodal T-cell lymphomas and T-cell lymphoma mimics. Am J Clin Pathol 2007; 127(4):511–27.
36. Kojima M, Nakamura S, Itoh H, et al. Acute viral lymphadenitis mimicking low-grade peripheral T-cell lymphoma. A clinicopathological study of nine cases. APMIS 2001;109(6):419–27.
37. Castleman B, Iverson L, Menendez VP. Localized mediastinal lymphnode hyperplasia resembling thymoma. Cancer 1956;9(4):822–30.
38. Keller AR, Hochholzer L, Castleman B. Hyaline-vascular and plasma-cell types of giant lymph node hyperplasia of the mediastinum and other locations. Cancer 1972;29(3):670–83.
39. McCarty MJ, Vukelja SJ, Banks PM, et al. Angiofollicular lymph node hyperplasia (Castleman's disease). Cancer Treat Rev 1995;21(4):291–310.
40. Nguyen DT, Diamond LW, Hansmann ML, et al. Castleman's disease. Differences in follicular dendritic network in the hyaline vascular and plasma cell variants. Histopathology 1994;24(5):437–43.
41. Maheswaran PR, Ramsay AD, Norton AJ, et al. Hodgkin's disease presenting with the histological features of Castleman's disease. Histopathology 1991;18(3):249–53.
42. Frizzera G. Castleman's disease and related disorders. Semin Diagn Pathol 1988; 5(4):346–64.
43. Soulier J, Grollet L, Oksenhendler E, et al. Molecular analysis of clonality in Castleman's disease. Blood 1995;86(3):1131–8.
44. Al-Maghrabi J, Kamel-Reid S, Bailey D. Immunoglobulin and T-cell receptor gene rearrangement in Castleman's disease: molecular genetic analysis. Histopathology 2006;48(3):233–8.
45. Leger-Ravet MB, Peuchmaur M, Devergne O, et al. Interleukin-6 gene expression in Castleman's disease. Blood 1991;78(11):2923–30.
46. Hsu SM, Waldron JA, Xie SS, et al. Expression of interleukin-6 in Castleman's disease. Hum Pathol 1993;24(8):833–9.
47. Smir BN, Greiner TC, Weisenburger DD. Multicentric angiofollicular lymph node hyperplasia in children: a clinicopathologic study of eight patients. Mod Pathol 1996;9(12):1135–42.
48. Chronowski GM, Ha CS, Wilder RB, et al. Treatment of unicentric and multicentric Castleman disease and the role of radiotherapy. Cancer 2001;92(3):670–6.

49. Frizzera G, Banks PM, Massarelli G, et al. A systemic lymphoproliferative disorder with morphologic features of Castleman's disease. Pathological findings in 15 patients. Am J Surg Pathol 1983;7(3):211–31.

50. Frizzera G, Peterson BA, Bayrd ED, et al. A systemic lymphoproliferative disorder with morphologic features of Castleman's disease: clinical findings and clinico-pathologic correlations in 15 patients. J Clin Oncol 1985;3(9):1202–16.

51. Dupin N, Diss TL, Kellam P, et al. HHV-8 is associated with a plasmablastic variant of Castleman disease that is linked to HHV-8-positive plasmablastic lymphoma. Blood 2000;95(4):1406–12.

52. Soulier J, Grollet L, Oksenhendler E, et al. Kaposi's sarcoma-associated herpes-virus-like DNA sequences in multicentric Castleman's disease. Blood 1995;86(4): 1276–80.

53. Du MQ, Liu H, Diss TC, et al. Kaposi sarcoma-associated herpesvirus infects monotypic (IgM lambda) but polyclonal naive B cells in Castleman disease and associated lymphoproliferative disorders. Blood 2001;97(7):2130–6.

54. Oksenhendler E, Boulanger E, Galicier L, et al. High incidence of Kaposi sarcoma-associated herpesvirus-related non-Hodgkin lymphoma in patients with HIV infection and multicentric Castleman disease. Blood 2002;99(7):2331–6.

55. Kikuchi M. Lymphadenitis showing focal reticulum cell hyperplasia with nuclear debris and phagocytosis. Nippon Ketsueki Gakkai Zasshi 1972;35:379–80.

56. Fujimoto Y, Kozima Y, Yamaguchi K. Cervical subacute necrotizing lymphadenitis. A new clinicopathological entity. Naika 1972;20:920–7.

57. Kuo TT. Kikuchi's disease (histiocytic necrotizing lymphadenitis). A clinicopatho-logic study of 79 cases with an analysis of histologic subtypes, immunohistology, and DNA ploidy. Am J Surg Pathol 1995;19(7):798–809.

58. Tsang WY, Chan JK, Ng CS. Kikuchi's lymphadenitis. A morphologic analysis of 75 cases with special reference to unusual features. Am J Surg Pathol 1994; 18(3):219–31.

59. Cho KJ, Lee SS, Khang SK. Histiocytic necrotizing lymphadenitis. A clinico-path-ologic study of 45 cases with in situ hybridization for Epstein-Barr virus and hepa-titis B virus. J Korean Med Sci 1996;11(5):409–14.

60. Chamulak GA, Brynes RK, Nathwani BN. Kikuchi-Fujimoto disease mimicking malignant lymphoma. Am J Surg Pathol 1990;14(6):514–23.

61. Pileri SA, Facchetti F, Ascani S, et al. Myeloperoxidase expression by histiocytes in Kikuchi's and Kikuchi-like lymphadenopathy. Am J Pathol 2001;159(3):915–24.

62. Felgar RE, Furth EE, Wasik MA, et al. Histiocytic necrotizing lymphadenitis (Kiku-chi's disease): in situ end-labeling, immunohistochemical, and serologic evidence supporting cytotoxic lymphocyte-mediated apoptotic cell death. Mod Pathol 1997;10(3):231–41.

63. Ohshima K, Shimazaki K, Kume T, et al. Perforin and Fas pathways of cyto-toxic T-cells in histiocytic necrotizing lymphadenitis. Histopathology 1998; 33(5):471–8.

64. Facchetti F, de Wolf-Peeters C, Mason DY, et al. Plasmacytoid T cells. Immunohis-tochemical evidence for their monocyte/macrophage origin. Am J Pathol 1988; 133(1):15–21.

65. Facchetti F, de Wolf-Peeters C, van den Oord JJ, et al. Plasmacytoid monocytes (so-called plasmacytoid T-cells) in Kikuchi's lymphadenitis. An immunohistologic study. Am J Clin Pathol 1989;92(1):42–50.

66. Scheffer E, Meijer CJ, Van Vloten WA. Dermatopathic lymphadenopathy and lymph node involvement in mycosis fungoides. Cancer 1980;45(1):137–48.

67. Burke JS, Colby TV. Dermatopathic lymphadenopathy. Comparison of cases associated and unassociated with mycosis fungoides. Am J Surg Pathol 1981; 5(4):343–52.
68. Colby TV, Burke JS, Hoppe RT. Lymph node biopsy in mycosis fungoides. Cancer 1981;47(2):351–9.
69. Weiss LM, Wood GS, Warnke RA. Immunophenotypic differences between dermatopathic lymphadenopathy and lymph node involvement in mycosis fungoides. Am J Pathol 1985;120(2):179–85.
70. Weiss LM, Hu E, Wood GS, et al. Clonal rearrangements of T-cell receptor genes in mycosis fungoides and dermatopathic lymphadenopathy. N Engl J Med 1985; 313(9):539–44.
71. Lynch JW Jr, Linoilla I, Sausville EA, et al. Prognostic implications of evaluation for lymph node involvement by T-cell antigen receptor gene rearrangement in mycosis fungoides. Blood 1992;79(12):3293–9.
72. Bakels V, Van Oostveen JW, Geerts ML, et al. Diagnostic and prognostic significance of clonal T-cell receptor beta gene rearrangements in lymph nodes of patients with mycosis fungoides. J Pathol 1993;170(3):249–55.
73. Kern DE, Kidd PG, Moe R, et al. Analysis of T-cell receptor gene rearrangement in lymph nodes of patients with mycosis fungoides. Prognostic implications. Arch Dermatol 1998;134(2):158–64.
74. Assaf C, Hummel M, Steinhoff M, et al. Early TCR-beta and TCR-gamma PCR detection of T-cell clonality indicates minimal tumor disease in lymph nodes of cutaneous T-cell lymphoma: diagnostic and prognostic implications. Blood 2005;105(2):503–10.

Hodgkin Lymphoma

Bertram Schnitzer, MD

KEYWORDS

- Hodgkin lymphoma • History • Classification • Pathology
- Immunophenotype • Molecular genetics

Hodgkin's disease was the name bestowed on this disorder by Sir Samuel Wilks in 1865. Known today as Hodgkin lymphoma (HL), it is an entity that has baffled and intrigued clinicians and pathologists for more than 175 years. Although first described by Dr. Thomas Hodgkin in his report of seven autopsies, the original author failed to give his entity a specific name.[1] It remained for Wilks to credit Dr. Hodgkin for his observation in his own publication of 15 cases similar to those described by Hodgkin, in an article entitled "Enlargement of the lymphatic glands and spleen (or Hodgkin's disease)."[2] If Wilks had not exhibited such generosity of spirit in giving credit to Hodgkin, the disease might today be known as Wilks disease or Wilks' lymphoma. Hodgkin's and Wilks' observations were made on gross examination only. Although Langhans in 1872 and Greenfield in 1878 described some of the histologic features of the disease, it remained for Carl Sternberg in Germany in 1898 and Dorothy Reed at Johns Hopkins in 1902 to describe in detail the giant cells that must be present for a diagnosis of Hodgkin lymphoma to be made.[3–6] These large cells, which are now recognized to be the malignant cells in Hodgkin lymphoma, are called Reed-Sternberg (RS) cells and Hodgkin (H) cells. Neither Sternberg nor Reed considered HL to be a malignant disorder. Sternberg theorized that the disease was related to tuberculosis, a disease prevalent at the time, whereas Reed believed it was an inflammatory process. It was not until 1967 that cytogenetic studies revealed that RS cells were aneuploid and of clonal derivation, thus indicating that they were malignant.[7] A confirmatory cytogenetic study was published in 1975.[8]

Clinically and histomorphologically, the features of HL are unusual for a lymphoma or for other malignancies. Patients may present with fever of unknown origin and drenching night sweats, which are symptoms resembling those of an infection, an autoimmune disorder, or an inflammatory process.[9] The search for an infectious agent as a cause, however, was never successful. Furthermore, the histologic picture differs from all other malignancies in that the malignant (Hodgkin and Reed-Sternberg) cells comprise less than 1% of the cells in the affected tissue. Most of the cells in the enlarged lymph nodes or masses are composed of inflammatory cells. In contrast, non-Hodgkin lymphomas (NHL) and other malignant tumors are composed almost exclusively of malignant cells.

Department of Pathology, University of Michigan, 1301 Catherine Street, Ann Arbor, MI 48109-5602, USA
E-mail address: raven@med.umich.edu

Hematol Oncol Clin N Am 23 (2009) 747–768
doi:10.1016/j.hoc.2009.04.013
0889-8588/09/$ – see front matter © 2009 Elsevier Inc. All rights reserved.

hemonc.theclinics.com

CLINICAL FEATURES

The incidence of HL is estimated to be 7400 new cases per year in the United States, resulting in an age-adjusted yearly rate of 2.7 per 100,000 per year.[10] This number accounts for approximately 30% of all lymphomas.[11] In industrial nations, classic Hodgkin lymphoma (CHL), in contrast to nodular lymphocyte predominant (NLP) HL, has a bimodal age distribution, the first peak being seen between the ages of 15 and 30 years, and the second peak occurring in the sixth decade.[12] The early peak is due to the high incidence of the nodular sclerosis (NS) subtype of HL in the younger age group. The incidence of NS HL in young adults has been linked to socioeconomic status, with occurrence, paradoxically, being greater in those individuals with a higher status.[10] Patients may be asymptomatic at presentation with the exception of enlarged, nontender lymph nodes that are most often localized in the cervical region (75% of cases).[13] Less frequently, axillary and inguinal lymphadenopathy is found at presentation. Sites that are rarely involved by Hodgkin lymphoma include Waldeyer's ring, mesenteric, epitrochlear and popliteal nodes. Infectious mononucleosis is a histologic mimicker of HL in tonsils;[14] therefore, in a young patient, a diagnosis of HL in the tonsillar region should be made with a great deal of caution. The initial manifestation of the disease, which may also occur in the mediastinum (NS HL), is occasionally found in an asymptomatic patient on a routine chest radiograph. Patients may also complain of symptoms such as chronic cough or discomfort/pain in the chest related to a large mediastinal mass. Superior vena cava syndrome is rare in HL. Occasionally, patients may complain of generalized pruritus, or following ingestion of alcoholic beverages, they may experience pain in the lymph nodes involved by HL.[15,16] They may also present with cyclic bouts of Pel-Ebstein fever, which is named after the two physicians who initially described it.[17,18] B symptoms in patients with HL include fevers, night sweats, and weight loss of greater than 10% of body weight.[19]

In contrast to NHL, HL spreads from one lymph node group to contiguous nodes in a nonrandom and highly predictable fashion through lymphatic channels.[20] The spleen becomes involved from para-aortic and splenic hilar lymph nodes. How the disease spreads to the spleen, which does not have afferent lymphatic channels, is unclear. If the spleen is involved, hematogenous spread to the liver and bone marrow may occur; however, the liver is not involved unless the spleen is. For unknown reasons, contiguous spread does not occur in HIV-positive patients.[21]

Treatment of CHL is based on the extent or stage of the disease and on prognostic factors independent of stage, such as bulky disease. Stage of disease is classified according to the Cotswold scheme, a modification of the Ann Arbor classification.[19] The pathologic staging that was used 30 to 40 years ago has been superceded by clinical staging techniques that include physical, laboratory, and a variety of imaging technologies.[22] In addition, bone marrow biopsies are now routinely performed.

Treatment of CHL consists of multiagent chemotherapy, radiation therapy, or both.[23–25] These modalities are most often effective, resulting in a cure in greater than 85% of cases.[26,27] Except for rare cases of high-stage disease, treatment of NLP HL differs from that of CHL. As previously stated, NLP HL is an indolent disease usually limited to a single peripheral lymph nodal region. It is rarely fatal with a 10-year survival of greater than 80%.[23,28] Therefore, it is recommended that patients with NLP HL should receive less intensive therapy than patients with CHL.[29,30] The aim of present-day therapy is to avoid the toxic complications that contribute to overall mortality.[31,32] Patients with localized NLP HL and favorable prognostic factors should be treated with involved-field radiotherapy without chemotherapy. Anti-CD20 (rituximab) has also been used in clinical trials in de novo and relapsed disease.[32–34]

A study performed by the French Society of Pediatric Oncology found that a watch and wait approach following excision of the affected lymph node in children with stage I NLP HL had no adverse effect on survival.[31] It is recommended that patients with high-stage disease or unfavorable prognostic factors receive treatment similar to that of patients with CHL.[35]

CLASSIFICATION OF HODGKIN LYMPHOMA

Although there have been numerous classifications of NHL over time, the organizational schemes of HL, on the other hand, have been stable. Following the publications by Sternberg and Reed, 45 years elapsed, during which other cases of HL were described, finally culminating in the first useful classification by Jackson and Parker in 1947.[36] Three histologic types were described: (1) paragranuloma, (2) granuloma, and (3) sarcoma. Although this classification was adhered to for almost 20 years, it was not useful in predicting the outcome of the disease. Most cases (approximately 90%) fell into the mixed cellularity (MC) type; the remaining cases were approximately equally divided among MC and lymphocyte depletion (LD) types. In 1966, Lukes and Butler introduced their morphologic classification, which divided the morphologic and prognostically heterogeneous MC type into MC and a new subtype called NS Hodgkin disease.[37] This subtype had been previously described in 1956 by Smetana and Cohen, who called it nodular mixed cellularity.[38] The remainder of the Jackson-Parker classification remained essentially intact except that the names were changed. Paragranuloma became the morphologically descriptive lymphocytic or histiocytic (L&H) type, which was further subdivided into the nodular and diffuse forms. The sarcoma group was split into the reticular and diffuse fibrosis types. This classification was condensed into four subtypes by a group of hematopathologists, hematologists, and oncologists, all experts in lymphomas, who met in Rye, NY, hence the name Rye classification.[39] The lymphocytic or histiocytic nodular and diffuse types were merged into an entity called lymphocytic predominance, and the diffuse fibrosis and reticular types were combined and renamed lymphocyte depletion (LD). As the names imply, lymphocyte predominance was composed of numerous benign lymphocytes and few malignant cells, whereas at the other end of the spectrum, LD contained few lymphocytes and many H/RS type cells. NS consisted of fibrous (sclerosing) bands forming nodules of HL, whereas MC was characterized by a mixture of inflammatory cells and H/RS cells. The lymphocyte predominance type was, in most cases, an indolent low-stage disease (I/II), whereas the LD type was often discovered in stages III and IV and had a more aggressive course. The Rye scheme was widely and fairly successfully used for almost 30 years until the introduction of the Revised European American Lymphoma (REAL) classification in 1994.[40] This scheme was based on the subtypes that had originally been described by Lukes and Butler.[37] The sole change in this new classification was the addition of a histologic type named lymphocyte-rich classic HL (LRC HL) as a provisional entity. Because in previous studies this subtype had usually been interpreted as representing NLP HL, immunohistochemistry was deemed necessary to differentiate this new entity from NLP HL.[41] In the third edition of the WHO classification published in 2001 (**Box 1**), which is an updated version of the REAL scheme, LRC HL was accepted as a distinct and separate entity and was divided into the more common nodular and diffuse categories.[42] Furthermore, four additional changes were made: (1) the name was changed from Hodgkin disease to Hodgkin lymphoma, because molecular studies had conclusively demonstrated that RS cells in NLP HL and CHL are derived from lymphocytes (see later discussion); (2) HL was divided into 2 major subgroups: NLP and CHL;[13,23,42]

Box 1
2001/2008 World Health Organization classification of Hodgkin lymphoma

Nodular lymphocyte predominant Hodgkin lymphoma

Classic Hodgkin lymphoma

    Nodular sclerosis classic Hodgkin lymphoma

    Mixed cellularity classic Hodgkin lymphoma

    Lymphocyte-rich classic Hodgkin lymphoma

    Lymphocyte-depleted classic Hodgkin lymphoma

---

(3) diffuse LP was no longer recognized as a distinct subgroup but may be a minor or even major component of NLP HL (NLP with diffuse areas); (4) the syncytial variant of NS was subclassified into 2 grades; however, grading is not required for routine diagnosis (see section on NS HL). A revised fourth edition of the WHO classification, published in 2008 (see **Box 1**), made the following changes; lymphocyte predominant (LP) cells replaced the terms L&H and popcorn cells.[43] Cases of CHL that could not be otherwise classified were placed into the mixed cellularity category.[44]

REED-STERNBERG CELLS

The RS cell or one of the variant RS cells must be present for a diagnosis of HL to be established. Not only must an RS cell be present, but it must be in the cellular milieu of one of the HL subtypes. The cellular background is important because H/RS mimickers that may be morphologically indistinguishable from classic RS cells may be present in benign proliferations and in NHL. With the exception of some peripheral T cell lymphomas (PTCL) and T cell/histiocyte-rich large B cell lymphomas (TC/HRLBCL), the background inflammatory cells in the mimickers are usually not consistent with those seen in CHL, which are T cells. The subtype of RS cells also varies according to the histologic subtype of CHL. Classic or "diagnostic" binucleate RS cells are most plentiful in MC HL. These cells, also referred to as "diagnostic" or "owl eye" cells, are binucleate or multinucleate, with each nucleus containing a large, inclusion-like nucleolus surrounded by a clear zone or halo (**Fig. 1**). Uninucleate cells with cytologic features identical to those of RS cells are referred to as Hodgkin cells. Hodgkin cells by themselves are insufficient for a definitive diagnosis of HL to be made on morphologic grounds on the initial biopsy, but are sufficient to establish a diagnosis of relapsed disease when the immunophenotype of these Hodgkin's cells is characteristic. Classic RS cells may occasionally be seen in NS and LD subtypes; however, they are usually absent in NLP HL. Lacunar cell variants of RS cells are characteristic of NS HL. They may occasionally be found in the recently described NLRC HL and, rarely, in MC HL. The appearance of these cells varies according to the fixative employed. In formalin-fixed tissue, a retraction artifact develops that aids in making a diagnosis. The cytoplasm pulls away from the cell membrane around the nucleus leaving a clear space or lacuna, hence the name lacunar cell. Wisps of cytoplasm still attach to the cell membrane and may be seen coursing through the lacuna. This fixation artifact is not observed in well-fixed, mercury-containing fixatives such as B5, in which copious amounts of clear cytoplasm are evident. The nucleus of lacunar cells differs from that seen in CHL and may vary considerably from case to case and area to area. The typical lacunar cell is hyperlobated and contains multiple nuclear segments. The morphologic variants of lacunar cells, however, are more numerous than is

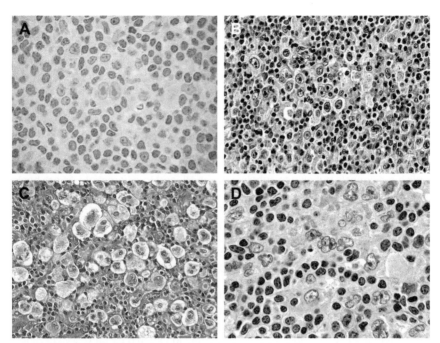

Fig. 1. Reed-Sternberg and Hodgkin cells. (*A*) Classic binucleate Reed-Sternberg cell. Each nucleus contains a prominent nucleolus surrounded by a halo. (*B*) Classic bilobed Reed-Sternberg cells and mononuclear (or Hodgkin) cells with the same cytologic features as the Reed-Sternberg cells in a case of mixed cellularity Hodgkin lymphoma. (*C*) Lacunar variants of Reed-Sternberg cells from a case of nodular sclerosis Hodgkin lymphoma. Some of the cells show wisps of cytoplasm traversing the lacunae. (*D*) Lymphocyte predominant (LP) cells from a case of lymphocyte predominant Hodgkin lymphoma. The cells have polylobated nuclei with nucleoli smaller than those in classic Hodgkin lymphoma.

generally appreciated (see later discussion), especially in the syncytial variant of NS. The nucleoli in the typical hyperlobated lacunar cells are not as large as those in classic RS cells and are found in most of the nuclear lobes. The typical RS cells in the LD type of HL, which are often bizarre, are referred to as pleomorphic, anaplastic, or sarcomatous. Occasional apoptotic cells may be found in all types of CHL. Also known as mummified or zombie cells, they are characterized by deeply staining eosinophilic or purplish cytoplasm and pyknotic nuclei with barely distinguishable nucleoli. The neoplastic cells in NLP HL are called lymphocytic and histiocytic (L&H) cells in the classification of Lukes and Butler, and are also known as popcorn cells because of their resemblance to an exploded kernel of corn (see **Fig. 1**).[45] As stated earlier, these RS variants were renamed lymphocyte predominant (LP) cells in the fourth edition of the WHO classification.[43] Cytologically, the lobated nuclei of LP cells contain nucleoli that are smaller than those in classic RS cells, although in some cases a subset of cells with prominent nucleoli may be present.

The lineage of RS cells remained obscure for many years. Immunophenotyping suggested an origin from a variety of nonlymphoid cells including follicular or dendritic reticulum cells, myeloid cells, and macrophages.[46–49] Recently, however, molecular studies have conclusively shown that, with rare exceptions, H/RS cells are clonal B lymphocytes of germinal center cell origin, and, as previously mentioned, the WHO classifications recognize HL as a true lymphoma.[50] In addition, HL is separated into two major subtypes: NLP and CHL.[13,40–42] NLP HL and CHL differ from one another in terms of clinical behavior, composition of their reactive cell populations, and the immunophenotype of their H/RS cells, as well as the presence or absence of their B lineage specific gene expression program.[51,52] The LP cells in NLP HL preserve the expression of a full B lineage specific program, whereas in classic H/RS cells the B cell program is lost.[52] There is evidence that classic RS cells in rare instances may also be of T cell origin.[53,54]

IMMUNOPHENOTYPE OF HODGKIN LYMPHOMA

Immunophenotyping in paraffin sections is useful and often essential not only to establish a diagnosis but also to subclassify the HL and to differentiate it from benign or other neoplastic lymphoid proliferations. Panels of antibodies are used to characterize the H/RS cells, because no single marker is sensitive or specific.[55] A short panel of antibodies that will usually result in diagnosing CHL include CD15, CD30, CD20, and CD3 (**Fig. 2**). If a definitive diagnosis cannot be established with these markers, the addition of fascin (see **Fig. 2**), 79a, CD45, in situ hybridization for Epstein-Barr virus (EBV)-encoded RNA (EBER), PAX-5 and B cell transcription factors Oct2, BOB1, PU.1 may be helpful.[56,57]

The immunophenotype of H/RS cells in all subtypes of CHL is essentially the same. CD15 is expressed by H/RS cells in 70% to 85% of cases; therefore, lack of CD15 expression does not exclude the diagnosis of CHL.[58–60] CD15 may be expressed by only a minor subset of H/RS cells, and the section should be carefully scrutinized for positive cells. CD30 and fascin are usually positive in virtually all cases and almost

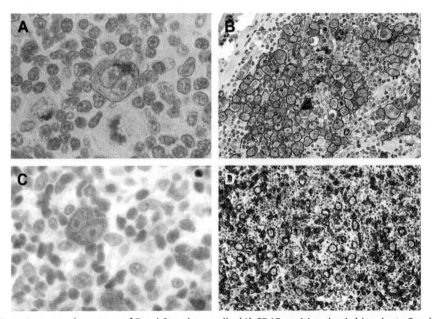

Fig. 2. Immunophenotype of Reed-Sternberg cells. (*A*) CD15 positive classic binucleate Reed-Sternberg cell staining the cell membrane and the Golgi region. (*B*) Lacunar cell from a case of syncytial nodular sclerosis Hodgkin lymphoma. CD30 stains the membrane and/or Golgi region. (*C*) Fascin stains the cytoplasm of a classic Reed-Sternberg cell. (*D*) CD20 stains the LP cells in a nodule of nodular lymphocyte predominant Hodgkin lymphoma.

all H/RS cells in a given case are positive.[59,61,62] However, none of these markers is specific for H/RS cells. CD15, CD30, as well as fascin, may also be expressed in a variety of cells of other lineages.[55,63,64] CD20 may be expressed by H/RS cells in about 30% to 40% of cases. The intensity of the expression of CD20 is usually variable and weak and found in only a subset of cells; in some cases, however, the expression may be intense. CD79a, another B cell associated antibody, may be expressed in H/RS cells but in only about 10% of cases. Whether CD20 expression by classic H/RS cells has prognostic implications is controversial.[65–68]

The immunophenotype of LP cells in NLP HL is completely different from that of classic H/RS cells. The LP cells are CD15 negative, CD30 negative, and fascin negative but strongly express CD20 and CD45. CD3 staining should always be performed because these T cells form rosettes around the LP cells, which is a characteristic feature of NLP HL; therefore, CD20 and CD3 are often sufficient to establish a diagnosis. The programmed death (PD-1) marker, which is expressed by germinal center-associated T cells in reactive germinal centers, is also an excellent immunomarker of T cell rosettes in NLP HL.[69,70] PD-1 may also be helpful in the differential diagnosis between NLP HL and TC/HRLBCL, because PD-1 rosettes are not found around large cells in the latter lymphoma.[70] Other antibodies expressed by LP cells that may, in some instances, be used to confirm the diagnosis, include the germinal center cell marker BCL-6 as well as epithelial membrane antigen (EMA), which is positive in approximately 20% to 50% of cases. Furthermore, LP cells are positive for the B cell transcription factors Bob1, OCT2, PU.1 and PAX-5. LP cells also express J chains.[56] CD57+ cells (occasionally forming rosettes around LP cells) are found scattered randomly within the nodules, and CD21/CD35 outlines an expanded follicular dendritic meshwork in the nodules. EBER is consistently negative in LP cells, although a rare case with EBER-positive LP cells has been reported.[71]

The immunophenotypes of the background benign lymphocytes of classic and NLP HL also differ. With the exception of NLRC HL, the lymphocytes in CHL are T cells, whereas the lymphocytes within the nodules of NLRC HL and of NLP HL are CD20 and CD79a positive B cells. T cell rosettes around H/RS are also readily identified against the B cell background of the nodules of NLRC HL. Rosettes are also present in all other types of CHL but are difficult to detect because the background lymphocytes are also T cells.

There has been a debate about the origin and lineage of RS cells for many years. The major reason for the delay in determining the lineage of RS cells was that they are scarce and scattered among the benign background milieu. Finally, with the availability of new techniques for isolating single RS cells from tissue sections by laser capture techniques and the application of the sensitive polymerase chain reaction (PCR) to isolated single RS cells in all subtypes of HL, it has unequivocally been demonstrated that in greater than 98% of cases, RS cells are clonal B cells of follicle center cell origin.[72–75] Additional evidence for the derivation of classic RS cells from germinal center cells is the finding that in composite lymphomas of follicular lymphoma and CHL, common germinal center B cell precursors were detected.[76,77] The clonal rearrangements are usually detectable only in DNA of isolated single RS cells rather than in whole tissue DNA. The rearranged IG genes of the RS cells and LP cells were shown to carry a high load of somatic hypermutations in the variable region of the IG heavy chain genes without signs of ongoing mutations in CHL, which is in contrast to the LP cells in NLP HL where ongoing mutations are found. The rearrangements in LP cells are usually functional, and IGmRNA transcripts are detectable in the LP cells in most cases, whereas IGmRNA transcripts are absent in RS cells of CHL.[77]

NODULAR LYMPHOCYTE PREDOMINANT HODGKIN LYMPHOMA

NLP HL is defined as a monoclonal B cell neoplasm histologically composed of a nodular or, less often, a nodular and diffuse growth pattern. Approximately 5% of all cases of HL are NLP HL.[78] The clinical features of NLP HL differ from those of CHL, except that in both these major types of HL the disease manifests itself most often in cervical lymph nodes.[13] There is a male predominance, and although this subtype is seen most often in the 30- to 50-year-old age group, it is not uncommon in children and teenagers. In addition to cervical lymph nodes, axillary and inguinal nodes may also be sites of presentation of the disease. Most often, patients first present with low-stage disease (I or II). Because patients are usually asymptomatic and because their lymph nodes enlarge slowly, the nodes often are significantly enlarged when medical attention, often delayed for months or even years, is finally sought. Another characteristic of this type of HL is the occurrence of multiple late relapses, especially following prolonged disease-free intervals. Despite multiple relapses, the disease remains indolent.[79] The number of relapses is probably overestimated, because these reports are often based on clinical findings and imaging studies; however, it is well known that patients with NLP HL often develop recurrent lymphadenopathies due to follicular hyperplasia with progressive transformation of germinal centers but without morphologic evidence of HL. The large nodules in LP HL may either be distinct from one another or else show molding together. However, in instances where they are indistinct, immunophenotyping with CD20 or CD79a may be helpful in defining them. If an uninvolved area remains, it is usually compressed beneath the nodal capsule. Such foci may contain reactive follicles or progressively transformed germinal centers. The macronodules contain a vast predominance of small lymphocytes and, often, a minor population of epithelial histiocytes and scattered neoplastic large cells known as LP variants of RS cells. A purely diffuse form of LP HL is not accepted as a definitive subtype in the WHO schemes but may be a minor or major component of the nodular type. The presence of a single nodule is sufficient to diagnose NLP HL, which is then called NLP HL with diffuse areas. Most cases that were called diffuse LP HL in the past were most likely examples of T cell/histiocyte-rich large B cell lymphoma (TC/HRLBCL). At the present time, an overlap between NLP HL and TC/HRLBCL cannot be excluded. Moreover, it is not clear if a diffuse form of LP exists.[43]

As stated earlier (see also the section on RS cells), antibodies against CD20, CD45, and CD3 are usually sufficient to establish a diagnosis. The small lymphocytes within the nodules in the typical case consist almost exclusively of CD20/CD79a positive B cells with scattered clusters of T cells, some forming rosettes around the LP cells[69,70] (see also the section on immunophenotypes). Staining with CD20/CD79a shows that the nodules have irregular contours, so-called "moth eaten" borders. This feature differs from that of progressive transformation of germinal centers (PTGC) in which the macronodules have a smooth perimeter.[80] CD21/CD35 shows large expansile follicular dendritic meshworks within the nodules. These meshworks are either entirely absent in diffuse areas or else exist only as remnants. With the passage of time, T cells may infiltrate the nodules, gradually replacing the B cells until the nodule is composed predominantly of small T lymphocytes.[41,81,82] This T cell infiltrate may progress and become a diffuse area. In contrast to the B cell nodules, the background infiltrate in diffuse areas consists of T cells. A variety of morphologic and immuno-architectural patterns have recently been identified: (1) "Classic" (B cell–rich) nodular; (2) serpinginous/interconnected nodular; (3) nodular with prominent extranodular L&H cells; (4) T cell–rich nodular; (5) diffuse with T cell–rich background (T cell–rich B cell lymphoma like); and (6) diffuse B cell–rich pattern.[83] CD21 staining is essential to reveal some of these patterns. Small germinal centers within nodules in NLP HL, a hitherto overlooked finding, may be present in approximately 15% of cases. These are, however, also commonly seen in NLRC HL, a situation that may cause a problem in differential diagnosis between the two entities. However, staining with CD15 and CD30 will clarify the distinction, that is, positive results in NLRC HL and negative in NLP HL.[41,65,78] Additional differential diagnostic considerations include (1) PTGC and (2) TC/HRLBCL. PTGC is a benign process that is always associated with follicular hyperplasia, whereas NLP HL is not. Furthermore, LP cells are absent in the former. When diffuse areas in NLP HL are present, this entity must be differentiated from TC/HRLBCL. Although immunostaining does not necessarily resolve the differential diagnosis, features favoring NLP HL are the presence of substantial numbers of small B lymphocytes, remnants of a follicular dendritic cell meshwork, or CD57 positive cells.[78,84] A combination of CD8+ and TIA1 positive cells with a paucity of B cells favors TC/HRLBCL.[43] In addition, the clinical history may also assist in differentiating the 2 lymphomas. TC/HRLBCL often involves the spleen and bone marrow at presentation, but NLP HL is usually localized.[85]

Progression to large cell lymphoma is reported to occur in 3% to 5% of cases.[86,87] The progression/transformation may occur when the HL is diagnosed or many years later. Both lymphomas may be found either in the same lymph node or in different sites.[88] This large cell lymphoma may or may not be clonally related to the LP cells of NLP HL.[89–91] If it is not clonally related, the large cell lymphoma represents a secondary entity. In many cases, the prognosis of the large cell lymphoma is favorable (similar to that of the HL) if it is localized, although other studies refute this finding.[86,88,92,93]

NODULAR SCLEROSIS CLASSIC HODGKIN LYMPHOMA

Nodular sclerosis classic Hodgkin lymphoma (NS CHL) is defined as a type of classic HL characterized by bands of fibrocollagenous tissue forming nodules of inflammatory background cells containing H/RS variants. It is the most common type of HL in industrialized nations, accounting for 60% to 80% of cases of CHL. It is the only subtype in which there is a slight female predominance and the median age at diagnosis is 28 years. Often found in adolescents, NS CHL may also occur in older individuals. A high percentage of patients present with a mediastinal mass (approximately 80%), and approximately one half have bulky mediastinal disease, which is an adverse risk factor.[94] A characteristic clinical history is that of a young woman with an enlarged supraclavicular lymph node, who is found to have a mediastinal mass on imaging studies. Most patients are found at presentation to have stage II disease, and B symptoms are present in approximately 40% of cases. Lung involvement by contiguous spread from the mediastinum is found in approximately 10% of patients. The spleen is positive in 10% of cases, and bone marrow spread in less than 5% of cases.[24,95]

As mentioned earlier, the histologic features of NS HL include sclerosis, nodules, and lacunar cell variants of classic RS cells. A minimum of one single nodule that is at least partially surrounded by a fibrous band should be present for this diagnosis to be made. The degree of fibrosis varies considerably from case to case and from one area to another, even in a single lymph node. Sometimes the sclerotic bands are thin and delicate, but they may also be thick; occasionally there will be subtotal fibrosis of the lymph node with only a minor component of HL. The inflammatory background may also vary from case to case and is similar to that seen in other types of HL (predominance of small lymphocytes or a mixed cellular infiltrate, or a reduction in the number of lymphocytes).[96] The number of lacunar cells also varies in that there may be a few scattered within the inflammatory infiltrate or, in some nodules, there may be sheets of these cells. In the latter instance, the disease is called the syncytial variant of NS, the one that is responsible for the greatest problems in differential diagnosis.[97] The RS cells in the nodular sclerosis type, especially in the syncytial variant, often do not resemble classic lacunar cell morphology but may look like the cells in large cell or immunoblastic lymphoma; alternatively, they may have a bizarre appearance, closely resembling the cells of anaplastic large cell lymphoma or even those of meta-static neoplasms.[40,52,96,98,99] Foci of central necrosis within these syncytia are common and may in some instances resemble necrotizing granulomas. The immuno-phenotype of NS HL is the same as that of other subtypes of CHL. EBV is associated with this subtype in 10% to 40% of cases.[100–102] A grading system for NS HL based on the proportion of H/RS cells or the type of background milieu has been devised by the REAL/WHO classifications; primarily, at the present time, using this system is not required for routine diagnosis; it is useful for data collection.[103–105]

Occasional cases have lacunar cells arranged in vague nodules that are not sur-rounded by fibrous bands; these cases have been referred to as the cellular phase of NS. These are most likely true cases of NS because in the days when pathologic staging was performed, some patients with this type of involvement, especially in abdominal nodes, had typical features of NS HL in the initial diagnostic cervical lymph node biopsy.

The differential diagnosis of syncytial NS includes (1) anaplastic large cell lymphoma (ALCL),[106,107] (2) primary mediastinal (thymic) large B cell lymphoma (PMBCL),[108–111] (3) mediastinal seminoma,[98] (4) metastatic carcinoma or melanoma,[99] or (5) necro-tizing granuloma, especially cat scratch disease.[112] These differential diagnostic considerations are particularly challenging if the biopsy is small and consists entirely of syncytial areas. Antibodies useful in differentiating ALCL from CHL include PAX-5 and EBER. The expression of one of these two markers is usually sufficient to exclude a diagnosis of ALCL, because both markers are consistently negative in this non-Hodgkin lymphoma. In addition, positivity of CD20 excludes a diagnosis of ALCL, whereas positivity for anaplastic lymphoma kinase (ALK), along with a T cell marker, favors a diagnosis of ALCL. PMBLCL and syncytial NS HL may be difficult or impos-sible to differentiate from one another because of overlapping clinical, morphologic, and immunophenotypic features.[113,114] These lymphomas, previously referred to as gray zone lymphomas, are now known as B cell lymphomas, unclassifiable, with features intermediate between diffuse large B cell lymphoma and classic HL.[115] Meta-static carcinomas and melanomas are readily differentiated from NS HL by immunos-taining with antikeratin antibodies for carcinoma and S-100 and melan A for melanoma.[99] The malignancy that may most closely resemble syncytial NS HL morphologically is metastatic undifferentiated nasopharyngeal carcinoma, which is often occult in the primary site and is initially discovered in laterocervical lymph nodes. The neoplastic cells are LMP1+, EBER+, EMA+, as well as keratin positive, but they are CD15 and CD30 negative.[116,117] Seminomas express placental alkaline phospha-tase.[98] The necrosis in syncytial NS HL may be coagulative or more often suppurative. Although the areas of necrosis are usually surrounded by lacunar cells, in some instances, most of the cells are epithelioid histiocytes, which palisade around the suppurative necrosis, resembling the histologic features of cat scratch disease. In the latter disease, CD15+, CD30+ large cells should not be present.

LYMPHOCYTE-RICH CLASSIC HODGKIN LYMPHOMA

Lymphocyte-rich classic HL is a distinct subtype of CHL with features of CHL and NLP HL.[24,41] It was a provisional entity in the REAL classification, in which only a diffuse subtype was recognized. In the 2001 and 2008 versions of the WHO classification, this entity was accepted as a distinct subtype and was divided into the diffuse lympho-cyte-rich (DLRC) and nodular (NLRC HL) subtypes, the latter being more common.[24,41,118,119] The nodular type has several clinical and histologic similarities to NLP HL.[23] Each subtype comprises approximately 4% to 6% of all cases of CHL.[24] NLRC HL differs from other types of CHL. Approximately 70% of patients are male, and patients tend to be older than those with CHL and NLP. They usually present with a lower stage of disease (I–II) than patients with MC and LD HL, and they rarely have mediastinal, bulky disease, or extranodal involvement. B symptoms in these patients are rare and relapses are more common, in contrast with patients with other types of CHL; but unlike patients with NLP HL, the prognosis is less favor-able when relapses do occur. Like NLP HL, NLRC HL is associated with an excellent prognosis when treated with current therapy regimens.[24] In a report by the German Hodgkin's Study Group trials, only 3 of 100 patients died, and all of the deaths were due to treatment-related toxicity.[24] Before the advent of immunophenotyping, NLR was most likely included in the NLP category.[13,23] LRC HL is the type of HL that frequently involves the nasopharynx, which is a rare site of disease in all other types of HL.[120]

The histologic features of this type of HL superficially mimic those of NLP HL.[41] Both have a nodular growth pattern composed predominantly of small B lymphocytes, and the nodules have irregular contours, best appreciated with CD20 and CD79a immu-nostaining. Some of the nodules contain atrophic germinal centers that are eccentri-cally placed within nodules, which are expanded mantle zones. Less often, the germinal centers are hyperplastic. Although small germinal centers may occasionally (15%) be seen in a subset of nodules of NLP HL, hyperplastic germinal centers are usually not found.[83] In occasional cases, many of the nodules in NLRC HL are devoid of germinal centers. Immunophenotyping should always be performed to differentiate NLRC from NLP HL, because therapy and prognosis of these 2 subtypes are different. The RS cells, which are usually few, are located within the nodules and may be of the classic type (binucleate), or there may be a mixture consisting of classic RS cells, lacunar cells, and LP types. However, the immunophenotype of these different types of RS cells is that of classic RS cells (CD15+/−, CD30+, CD20−/+, CD45−). This im-munophenotype definitively differentiates NLRC HL from NLP HL.[41] Small numbers of eosinophils and, rarely, plasma cells may be present. The nodular type of LRC HL was originally reported as follicular HL, but the name was changed by the WHO classifica-tion.[118,119] A feature readily identified in NLRC HL and NLP HL is the rosetting of T cells around RS cells, a pattern readily detected under low magnification (see differential diagnosis of NLP HL). EBV is present in H/RS cells more frequently than in NS HL.

The diffuse type of LRC HL (DLRC HL) is much less common than the nodular type. It consists of a diffuse proliferation of small lymphocytes, which in contrast to the background lymphocytes in the nodular type, are T cells. As in the nodular type, scat-tered, classic, binucleate RS cells, or, less often, lacunar or LP-like cells, are present. Some histiocytes, eosinophils, and, rarely, plasma cells may be admixed with the T cells. Necrosis and fibrosis are absent. In the Lukes and Butler classification, such cases were probably diagnosed as diffuse lymphocyte predominant or, if eosinophils and plasma cells were present, as MC HL.[41]

The differential diagnosis of DLRC HL, which may be difficult to make, includes (1) diffuse areas of NLP HL, especially in a small needle core biopsy in which only diffuse areas are present, (2) TC/HRLBCL, and (3) MC HL if eosinophils are present. Immuno-phenotyping will, in most, but not all instances, result in a definitive diagnosis. The im-munophenotype of the H/RS cells of DLRC HL (CD15+/−, CD30+, CD45−) differs from that of LP cells of NLP HL (CD20+, CD45+, CD15−, and CD30−). The large cells in TC/HRLBCL strongly express CD20 and are CD15− and CD30−.

MIXED CELLULARITY CLASSIC HODGKIN LYMPHOMA

Mixed cellularity HL is defined as a type of CHL with classic H/RS cells scattered among a polymorphous diffuse or vaguely nodular infiltrate. It includes not only cases that are characteristic of MC but also cases that cannot be classified as one of the other subtypes of HL.[44] In industrialized nations, MC comprises approximately 15% to 25% of cases, whereas in developing countries about 50% are of this subtype. The median age at diagnosis is approximately 37 years, and there is a male to female ratio of 3:1. Patients often present in an advanced stage (III/IV), and most have B symptoms. The spleen is involved in approximately 20% to 30% of cases, the liver in 3%, and the bone marrow in about 5% to 10% of cases at the time of initial diagnosis.[44] MC and LD HL are the major subtypes found in HIV/AIDS patients.[121]

As the name MC implies, the histologic features are characterized by a predominance of small T lymphocytes together with varying numbers of eosinophils, plasma cells, epithelioid histiocytes, neutrophils, and fibroblasts. Classic binucleate RS cells, occasional multinucleate RS cells, and Hodgkin cells are usually easily found. Foci of necrosis are not uncommon. EBER+ H/RS cells are found in up to 75% of cases of MC HL.[44] In some cases, numerous epithelioid histiocytes are present. Such cases must be differentiated from lymphoepithelioid cell (Lennert) lymphoma, which is currently classified as peripheral T cell lymphoma, not otherwise specified.[122,123] This non-Hodgkin lymphoma contains numerous epithelioid histiocytes and often scattered H/RS-like cells. Like other peripheral T cell lymphomas, it is aggressive and thus requires aggressive therapy.

The differential diagnosis includes non-Hodgkin lymphomas and benign lymphoid proliferations: (1) peripheral T cell lymphoma (PTCL), and (2) T cell/histiocyte–rich large B cell lymphoma, which are the non-Hodgkin lymphomas. The benign entities include (1) viral disorders such as infectious mononucleosis, and (2) drug-induced hypersensitivity reactions (see section on interfollicular HL). Immunophenotyping and clinical correlation will usually differentiate these entities. PTCL may contain a polymorphous infiltrate similar to that seen in MC HL with cells resembling H/RS cells. Although H/RS-like cells in PTCL are usually CD15−, they may also occasionally express this marker.[124] In contrast to the small lymphocytes in HL, those in PTCL usually have a spectrum of sizes ranging from small to large, and they often have irregular, angulated nuclear contours.[125] The presence of an aberrant T cell phenotype that is found in most cases of PTCL further supports this diagnosis.[126] A clonal T cell population demonstrated by PCR on a whole tissue section supports a diagnosis of peripheral T cell lymphoma. Lennert (lymphoepithelioid) lymphoma also contains numerous epithelioid histiocytes and often scattered H/RS-like cells, and thus must also be distinguished from MC HL.

LYMPHOCYTE-DEPLETED CLASSIC HODGKIN LYMPHOMA

Lymphocyte-depleted classic Hodgkin lymphoma (LD HL) is a rare type of CHL (less than 1% of cases in Western countries but common in developing countries) characterized by decreased numbers of lymphocytes and either many or few H/RS cells.[37,127] Before immunophenotyping was available, this type of HL was overdiagnosed, and because it is so rare today, the clinical reports of true cases of this entity are unreliable. Cases previously diagnosed as LD HL in industrialized nations are now known to be examples of non-Hodgkin lymphoma, especially anaplastic large cell lymphoma or the syncytial variant of NS HL. The median age at diagnosis was reported to be 37 years, and approximately 75% of patients were male.[24,128] These patients usually had B symptoms, stage IV disease with abdominal involvement, and frequent splenic, liver, and bone marrow disease at diagnosis.[24,129] Peripheral lymph node involvement was found to be rare. With modern chemotherapy, LD now has a clinical course similar to that of other types of CHL at a similar stage of disease. LD and MC HL are the types most often seen in HIV-positive individuals.[121,127,130]

There are two histologic types of LD HL. Originally described by Lukes and Butler, these consist of the reticular and diffuse fibrosis types.[131,132] In both types, the architecture of the lymph node is totally effaced. The reticular type consists predominantly of pleomorphic large cells, some of which are classic H/RS cells. Some of the large cells are multinucleate, whereas others have features of anaplastic large cell lymphoma. Still other cases may resemble a sarcoma. Necrosis is common, and disorderly fibrosis as well as a fibrillary matrix are often present. If there are fibrous bands (even a single band), a diagnosis of syncytial nodular sclerosis HL should be seriously considered. In addition to scant lymphocytes, eosinophils and plasma cells are also sparse. In contrast to the reticular type, the diffuse fibrosis pattern is characterized by disorderly fibrosis (rather than a nodular sclerosis pattern) or a proliferation of fibroblasts/myofibroblasts with a few H/RS cells. Other areas may be composed of pink-staining proteinaceous material with reticulin fibrosis surrounding single cells. Few inflammatory cells are present, and areas of necrosis are common. The reticular and diffuse fibrosis types may be present in the same node. The diagnosis of LD HL should never be made without immunophenotypic confirmation. The large cells should express CD15 and CD30 but should be negative for CD45, CD20 and CD3. In HIV-positive patients, the H/RS cells are usually EBV positive.[133,134] The differential diagnosis of the reticular type includes (1) anaplastic large cell lymphoma (see differential diagnosis of NS HL), (2) pleomorphic large B or T cell lymphoma (positive with B and T cell antibodies), and (3) the syncytial variant of NS HL (which contains fibrous bands). Immunohistochemistry in most instances differentiates between these lymphomas.

INTERFOLLICULAR HODGKIN LYMPHOMA

NS or MC HL may involve interfollicular areas of lymph nodes with follicular hyperplasia.[135] The follicular hyperplasia may be pronounced and may mask small foci of HL. Therefore, interfollicular areas in cases of follicular hyperplasia should be scrutinized for evidence of CHL. Although such cases usually cannot be subclassified, subsequent biopsies will reveal that the cases are either of the NS or MC type. Histologically, the interfollicular areas may be expanded by a mixture of cell types including eosinophils, plasma cells and histiocytes, in addition to occasional H/RS cells. Such cases must be differentiated from benign proliferations such as viral infections, especially infectious mononucleosis, as well as drug-induced hypersensitivity reactions.[14,136–138] These two benign proliferations are similar; however, when eosinophils are present in the infiltrate, a drug-induced hypersensitivity reaction is favored. In both disorders, there is a proliferation of immunoblasts that may resemble Hodgkin cells in interfollicular areas; some may be binucleate, resembling H/RS cells. Although these immunoblasts are often CD30-positive, they never express CD15 but are usually a mixture of B and T cells, whereas true H/RS cells, even if they are CD15 negative, do not express mixtures of B and T cell markers. A proliferation of high endothelial venules is characteristically present among the immunoblasts; however, such a vascular proliferation is usually not found in HL. In situ hybridization for EBV (EBER) is positive in immunoblasts in cases of infectious mononucleosis but may also be positive in H/RS cells in a subset of CHL cases. Clinical correlation should be performed to confirm the histologic impression.

FIBROBLASTIC VARIANT OF HODGKIN LYMPHOMA

The fibroblastic variant of HL is most often seen in cases of NS HL. Nodules in such cases may be composed of numerous fibroblasts usually accompanied by varying numbers of histiocytes.[95] Such cases may resemble and be mistaken for malignant fibrous histiocytoma;[139] however, immunostains for CD15 and CD30 are helpful in identifying H/RS cells that may be obscured in this proliferation.

HODGKIN LYMPHOMA AND HUMAN IMMUNODEFICIENCY VIRUS INFECTION

It is well documented that the incidence of NHL and HL is increased in patients with HIV/AIDS.[121] Although the histologic features of HL are similar in HIV/AIDS and immunocompetent individuals, there are several clinical differences. Patients with HIV/AIDS have advanced stage disease at the time of diagnosis, an aggressive clinical course, poor response to conventional therapy, noncontiguous spread, frequent involvement of bone marrow and other extranodal sites, more cases of MC and LD, and a strong association with EBV (80%–100%).[121] There is no increase in the incidence of cases of NLP HL associated with HIV/AIDS. There are few cases of NS HL in immunocompromised patients, in contrast to the general population in which 70% to 80% of patients with CHL have the NS type. The introduction and widespread use of highly active antiretroviral therapy (HAART) has resulted in a spectacular decrease in the development of full-blown AIDS, and a decline in the incidence and mortality of non-Hodgkin lymphoma and Kaposi sarcoma.[140] Paradoxically, however, the number of cases of CHL increased in patients treated with HAART.[121,141] It has been suggested that the improved immunity related to an increased number of CD4+ lymphocytes in peripheral blood and within the tissue in patients treated with HAART results in the increased incidence of HL, especially the NS type. Furthermore, HAART may have put AIDS patients at an increased risk for the development of HL.[121]

Although the histologic features and immunophenotype of H/RS cells are identical in patients with and without HIV/AIDS, the background lymphocyte populations differ. In contrast with immunocompetent patients, in whom there is a predominance of CD4+ cells, CD8+ lymphocytes predominate in HIV patients.[142] Furthermore, H/RS cells in MC and LD are usually EBV positive, whereas in NS they are usually not. The prognosis in HIV-positive patients is not favorable, although it has improved in patients who receive combined antineoplastic therapy and HAART.[121]

REFERENCES

1. Hodgkin T. On some morbid experiences of the absorbent glands and spleen. Med Clir Trans 1832;17:69–97.
2. Wilks S. Cases of enlargement of the lymphatic glands and spleen (or Hodgkin's disease), with remarks. Guys Hosp Rep 1865;11:56–67.
3. Sternberg C. Ueber eine Eigenartige unter dem Bilde der Pseudoleukaemie verlaufende Tuberculosis des lymphatischen Apparates. Ztschr Heilk 1898;19:21–30.
4. Reed DM. On the pathological changes in Hodgkin's disease with especial reference to its relation to tuberculosis. Johns Hopkins Hosp Rep 1902;10:133–6.
5. Langhans T. Das maligne Lymphosarkum Pseudoleukamie. Virchows Pathol Anat 1872;54:509–36 [in German].

6. Greenfield WS. Specimens illustrative of the pathology of lymphadenoma and leucothemia. Trans Pathol Soc London 1878;29:272–304.

7. Seif GS, Spriggs AI. Chromosome changes in Hodgkin's disease. J Natl Cancer Inst 1967;39(3):557–70.

8. Boecker WR, Hossfeld DK, Gallmeier WM, et al. Clonal growth of Hodgkin cells. Nature 1975;258(5532):235–6.

9. Wolf J, Diehl V. Is Hodgkin's disease an infectious disease? Ann Oncol 1994; 5(Suppl 1):105–11.

10. National Cancer Institute. Surveillance, Epidemiology and, End Results Program. Stat Fact Sheet. Cancer Statistics. Available at: http://www.seers.cancer.gov/statfacts/html/lymph.html. 2005. Accessed January 29, 2009.

11. Stein H. Introduction. In: Swerdlow S, Campo E, Harris N, et al, editors. WHO classifications of tumours of haematopoietic and lymphoid tissues. 4th edition. Lyon, France: IARC Press; 2008. p. 322.

12. MacMahon B. Epidemiology of Hodgkin's disease. Cancer Res 1966;26(6): 1189–201.

13. Nogova L, Reineke T, Brillant C, et al. Lymphocyte-predominant and classical Hodgkin's lymphoma: a comprehensive analysis from the German Hodgkin Study Group. J Clin Oncol 2008;26(3):434–9.

14. Tindle BH, Parker JW, Lukes RJ. "Reed-Sternberg cells" in infectious mononucleosis? Am J Clin Pathol 1972;58(6):607–17.

15. Gobbi PG, Cavalli C, Gendarini A, et al. Reevaluation of prognostic significance of symptoms in Hodgkin's disease. Cancer 1985;56(12):2874–80.

16. Atkinson K, Austin DE, McElwain TJ, et al. Alcohol pain in Hodgkin's disease. Cancer 1976;37(2):895–9.

17. Pel PK. Pseudoleukaemie oder chronisches Ruckfallfieber? Berlin Klin Wochenschr 1887;24:644–6 [in German].

18. Ebstein W. Das chronische Ruckfallfieber, eine neue Infectionskrankheit. Berlin Klin Wochenschr 1887;24:565–8 [in German].

19. Lister TA, Crowther D, Sutcliffe SB, et al. Report of a committee convened to discuss the evaluation and staging of patients with Hodgkin's disease: Cotswolds meeting. J Clin Oncol 1989;7(11):1630–6.

20. Rosenberg SA, Kaplan HS. Evidence for an orderly progression in the spread of Hodgkin's disease. Cancer Res 1966;26(6):1225–31.

21. Errante D, Zagonel V, Vaccher E, et al. Hodgkin's disease in patients with HIV infection and in the general population: comparison of clinicopathological features and survival. Ann Oncol 1994;5(Suppl 2):37–40.

22. Wolkov H, Constine L, Yahalom J, et al. Staging evaluation – Hodgkin's disease. Reston (VA): American College of Radiology (ACR); 2005. p. 15.

23. Diehl V, Sextro M, Franklin J, et al. Clinical presentation, course, and prognostic factors in lymphocyte-predominant Hodgkin's disease and lymphocyte-rich classical Hodgkin's disease: report from the European Task Force on Lymphoma Project on Lymphocyte-Predominant Hodgkin's Disease. J Clin Oncol 1999; 17(3):776–83.

24. Shimabukuro-Vornhagen A, Haverkamp H, Engert A, et al. Lymphocyte-rich classical Hodgkin's lymphoma: clinical presentation and treatment outcome in 100 patients treated within German Hodgkin's Study Group trials. J Clin Oncol 2005;23(24):5739–45.

25. Nogova L, Reineke T, Eich HT, et al. Extended field radiotherapy, combined modality treatment or involved field radiotherapy for patients with stage IA

lymphocyte-predominant Hodgkin's lymphoma: a retrospective analysis from the German Hodgkin Study Group (GHSG). Ann Oncol 2005;16(10):1683–7.

26. Connors JM. State-of-the-art therapeutics: Hodgkin's lymphoma. J Clin Oncol 2005;23(26):6400–8.

27. Josting A, Wolf J, Diehl V. Hodgkin disease: prognostic factors and treatment strategies. Curr Opin Oncol 2000;12(5):403–11.

28. Diehl V, Franklin J, Sextro M, et al. Clinical presentation and treatment of lymphocyte predominance Hodgkin's disease. In: Mauch P, Armitage JO, Diehl V, editors. Hodgkin's disease. Philadelphia: Lippincott Williams & Wilkins; 1999. p. 563–82.

29. Murphy SB, Morgan ER, Katzenstein HM, et al. Results of little or no treatment for lymphocyte-predominant Hodgkin disease in children and adolescents. J Pediatr Hematol Oncol 2003;25(9):684–7.

30. Mason DY, Banks PM, Chan J, et al. Nodular lymphocyte predominance Hodgkin's disease. A distinct clinicopathological entity. Am J Surg Pathol 1994;18(5):526–30.

31. Pellegrino B, Terrier-Lacombe MJ, Oberlin O, et al. Lymphocyte-predominant Hodgkin's lymphoma in children: therapeutic abstention after initial lymph node resection – a study of the French Society of Pediatric Oncology. J Clin Oncol 2003;21(15):2948–52.

32. Dores GM, Metayer C, Curtis RE, et al. Second malignant neoplasms among long-term survivors of Hodgkin's disease: a population-based evaluation over 25 years. J Clin Oncol 2002;20(16):3484–94.

33. Ekstrand BC, Lucas JB, Horwitz SM, et al. Rituximab in lymphocyte-predominant Hodgkin disease: results of a phase 2 trial. Blood 2003;101(11):4285–9.

34. Azim HA Jr, Pruneri G, Cocorocchio E, et al. Rituximab in lymphocyte-predominant Hodgkin disease. Oncology 2008;76(1):26–9.

35. Pappa VI, Norton AJ, Gupta RK, et al. Nodular type of lymphocyte predominant Hodgkin's disease. A clinical study of 50 cases. Ann Oncol 1995;6(6):559–65.

36. Jackson H, Parker F. Hodgkin's disease and allied disorders. New York: Oxford University Press; 1947.

37. Lukes R, Butler J, Hicks E. Natural history of Hodgkin's disease as related to its pathological picture. Cancer 1966;19:317–44.

38. Smetana HF, Cohen BM. Mortality in relation to histologic type in Hodgkin's disease. Blood 1956;11(3):211–24.

39. Lukes R, Craver L, Hall T, et al. Report of the nomenclature committee. Cancer Res 1966;26:1311.

40. Harris NL, Jaffe ES, Stein H, et al. A revised European-American classification of lymphoid neoplasms: a proposal from the International Lymphoma Study Group. Blood 1994;84(5):1361–92.

41. Anagnostopoulos I, Hansmann ML, Franssila K, et al. European Task Force on Lymphoma project on lymphocyte predominance Hodgkin disease: histologic and immunohistologic analysis of submitted cases reveals 2 types of Hodgkin disease with a nodular growth pattern and abundant lymphocytes. Blood 2000;96(5):1889–99.

42. Jaffe E, Harris N, Stein H, et al. World Health Organization classification of tumours: pathology and genetics of tumours of hematopoietic and lymphoid tissues. Lyon, France: IARC Press; 2001.

43. Poppema S, Delsol G, Pileri S, et al. Nodular lymphocyte predominant Hodgkin lymphoma. In: Swerdlow S, Campo E, Harris N, et al, editors. WHO classifications of tumours of haematopoietic and lymphoid tissues. 4th edition. Lyon, France: IARC Press; 2008. p. 323–5.

44. Weiss LM, Von Wasielewski R, Delsol G, et al. Mixed cellularity classical Hodgkin lymphoma. In: Swerdlow S, Campo E, Harris N, et al, editors. WHO classifications of tumours of haematopoietic and lymphoid tissues. 4th edition. Lyon, France: IARC Press; 2008. p. 331.

45. Neiman RS. Current problems in the histopathologic diagnosis and classification of Hodgkin's disease. Pathol Annu 1978;13(Pt 2):289–328.

46. Delsol G, Meggetto F, Brousset P, et al. Relation of follicular dendritic reticulum cells to Reed-Sternberg cells of Hodgkin's disease with emphasis on the expression of CD21 antigen. Am J Pathol 1993;142(6):1729–38.

47. Kadin ME. Possible origin of the Reed-Sternberg cell from an interdigitating reticulum cell. Cancer Treat Rep 1982;66(4):601–8.

48. Kadin ME, Stites DP, Levy R, et al. Exogenous immunoglobulin and the macrophage origin of Reed-Sternberg cells in Hodgkin's disease. N Engl J Med 1978; 299(22):1208–14.

49. Soderstrom KO, Rinne R, Hopsu-Havu VK, et al. Hodgkin's disease: a malignancy of follicular dendritic cells? Lancet 1994;343(8894):422–3.

50. Stein H, Hummel M. Cellular origin and clonality of classic Hodgkin's lymphoma: immunophenotypic and molecular studies. Semin Hematol 1999; 36(3):233–41.

51. Schwering I, Brauninger A, Klein U, et al. Loss of the B-lineage-specific gene expression program in Hodgkin and Reed-Sternberg cells of Hodgkin lymphoma. Blood 2003;101(4):1505–12.

52. Stein H, Del sol G, Pileri S, et al. Classical Hodgkin lymphoma introduction WHO. In: Swerdlow S, Campo E, Harris N, et al, editors. WHO classifications of tumours of haematopoietic and lymphoid tissues. 4th edition. Lyon, France: IARC Press; 2008. p. 326–9.

53. Muschen M, Rajewsky K, Brauninger A, et al. Rare occurrence of classical Hodgkin's disease as a T cell lymphoma. J Exp Med 2000;191(2):387–94.

54. Seitz V, Hummel M, Marafioti T, et al. Detection of clonal T-cell receptor gamma-chain gene rearrangements in Reed-Sternberg cells of classic Hodgkin disease. Blood 2000;95(10):3020–4.

55. Sheibani K, Battifora H, Burke JS, et al. Leu-M1 antigen in human neoplasms. An immunohistologic study of 400 cases. Am J Surg Pathol 1986;10(4):227–36.

56. Stein H, Hansmann ML, Lennert K, et al. Reed-Sternberg and Hodgkin cells in lymphocyte-predominant Hodgkin's disease of nodular subtype contain J chain. Am J Clin Pathol 1986;86(3):292–7.

57. Stein H, Marafioti T, Foss HD, et al. Down-regulation of BOB.1/OBF.1 and Oct2 in classical Hodgkin disease but not in lymphocyte predominant Hodgkin disease correlates with immunoglobulin transcription. Blood 2001;97(2):496–501.

58. Hsu SM, Jaffe ES. Leu M1 and peanut agglutinin stain the neoplastic cells of Hodgkin's disease. Am J Clin Pathol 1984;82(1):29–32.

59. Stein H, Mason DY, Gerdes J, et al. The expression of the Hodgkin's disease associated antigen Ki-1 in reactive and neoplastic lymphoid tissue: evidence that Reed-Sternberg cells and histiocytic malignancies are derived from activated lymphoid cells. Blood 1985;66(4):848–58.

60. Stein H, Uchanska-Ziegler B, Gerdes J, et al. Hodgkin and Sternberg-Reed cells contain antigens specific to late cells of granulopoiesis. Int J Cancer 1982;29(3): 283–90.

61. Pinkus GS, Pinkus JL, Langhoff E, et al. Fascin, a sensitive new marker for Reed-Sternberg cells of Hodgkin's disease. Evidence for a dendritic or B cell derivation? Am J Pathol 1997;150(2):543–62.

62. Schwarting R, Gerdes J, Durkop H, et al. BER-H2: a new anti-Ki-1 (CD30) monoclonal antibody directed at a formol-resistant epitope. Blood 1989;74(5): 1678–89.

63. Fan G, Kotylo P, Neiman RS, et al. Comparison of fascin expression in anaplastic large cell lymphoma and Hodgkin disease. Am J Clin Pathol 2003;119(2):199–204.

64. Bakshi NA, Finn WG, Schnitzer B, et al. Fascin expression in diffuse large B-cell lymphoma, anaplastic large cell lymphoma, and classical Hodgkin lymphoma. Arch Pathol Lab Med 2007;131(5):742–7.

65. von Wasielewski R, Mengel M, Fischer R, et al. Classical Hodgkin's disease. Clinical impact of the immunophenotype. Am J Pathol 1997;151(4):1123–30.

66. Portlock CS, Donnelly GB, Qin J, et al. Adverse prognostic significance of CD20 positive Reed-Sternberg cells in classical Hodgkin's disease. Br J Haematol 2004;125(6):701–8.

67. Rassidakis GZ, Medeiros LJ, Viviani S, et al. CD20 expression in Hodgkin and Reed-Sternberg cells of classical Hodgkin's disease: associations with presenting features and clinical outcome. J Clin Oncol 2002;20(5):1278–87.

68. Tzankov A, Krugmann J, Fend F, et al. Prognostic significance of CD20 expression in classical Hodgkin lymphoma: a clinicopathological study of 119 cases. Clin Cancer Res 2003;9(4):1381–6.

69. Dorfman DM, Brown JA, Shahsafaei A, et al. Programmed death-1 (PD-1) is a marker of germinal center-associated T cells and angioimmunoblastic T-cell lymphoma. Am J Surg Pathol 2006;30(7):802–10.

70. Nam-Cha SH, Roncador G, Sanchez-Verde L, et al. PD-1, a follicular T-cell marker useful for recognizing nodular lymphocyte-predominant Hodgkin lymphoma. Am J Surg Pathol 2008;32(8):1252–7.

71. Khalidi HS, Lones MA, Zhou Y, et al. Detection of Epstein-Barr virus in the L & H cells of nodular lymphocyte predominance Hodgkin's disease: report of a case documented by immunohistochemical, in situ hybridization, and polymerase chain reaction methods. Am J Clin Pathol 1997;108(6):687–92.

72. Braeuninger A, Kuppers R, Strickler JG, et al. Hodgkin and Reed-Sternberg cells in lymphocyte predominant Hodgkin disease represent clonal populations of germinal center-derived tumor B cells. Proc Natl Acad Sci U S A 1997;94(17):9337–42.

73. Marafioti T, Hummel M, Anagnostopoulos I, et al. Origin of nodular lymphocyte-predominant Hodgkin's disease from a clonal expansion of highly mutated germinal-center B cells. N Engl J Med 1997;337(7):453–8.

74. Ohno T, Stribley JA, Wu G, et al. Clonality in nodular lymphocyte-predominant Hodgkin's disease. N Engl J Med 1997;337(7):459–65.

75. Kanzler H, Kuppers R, Hansmann ML, et al. Hodgkin and Reed-Sternberg cells in Hodgkin's disease represent the outgrowth of a dominant tumor clone derived from (crippled) germinal center B cells. J Exp Med 1996;184(4):1495–505.

76. Brauinger A, Hansmann ML, Strickler JG, et al. Identification of common germinal-center B-cell precursors in two patients with both Hodgkin's disease and non-Hodgkin's lymphoma. N Engl J Med 1999;340(16):1239–47.

77. Marafioti T, Hummel M, Anagnostopoulos I, et al. Classical Hodgkin's disease and follicular lymphoma originating from the same germinal center B cell. J Clin Oncol 1999;17(12):3804–9.

78. Boudova L, Torlakovic E, Delabie J, et al. Nodular lymphocyte-predominant Hodgkin lymphoma with nodules resembling T-cell/histiocyte-rich B-cell lymphoma: differential diagnosis between nodular lymphocyte-predominant Hodgkin lymphoma and T-cell/histiocyte-rich B-cell lymphoma. Blood 2003; 102(10):3753–8.

79. Orlandi E, Lazzarino M, Brusamolino E, et al. Nodular lymphocyte predominance Hodgkin's disease: long-term observation reveals a continuous pattern of recurrence. Leuk Lymphoma 1997;26(3–4):359–68.
80. Nguyen PL, Ferry JA, Harris NL. Progressive transformation of germinal centers and nodular lymphocyte predominance Hodgkin's disease: a comparative immunohistochemical study. Am J Surg Pathol 1999;23(1):27–33.
81. Hansmann ML, Wacker HH, Radzun HJ. Paragranuloma is a variant of Hodgkin's disease with predominance of B-cells. Virchows Arch A Pathol Anat Histopathol 1986;409(2):171–81.
82. Hansmann ML, Kuppers R. Pathology and "molecular histology" of Hodgkin's disease and the border to non-Hodgkin's lymphomas. Baillieres Clin Haematol 1996;9(3):459–77.
83. Fan Z, Natkunam Y, Bair E, et al. Characterization of variant patterns of nodular lymphocyte predominant Hodgkin lymphoma with immunohistologic and clinical correlation. Am J Surg Pathol 2003;27(10):1346–56.
84. Kamel OW, Gelb AB, Shibuya RB, et al. Leu 7 (CD57) reactivity distinguishes nodular lymphocyte predominance Hodgkin's disease from nodular sclerosing Hodgkin's disease, T-cell-rich B-cell lymphoma and follicular lymphoma. Am J Pathol 1993;142(2):541–6.
85. Khoury JD, Jones D, Yared MA, et al. Bone marrow involvement in patients with nodular lymphocyte predominant Hodgkin lymphoma. Am J Surg Pathol 2004; 28(4):489–95.
86. Huang JZ, Weisenburger DD, Vose JM, et al. Diffuse large B-cell lymphoma arising in nodular lymphocyte predominant Hodgkin lymphoma: a report of 21 cases from the Nebraska Lymphoma Study Group. Leuk Lymphoma 2004; 45(8):1551–7.
87. Fanale MA, Younes A. Nodular lymphocyte predominant Hodgkin's lymphoma. Cancer Treat Res 2008;142:367–81.
88. Grossman DM, Hanson CA, Schnitzer B. Simultaneous lymphocyte predominant Hodgkin's disease and large-cell lymphoma. Am J Surg Pathol 1991;15(7): 668–76.
89. Greiner TC, Gascoyne RD, Anderson ME, et al. Nodular lymphocyte-predominant Hodgkin's disease associated with large-cell lymphoma: analysis of Ig gene rearrangements by V-J polymerase chain reaction. Blood 1996;88(2):657–66.
90. Wickert RS, Weisenburger DD, Tierens A, et al. Clonal relationship between lymphocytic predominance Hodgkin's disease and concurrent or subsequent large-cell lymphoma of B lineage. Blood 1995;86(6):2312–20.
91. Hell K, Hansmann ML, Pringle JH, et al. Combination of Hodgkin's disease and diffuse large cell lymphoma: an in situ hybridization study for immunoglobulin light chain messenger RNA. Histopathology 1995;27(6):491–9.
92. Hansmann ML, Stein H, Fellbaum C, et al. Nodular paragranuloma can transform into high-grade malignant lymphoma of B type. Hum Pathol 1989;20(12): 1169–75.
93. Chittal SM, Alard C, Rossi JF, et al. Further phenotypic evidence that nodular, lymphocyte-predominant Hodgkin's disease is a large B-cell lymphoma in evolution. Am J Surg Pathol 1990;14(11):1024–35.
94. Specht L, Hasenclever D. Prognostic factors of Hodgkin's disease. In: Mauch P, Armitage JO, Diehl V, editors. Hodgkin's disease. Philadelphia: Lippincott Williams & Wilkins; 1999. p. 295–325.
95. Colby TV, Hoppe RT, Warnke RA. Hodgkin's disease: a clinicopathologic study of 659 cases. Cancer 1982;49(9):1848–58.

96. Pileri SA, Ascani S, Leoncini L, et al. Hodgkin's lymphoma: the pathologist's viewpoint. J Clin Pathol 2002;55(3):162–76.
97. Strickler JG, Michie SA, Warnke RA, et al. The "syncytial variant" of nodular sclerosing Hodgkin's disease. Am J Surg Pathol 1986;10(7):470–7.
98. Moran CA, Suster S, Przygodzki RM, et al. Primary germ cell tumors of the mediastinum: II. Mediastinal seminomas – a clinicopathologic and immunohistochemical study of 120 cases. Cancer 1997;80(4):691–8.
99. Mangini J, Li N, Bhawan J. Immunohistochemical markers of melanocytic lesions: a review of their diagnostic usefulness. Am J Dermatopathol 2002;24(3):270–81.
100. Herbst H, Dallenbach F, Hummel M, et al. Epstein-Barr virus latent membrane protein expression in Hodgkin and Reed-Sternberg cells. Proc Natl Acad Sci U S A 1991;88(11):4766–70.
101. Weiss LM. Epstein-Barr virus and Hodgkin's disease. Curr Oncol Rep 2000;2(2):199–204.
102. Weiss LM, Movahed LA, Warnke RA, et al. Detection of Epstein-Barr viral genomes in Reed-Sternberg cells of Hodgkin's disease. N Engl J Med 1989;320(8):502–6.
103. van Spronsen DJ, Vrints LW, Hofstra G, et al. Disappearance of prognostic significance of histiopathologic grading of nodular sclerosing Hodgkin's disease for unselected patients, 1927–92. Br J Haematol 1997;96:322–7.
104. Stein H, Von Wasielewski R, Poppema S, et al. Nodular sclerosis classical Hodgkin lymphoma. In: Swerdlow S, Campo E, Harris N, editors. WHO classifications of tumours of haematopoietic and lymphoid tissues. 4th edition. Lyon, France: IARC Press; 2008. p. 330.
105. Hess JL, Bodis S, Pinkus G, et al. Histopathologic grading of nodular sclerosis Hodgkin's disease. Lack of prognostic significance in 254 surgically staged patients. Cancer 1994;74(2):708–14.
106. Delsol G, Al Saati T, Gatter KC, et al. Coexpression of epithelial membrane antigen (EMA), Ki-1, and interleukin-2 receptor by anaplastic large cell lymphomas. Diagnostic value in so-called malignant histiocytosis. Am J Pathol 1988;130(1):59–70.
107. Del sol G, Falini B, Muller-Hermelink HK. Anaplastic large cell lymphoma (ALCL) ALK-positive. In: Swerdlow S, Campo E, Harris N, et al, editors. WHO classifications of tumours of haematopoietic and lymphoid tissues. 4th edition. Lyon, France: IARC Press; 2008. p. 312–9.
108. Cazals-Hatem D, Lepage E, Brice P, et al. Primary mediastinal large B-cell lymphoma. A clinicopathologic study of 141 cases compared with 916 nonmediastinal large B-cell lymphomas, a GELA ("Groupe d'Etude des Lymphomes de l'Adulte") study. Am J Surg Pathol 1996;20(7):877–88.
109. Lazzarino M, Orlandi E, Paulli M, et al. Treatment outcome and prognostic factors for primary mediastinal (thymic) B-cell lymphoma: a multicenter study of 106 patients. J Clin Oncol 1997;15(4):1646–53.
110. Savage KJ, Al-Rajhi N, Voss N, et al. Favorable outcome of primary mediastinal large B-cell lymphoma in a single institution: the British Columbia experience. Ann Oncol 2006;17(1):123–30.
111. Zinzani PL, Martelli M, Bertini M, et al. Induction chemotherapy strategies for primary mediastinal large B-cell lymphoma with sclerosis: a retrospective multinational study on 426 previously untreated patients. Haematologica 2002;87(12):1258–64.
112. Carithers HA. Cat-scratch disease. An overview based on a study of 1,200 patients. Am J Dis Child 1985;139(11):1124–33.

113. Traverse-Glehen A, Pittaluga S, Gaulard P, et al. Mediastinal gray zone lymphoma: the missing link between classic Hodgkin's lymphoma and mediastinal large B-cell lymphoma. Am J Surg Pathol 2005;29(11):1411–21.

114. Calvo KR, Traverse-Glehen A, Pittaluga S, et al. Molecular profiling provides evidence of primary mediastinal large B-cell lymphoma as a distinct entity related to classic Hodgkin lymphoma: implications for mediastinal gray zone lymphomas as an intermediate form of B-cell lymphoma. Adv Anat Pathol 2004;11(5):227–38.

115. Jaffe E, Stein H, Swerdlow S, et al. B-Cell lymphoma, unclassifiable, with features intermediate between diffuse large B-cell lymphoma and classical Hodgkin lymphoma. In: Swerdlow S, Campo E, Harris N, editors. WHO classifications of tumours of haematopoietic and lymphoid tissues. Lyon, France: IARC Press; 2008. p. 267–8.

116. Bacchi CE, Dorfman RF, Hoppe RT, et al. Metastatic carcinoma in lymph nodes simulating "syncytial variant" of nodular sclerosing Hodgkin's disease. Am J Clin Pathol 1991;96(5):589–93.

117. Zarate-Osorno A, Jaffe ES, Medeiros LJ. Metastatic nasopharyngeal carcinoma initially presenting as cervical lymphadenopathy. A report of two cases that resembled Hodgkin's disease. Arch Pathol Lab Med 1992;116(8):862–5.

118. Ashton-Key M, Thorpe PA, Allen JP, et al. Follicular Hodgkin's disease. Am J Surg Pathol 1995;19(11):1294–9.

119. Kansal R, Singleton TP, Ross CW, et al. Follicular Hodgkin lymphoma: a histopathologic study. Am J Clin Pathol 2002;117(1):29–35.

120. Quinones-Avila Mdel P, Gonzalez-Longoria AA, Admirand JH, et al. Hodgkin lymphoma involving Waldeyer ring: a clinicopathologic study of 22 cases. Am J Clin Pathol 2005;123(5):651–6.

121. Biggar RJ, Jaffe ES, Goedert JJ, et al. Hodgkin lymphoma and immunodeficiency in persons with HIV/AIDS. Blood 2006;108(12):3786–91.

122. Patsouris E, Noel H, Lennert K. Cytohistologic and immunohistochemical findings in Hodgkin's disease, mixed cellularity type, with a high content of epithelioid cells. Am J Surg Pathol 1989;13(12):1014–22.

123. Pileri S, Weisenburger DD, Sng I, et al. Peripheral T-cell lymphoma, not otherwise specified. In: Swerdlow S, Campo E, Harris N, et al, editors. WHO classifications of tumours of haematopoietic and lymphoid tissues. 4th edition. Lyon, France: IARC Press; 2008. p. 306–8.

124. Barry TS, Jaffe ES, Sorbara L, et al. Peripheral T-cell lymphomas expressing CD30 and CD15. Am J Surg Pathol 2003;27(12):1513–22.

125. Banks PM. The distinction of Hodgkin's disease from T cell lymphoma. Semin Diagn Pathol 1992;9(4):279–83.

126. Hastrup N, Ralfkiaer E, Pallesen G. Aberrant phenotypes in peripheral T cell lymphomas. J Clin Pathol 1989;42(4):398–402.

127. Vassallo J, Paes RP, Soares FA, et al. Histological classification of 1,025 cases of Hodgkin's lymphoma from the State of Sao Paulo, Brazil. Sao Paulo Med J 2005; 123(3):134–6.

128. Allemani C, Sant M, De Angelis R, et al. Hodgkin disease survival in Europe and the U.S.: prognostic significance of morphologic groups. Cancer 2006;107(2):352–60.

129. Neiman RS, Rosen PJ, Lukes RJ. Lymphocyte-depletion Hodgkin's disease. A clinicopathological entity. N Engl J Med 1973;288(15):751–5.

130. Glaser SL, Clarke CA, Gulley ML, et al. Population-based patterns of human immunodeficiency virus-related Hodgkin lymphoma in the Greater San Francisco Bay Area, 1988–1998. Cancer 2003;98(2):300–9.

131. Lukes RJ, Butler JJ. The pathology and nomenclature of Hodgkin's disease. Cancer Res 1966;26(6):1063–83.

132. Lukes RJ. Criteria for involvement of lymph node, bone marrow, spleen, and liver in Hodgkin's disease. Cancer Res 1971;31(11):1755–67.

133. Herndier BG, Sanchez HC, Chang KL, et al. High prevalence of Epstein-Barr virus in the Reed-Sternberg cells of HIV-associated Hodgkin's disease. Am J Pathol 1993;142(4):1073–9.

134. Uccini S, Monardo F, Stoppacciaro A, et al. High frequency of Epstein-Barr virus genome detection in Hodgkin's disease of HIV-positive patients. Int J Cancer 1990;46(4):581–5.

135. Doggett RS, Colby TV, Dorfman RF. Interfollicular Hodgkin's disease. Am J Surg Pathol 1983;7(2):145–9.

136. Fellbaum C, Hansmann ML, Lennert K. Lymphadenitis mimicking Hodgkin's disease. Histopathology 1988;12(3):253–62.

137. Yates P, Stockdill G, McIntyre M. Hypersensitivity to carbamazepine presenting as pseudolymphoma. J Clin Pathol 1986;39(11):1224–8.

138. Schnitzer B. Reactive lymphadenopathies. In: Knowles DM, editor. Neoplastic hematopathology. Philadelphia: Lippincott Williams and Williams; 2001. p. 537–68.

139. Weiss SW, Enzinger FM. Malignant fibrous histiocytoma: an analysis of 200 cases. Cancer 1978;41(6):2250–66.

140. Biggar RJ, Chaturvedi AK, Goedert JJ, et al. AIDS-related cancer and severity of immunosuppression in persons with AIDS. J Natl Cancer Inst 2007;99(12):962–72.

141. Clifford GM, Polesel J, Rickenbach M, et al. Cancer risk in the Swiss HIV Cohort Study: associations with immunodeficiency, smoking, and highly active antiretroviral therapy. J Natl Cancer Inst 2005;97(6):425–32.

142. Grogg KL, Miller RF, Dogan A. HIV infection and lymphoma. J Clin Pathol 2007;60(12):1365–72.

Indolent Lymphomas of Mature B Lymphocytes

Paul J. Kurtin, MD

KEYWORDS

- B cell • Lymphoma • Follicular • Mantle cell • Marginal zone
- Lymphoplasmacytic • Mucosa-associated lymphoid tissue

This article covers the relatively indolent lymphomas of mature B lymphocytes: B-cell small lymphocytic lymphoma (SLL)/chronic lymphocytic leukemia (CLL), mantle cell lymphoma (MCL), follicular lymphoma (FL), extranodal marginal zone B-cell lymphoma of mucosa-associated lymphoid tissue (MALT), nodal marginal zone B-cell lymphoma, splenic marginal zone lymphoma (SMZL), and lymphoplasmacytic lymphoma (LPL). Though morphologically somewhat similar to one another, these tumors are characterized by wide differences in clinical presentation, phenotype, genetic features, and outcome. **Tables 1–3** summarize the morphologic, phenotypic, and genetic features of these lymphoma types.

B-CELL SMALL LYMPHOCYTIC LYMPHOMA

B-cell SLL is an indolent B-cell non-Hodgkin lymphoma that is treated in the World Health Organization (WHO) classification as a single entity along with B-cell CLL.[1] Historically, the term "SLL" was used for lymphomas that are morphologically and immunophenotypically indistinguishable from CLL but that lacked lymphocytosis. However, most patients with "pure SLL" develop bone marrow involvement and lymphocytosis over the course of their disease. SLL in its "pure" form accounts for less than 10% of CLL/SLL and about 5% to 10% of all non-Hodgkin's lymphomas. Many early studies on the features of SLL did not exclude blood involvement, and thus accurate information about the presentation, prognosis, and treatment of "pure" SLL is lacking. The morphologic, phenotypic, and genetic features of B-cell CLL and SLL are almost identical.

In lymph nodes, SLL/CLL initially involves the interfollicular zones[2] and then spreads to efface the architecture (**Fig. 1**A).[3] Though most of the cells of the infiltrates are small with round nuclei, clumped chromatin, and sparse cytoplasm (**Fig. 1**B), ill-defined clusters of larger cells with single nucleoli (**Fig. 1**C) are also present in most cases. These larger cell clusters are variably termed proliferation centers, growth centers,

Division of Hematopathology, Department of Laboratory Medicine and Pathology, Mayo Clinic, 200 First Street SW, Rochester, MN 55906, USA
E-mail address: kurtin.paul@mayo.edu

Hematol Oncol Clin N Am 23 (2009) 769–790
doi:10.1016/j.hoc.2009.04.010
0889-8588/09/$ – see front matter

Table 1
Differential diagnosis of small B-cell lymphomas: morphology

Disease	Lymph Node	Spleen	Bone Marrow	Cytology
B-cell small lymphocytic/CLL	Diffuse pattern, proliferation centers	Red pulp; cords, sinuses; white pulp	Intertrabecular nodules, interstitial; not paratrabecular	Small lymphocytes, prolymphocytes & paraimmunoblasts
Mantle cell	Diffuse or nodular	White pulp; atrophic germinal centers, obliterated marginal zones	Intertrabecular nodules, paratrabecular aggregates	Small lymphocytes with nuclear irregularity; No large cells
MALT lymphoma	Paracortical infiltrates; surrounding germinal centers	White pulp marginal zones	Intertrabecular nodules, paratrabecular; intrasinusoidal	Centrocyte-like cells; plasma cells, large transformed lymphocytes; non-neoplastic germinal centers
Splenic marginal zone lymphoma	Surrounds primary and secondary follicles, interfollicular	White pulp expanded with neoplastic cells spilling into red pulp	Intertrabecular nodules, paratrabecular; intrasinusoidal	Medium-size cells; irregular nuclei, abundant pale cytoplasm; occasional large transformed cells
Nodal marginal zone lymphoma	Perisinusoidal or surrounding benign germinal centers and mantle zones	White pulp; small germinal centers, residual non-neoplastic mantle cells	Intertrabecular nodules, paratrabecular; intrasinusoidal	Medium-size cells; irregular nuclei, abundant pale cytoplasm; occasional large transformed cells
Follicular lymphoma	True follicular nodularity	White pulp; neoplastic germinal centers, benign mantle and marginal zones	Intertrabecular nodules, paratrabecular	Small centrocytes and large centroblasts in varying proportions
Lymphoplasmacytic lymphoma	Paracortical and hilar infiltrates, open sinuses	Red pulp and occasionally white pulp	Intertrabecular nodules, paratrabecular, interstitial	Small lymphocyte–plasma cell spectrum; varying large cells

Table 2
Differential diagnosis of small B-cell lymphomas: typical phenotypes

Disease	SIg	CD19	CD20	CD23	CD10/BCL6	CD5	CD3	Cyclin D1
B-cell SLL / CLL	Monoclonal (dim)	+	+ (dim)	+	–	+	–	–
MCL	Monoclonal (bright)	+	+ (bright)	–	–	+	–	+
Marginal zone lymphoma (MALT, nodal and splenic)	Monoclonal (bright)	+	+ (bright)	–	–	–	–	–
Follicular lymphoma	Monoclonal (bright)	+	+ (bright)	±	+	–	–	–
Lymphoplasmacytic lymphoma	Monoclonal (also monoclonal plasma cells)	+	+	±	–	–	–	–

Table 3
Differential diagnosis of small B-cell lymphomas: genetics

Disease	Chromosome Abnormality	Genes Involved
B cell SLL/CLL	+12	—
	del (6q)	—
	del(11q)	—
	del(13q)	—
	del (17p)	p53
MCL	t(11;14)(q13;q32)	CCND1/IGH
MALT lymphoma	t(11;18)(q21;q32)	API2/MALT1
	t(14;18)(q32;q21)	IGH/MALT1
	t(1;14)(p22;q32)	BCL10/IGH
	t(3;14)(p12.1;q32)	FOXP3/IGH
	+3, +18	—
Nodal marginal zone	+3	—
Splenic marginal zone lymphoma	del(7q)	—
Follicular lymphoma	t(14;18)(q32;q21)	BCL2
Lymphoplasmacytic lymphoma	del(6q21)	—

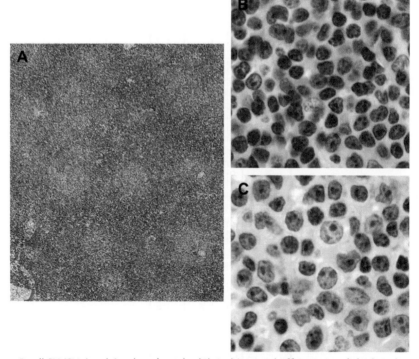

Fig. 1. B cell SLL/CLL involving lymph node. (*A*) Architectural effacement of the lymph node with dark zones alternating with pale zones (proliferation centers). (*B*) Cytology of SLL/CLL in dark zones. Small lymphocytes with round nuclei, clumped chromatin, inconspicuous nucleoli, and sparse cytoplasm predominate. (*C*) Cytology within the proliferation centers showing larger cells with nucleoli and dispersed chromatin.

or pseudofollicles. They have a high diagnostic sensitivity and specificity for SLL/CLL, but their prominence does not affect prognosis. A complete discussion of B CLL/SLL, including clinical and phenotypic findings, can be found elsewhere in this issue.

MANTLE CELL LYMPHOMA

MCLs represent 2% to 8% of non-Hodgkin lymphomas in the United States.[4] They occur in older individuals (median age, 63 years) with a decidedly male predominance (75% of patients). Most patients present with progressive adenopathy involving multiple sites, and there is a relatively high frequency of Waldeyer's ring involvement. Subsets of patients present with splenic involvement in the absence of lymphadenopathy, with multiple intestinal lymphomatous polyps[5] or with a leukemic phase resembling CLL. The staging bone marrows from MCL patients are frequently positive (70%), and 20% to 30% have morphologically recognizable blood involvement.[6,7] Thus, this disease is almost always widespread (Ann Arbor stage III or IV) with approximately one-third of patients having B symptoms at the time of diagnosis.

Morphology

MCLs are characterized by three growth patterns:[8,9] mantle zone, nodular (**Fig. 2**A), and diffuse (**Fig. 2**B) in increasing order of frequency. In the mantle zone pattern, the neoplastic cells surround reactive germinal centers. Numerous coalescing nodules of tumor cells devoid of germinal centers are characteristics of the nodular pattern, whereas a diffusely growing lymphoma cell population that effaces the architecture of the involved tissue defines the diffuse pattern. Hyalinized small blood vessels course through the lymphoma infiltrates in a substantial fraction of diffuse pattern MCL. Scattered mitotic figures and epithelioid histiocytes are also common.

Classical MCL is composed of monomorphous small lymphocytes with spheroidal nuclei, with irregularities, cleaves, and grooves. The chromatin is clumped, nucleoli are inconspicuous, and cytoplasm is sparse (**Fig. 2**C). Proliferation centers and intermixed centroblasts or immunoblasts are absent.[10]

Several cytologic variants of MCL have been described. In a small number of cases, MCLs are composed of small lymphocytes similar to those in SLL/CLL (but lacking proliferation centers) or marginal zone-like cells with slightly larger nuclei, more dispersed chromatin, and voluminous pale cytoplasm. Clinically aggressive MCL variants are collectively termed "blastoid" variants[9,11] and include cases composed of cells that resemble lymphoblasts (**Fig. 2**D), cases composed of cells with highly pleomorphic nuclei (**Fig. 2**E), and cases with cells resembling centroblasts.

The bone marrow is positive in 70% of MCL patients at diagnosis. Paratrabecular, intertrabecular nodular, and/or interstitial infiltrates are found in involved bone marrow biopsy specimens. In the spleen, MCL involves the white pulp, and, in a subset of cases, marginal zone differentiation is seen toward the periphery of the white pulp nodules. MCL is one of the lymphoma types that can cause multiple intestinal lymphomatous polyposis (**Fig. 2**F).

Phenotype

MCL cells express[9] CD19, CD20 (**Fig. 3**A), CD79a, CD79b, PAX-5, and surface immunoglobulin light chain. More MCL cases express lambda light chain than kappa light chain. Greater than 95% are positive for CD5 (**Fig. 3**B), and most either completely lack CD23 (**Fig. 3**C) expression or show weak CD23 marking in a subset of the tumor cells. They are usually negative for CD10 and BCL6. Notable exceptions include rare

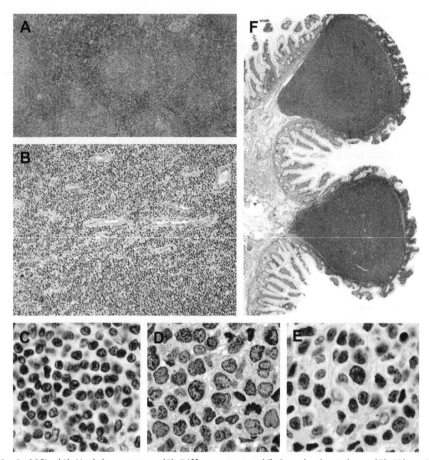

Fig. 2. MCL. (A) Nodular pattern, (B) Diffuse pattern. (C) Standard cytology. (D) "Blastoid variant"—the neoplastic lymphocytes resemble lymphoblasts. (E) "Blastoid variant"—the neoplastic cells have pleomorphic nuclei. (F) MCL involving small intestine in the pattern typically seen with multiple intestinal lymphomatous polyposis.

CD5 negativity or CD10 and /or BCL6 positivity. As a consequence of the t(11;14)(q13;q32) (see later section), the nuclei of almost all cases are positive for cyclin D1 (**Fig. 3**D).[12]

Genetics

Almost all cases of MCL contain a balanced translocation involving the cyclin D1 gene (*CCND1*) on chromosome 11q13.[13] The immunoglobulin heavy chain gene (*IGH*) on chromosome 14q32 is the most frequent partner in the translocation, but, in a small subset of cases, the kappa (2p11) or the lambda (22q11) immunoglobulin light chain genes are the partner loci. Because the morphology and phenotype of MCL overlap with other small B-cell lymphomas, demonstrating cyclin D1 positivity in the neoplastic cells by paraffin section immunohistochemistry (preferred method for fixed tissue samples) or detecting (*CCND1/IGH*) fusion by fluorescence in situ hybridization (**Fig. 3**E)[14] (preferred method for liquid bone marrow and blood samples) is essential to confirm the diagnosis. Other notable genetic findings in MCL include a high

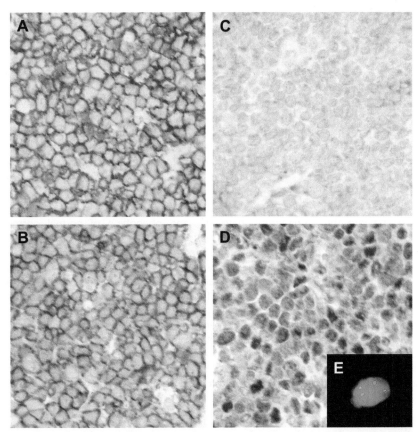

Fig. 3. Immunoperoxidase stains of MCL, illustrating the characteristic phenotype. (*A*) CD20 positive. (*B*) CD5 positive. (*C*) CD23 negative. (*D*) Cyclin D1 positive—nuclear staining. (*E*) (*inset*). Fluorescence in situ hybridization in MCL. There is a single signal for the normal *CCND1* (*red*), a single signal for the normal *IGH* (*green*), and two fusion signals (*yellow*) indicating the *CCND1/IGH* translocation.

frequency of nonrandom secondary chromosomal abnormalities, deletion (del)(17p) or mutations in the p53 gene, p16 deletion or hypermethylation, mutations in the *ATM* gene, and tetraploidy. Rare examples of cyclin D1–negative *CCND1/IGH* nontranslocated MCL case have been described. Morphologically and phenotypically identical to their *CCND1* translocated counterparts, they express cyclin D2, D3, or E with or without translocations involving these genes and are negative for p27.[15,16]

Clonal immunoglobulin heavy and light chain gene rearrangements can be demonstrated in virtually all cases of MCL. Most cases have no point mutations of *IGH* or in noncoding sequences of *BCL6*. However, in approximately one-third of cases, point mutations in the immunoglobulin heavy chain genes can be detected, indicating somatic hypermutation of the immunoglobulin genes and a postgerminal center cell genotype.[17]

FOLLICULAR LYMPHOMA

Accounting for approximately 20% of all non-Hodgkin lymphomas, FLs are the second most common lymphoma type in the United States and Western Europe.[4,18] The disease occurs with a median age of 60 years and with a slight female predominance; pediatric cases are rare. Patients usually present with gradually progressive or waxing and waning, painless lymph node enlargement involving cervical, supraclavicular, axillary, and/or inguinal regions. Isolated splenomegaly, multiple intestinal lymphomatous polyps, and a peripheral blood leukemic phase, superficially resembling CLL are rare initial manifestations of FL. At diagnosis, FL patients are usually found to have widespread disease; 40% of patients have spleen involvement, 50% have liver involvement, and 55% to 70% have bone marrow involvement. Thus, most patients present in Ann Arbor stage III or IV. Only 20% have B symptoms (fever, weight loss, night sweats) or elevated lactate dehydrogenase levels. Outcome and treatment of FL are determined by the grade of the lymphoma (see later section) and the FL international prognostic index.[19]

Morphology

FLs recapitulate the architecture, cytology, and phenotype of normal germinal centers.[18] Thus, most grow in a nodular pattern (**Fig. 4**A). The nodules efface the lymph node architecture, overrunning the sinuses and invading beyond the capsule of the lymph node into the perinodal soft tissue (**Fig. 4**B). The neoplastic follicles are crowded together, may coalesce (**Fig. 5**A), and tend to be smaller and have less prominent mantle zones than those of reactive follicles.[20] In many cases, the neoplastic nodules are accompanied by a diffusely growing component. Rarely, FLs grow in a purely diffuse pattern (**Fig. 4**C) and are termed "diffuse FL" by WHO convention.[18] This diagnosis requires phenotypic or genetic confirmation.

FLs vary in their cytologic composition from case to case or from area to area.[18,20] Centrocytes predominate in most FLs (**Fig. 5**C). They have ovoid nuclei with irregular, angulated contours and superimposed notches, grooves, and cleaves. Centroblasts

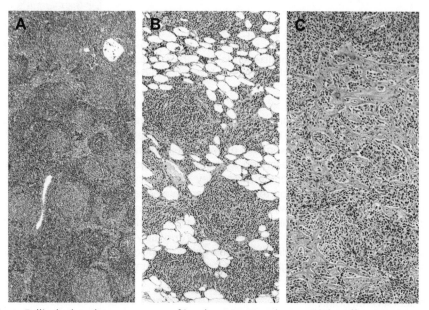

Fig. 4. Follicular lymphoma, patterns of involvement. Neoplastic nodules efface lymph node architecture (*A*) and extend outside the lymph node into the perinodal fat (*B*). (*C*) A diffuse pattern of involvement associated with collagen fibrosis.

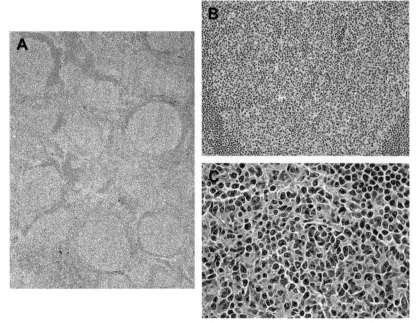

Fig. 5. Follicular lymphoma. (*A*) Coalescence of neoplastic nodules is an architectural feature of this case, which is composed of a monomorphous population of centrocytes (follicular lymphoma, grade 1) illustrated in panels (*B*) and (*C*).

comprise the second cell population in most FLs. They have round nuclei, dispersed chromatin, nucleoli that are usually multiple and adjacent to the nuclear membranes, and moderately abundant basophilic cytoplasm. Monocytoid-appearing lymphocytes, often at the margins of the neoplastic follicles ("marginal zone differentiation"),[21] monotypic plasma cells ("plasma cell differentiation"),[22] and centrocytes containing intranuclear immunoglobulin inclusions ("signet ring cell lymphoma") are present in a minority of FLs.

The relative proportions of centrocytes and centroblasts in individual cases form the basis for FL grading.[18,23] Grade 1 is assigned to those cases in which there are less than five large centroblasts per 400X field (**Fig. 5C**). Grade 2 is assigned to those cases with between 5 and 15 centroblasts per 400X field (**Fig. 6A**), and grade 3 FLs have more than 15 centroblasts per 400X field (**Fig. 6B**). Grade 3 is further subdivided into grade 3a and 3b. If virtually all of the cells in the neoplastic follicles are centroblasts, the tumor is assigned grade 3b. If there is a mixture of centrocytes together with the centroblasts, the lymphoma is graded 3a.

At diagnosis, the bone marrow is involved in approximately 55% to 70% of cases. A paratrabecular distribution is most characteristic, but intertrabecular nodules and interstitial infiltrates also occur. FLs in bone marrow may be of lower grade than that in concurrent lymph node specimens. Therefore, except in instances of grade 3 FL, grading is most prudently applied to specimens other than bone marrow.

In the spleen, FLs preferentially involve the white pulp.[24] Neoplastic centrocytes and/or centroblasts are present in the centers of white pulp nodules, and from there, they can irregularly infiltrate the splenic red pulp.

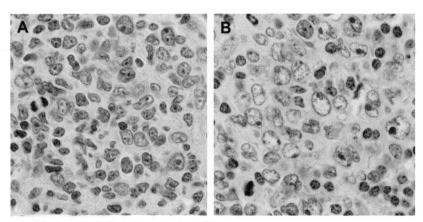

Fig. 6. Follicular lymphoma. (*A*) Grade 2 and (*B*) Grade 3.

Similar to MCL, FLs can present with widespread intestinal involvement (multiple intestinal lymphomatoid polyposis), often accompanied by enlarged mesenteric lymph nodes, and spread to other sites.[5] By contrast, a small number of patients with incidental FL of the duodenum as an isolated site of disease and an excellent outcome even without treatment have been described in 2008.[25]

Skin involvement can occur in systemic FLs, and in this situation, they are morphologically, phenotypically, and genetically similar to their nodal counterparts. However, when FLs arise primarily in the skin and involve only this organ, they exhibit important clinical and biologic differences from those that arise in lymph nodes.[26–29] They produce single or grouped erythematous papules and nodules often in the head and neck, shoulder girdle, upper chest, and back regions. Though morphologically similar to nodal FLs, the neoplastic cells in primary cutaneous FLs are often immunoglobulin negative and do not have *BCL2/IGH* translocations or BCL2 protein overexpression. Treated locally, they rarely disseminate or cause the death of the patient, regardless of grade. Thus, they are separately classified by the WHO as "primary cutaneous follicle center lymphomas" and are not graded.

Finally, FLs in children can be similar to those in adults.[18,30] However, more often they are localized to single lymph node sites or to Waldeyer's ring at diagnosis, contain very large, expansive follicles, lack *BCL2/IGH* translocations and BCL2 protein expression (see later section), and appear to have an excellent prognosis.

Phenotype

FL cells express CD19, CD20 (**Fig. 7**A), CD22, CD79a, CD79b, PAX-5, and light chain chain–restricted surface immunoglobulin. They are positive for CD10 (**Fig. 7**B) and/or BCL6 (**Fig. 7**C) in 90% of cases.[18,31] As a consequence of the t(14;18)(q21;q32) (see later), cytoplasmic BCL2 protein expression is a hallmark of most FL cases (**Fig. 7**D).[32] Though positive in nearly 100% of grade 1 FLs, only 75% of grade 3 FLs and lower percentages of pediatric, primary cutaneous, thyroid, splenic, and testicular FLs express BCL2. Because normal follicular center cells lack BCL2 protein expression, BCL2 is a useful marker to distinguish FL from follicular lymphoid hyperplasia.

Genetics

The genetic hallmark of FL, present in 85% of cases, is t(14;18)(q32;q21). This abnormality translocates *BCL2* (18q21) into the immunoglobulin heavy chain gene (*IGH* at

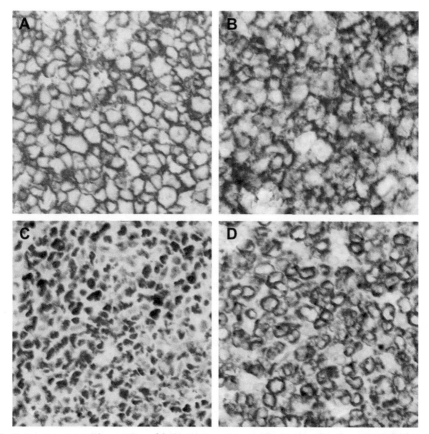

Fig. 7. Immunoperoxidase stains of follicular lymphoma, illustrating the characteristic phenotype. The neoplastic cells are positive for (*A*) CD20, (*B*) CD10, (*C*) bcl-6, and (*D*) bcl-2.

14q32), causing overexpression of BCL2 protein. Additional chromosomal gains and losses, none of which is specific for FL, but which may be of prognostic importance, usually accompany the t(14;18)(q32;q21).[33] In a subset of FLs (5%–15%), usually grade 3b and BCL2 negative, *BCL6* gene (3q27) translocations are present.[34,35] *IGH* is usually the partner genetic locus, in these situations, that is, t(3;14)(q27;q32).

Transformation of Follicular Lymphomas

Transformation of FL to diffuse large B-cell lymphoma (DLBCL) or less commonly to a lymphoma that morphologically resembles Burkitt lymphoma (BL) occurs in 25% to 50% of cases. This situation is associated with a change to more aggressive clinical behavior and is usually accompanied by progressive cytogenetic abnormalities in the transformed lymphoma.[36] When the lymphoma to which FL transforms resembles BL morphologically, there is often acquisition of a translocation of *MYC* in addition to the preexisting *BCL2* translocation from the original FL. These "dual translocation" cases virtually always express bcl-2 protein and are now typically reported as unclassifiable B-cell lymphomas with features intermediate between DLBCL and BL in the new 2008 WHO classification. The combination of both *MYC* and *BCL2* translocations in the same tumor is associated with a particularly poor prognosis.

EXTRANODAL MARGINAL ZONE B-CELL LYMPHOMA OF MUCOSA-ASSOCIATED LYMPHOID TISSUE

Extranodal marginal zone B-cell lymphoma of MALT comprises 7% to 8% of all B-cell lymphomas, and although it may occur in children or young adults, it is most frequently a disease of older individuals with a median age of 60 years.[4,37] There is a slight female predominance. MALT lymphomas preferentially arise in extranodal sites. They are most common in the stomach, the salivary glands, the lungs, the orbit and ocular adnexae, the thyroid, skin, and breast. The epidemiology of MALT lymphomas varies by anatomic site. In general, MALT lymphomas arise in organs devoid of or sparsely populated by lymphoid tissue. An inflammatory stimulus, either autoimmune or infectious, recruits lymphocytes and immune accessory cells to these sites, and it is within this inflammatory milieu that MALT lymphomas arise (**Table 4**).[38] The inflammatory disorders linked to MALT lymphomas in various anatomic sites are listed in **Table 4**.

The initial manifestations of MALT-type lymphomas vary by the organ primarily involved by the tumor.[39,40] For the stomach, nonspecific dyspepsia and epigastric pain are common symptoms.[41,42] For the lung, cough and chest pain herald the symptomatic onset of the disease.[43] For the salivary glands, thyroid, orbit, and skin, tumors involving those sites in association with symptoms of the salient associated autoimmune disease are present. Thus, the presenting manifestations of MALT lymphomas are quite nonspecific.

At the time of diagnosis, MALT lymphomas are usually localized to the organ in which they arise. For all primary anatomic sites, aggressive staging will uncover bone marrow involvement in 20% of patients, spread to another non-nodal site in 12% of patients, and involvement of lymph nodes in 7.5% of patients.[44]

Morphology

Regardless of the extranodal organ involved by the MALT lymphoma, five elements arranged architecturally in a manner that resembles Peyer's patches are present (**Fig. 8A, B**):[37,38] (1) The neoplastic marginal zone B cells, termed "centrocyte-like cells" are usually small to medium sized with irregular nuclear contours, partially clumped chromatin, and moderately abundant pale cytoplasm (**Fig. 8C**). (2) Varying numbers of transformed lymphocytes that resemble immunoblasts or centroblasts are present. (3) Plasma cells when present are polarized toward epithelial surfaces and can be polyclonal or clonally related to the neoplastic B cells. (4) Lymphoepithelial lesions are complexes of altered epithelial cells infiltrated by the neoplastic lymphocytes (**Fig. 8D**). (5) Non-neoplastic germinal centers are often surrounded by the tumor.

Table 4
Site-specific inflammatory disorders related to the pathogenesis of MALT lymphomas

Anatomic Site	Associated Condition
Stomach	*Helicobacter pylori* gastritis
Salivary gland	Sjøgren syndrome
Thyroid	Hashimoto thyroiditis
Lacrimal gland	*Chlamydia psittaci* infection
Skin	*Borrelia burgdorferi* infection
Immunoproliferative small intestinal disease	*Campylobacter jejuni* infection

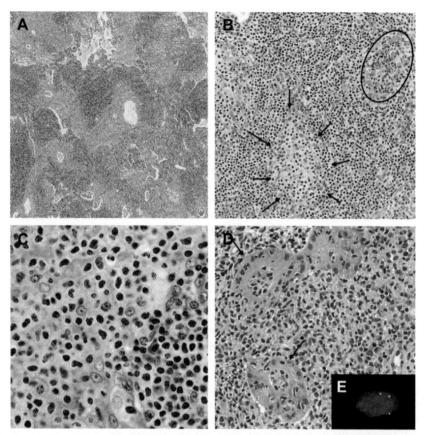

Fig. 8. MALT lymphoma involving lung (*A–C*) and stomach (*D*). (*A*) Note the architectural effacement of the lung with the neoplastic cells tracking along the bronchovascular septa. (*B*) MALT lymphomas recapitulate Peyer's patches with benign germinal centers (*oval*) and lymphoepithelial lesions (*arrows*). (*C*) Cytologic features of MALT lymphoma include medium size cells with irregular nuclei and abundant cytoplasm. (*D*) Lymphoepithelial lesions formed by neoplastic lymphocytes infiltrating the gastric glands (*arrows*). (*E*) Fluorescence in situ hybridization in MALT lymphoma. There is a single signal for the normal *API2* (*red*), a single signal for the normal *MALT1* (*green*) and 2 fusion signals (*yellow*) indicating the *API2/MALT1* translocation.

Phenotype

The cells of MALT lymphoma express CD19, CD20, CD22, CD79a, CD79b, and PAX-5 and show either kappa or lambda immunoglobulin light chain restriction. When the intermixed plasma cells are part of the lymphoma, they express the same immunoglobulin light chain as the neoplastic small lymphocytes. Typically, but not exclusively, the cells of MALT lymphoma are negative for CD5, CD10, and BCL6. CD43 is aberrantly expressed by a subset of MALT lymphomas.

Genetics

Four translocations with different frequencies in MALT lymphomas arising from different anatomic sites are highly characteristic. T(11;18)(q21;q21) results in fusion of *API2* from 11q21 and *MALT1* from 18q21(**Fig. 8**E) and production of a chimeric api2/malt1 protein.[45,46] In the t(14;18)(q32;q21), t(1;14)(p22;q32), and t(3;14)(p12.1; q32), *MALT1*, *BCL10*, and *FOX P3*, respectively, are involved in translocations with *IGH* resulting in overexpression of the relevant proteins.[47–51] The translocations are mutually exclusive and result in nonphysiologic activation of the canonical nuclear factor kappa B pathway. Trisomies of chromosomes 3 and 18, also common in MALT lymphomas, are mutually exclusive of the translocations.[52]

SPLENIC MARGINAL ZONE LYMPHOMA

SMZLs are rare, accounting for no more than 1% to 2% of all non-Hodgkin lymphomas.[53–57] They occur in older individuals (median age is 68 years) with an equal gender distribution. Most patients present with either symptomatic splenomegaly or lymphocytosis associated with an enlarged spleen (splenic lymphoma with villous lymphocytes, now considered synonymous with SMZL).[53] The bone marrow is positive for lymphoma in at least 80% of patients at diagnosis, and in 30% the liver is involved. Abdominal adenopathy is present in up to 25% of patients, but peripheral and mediastinal adenopathy are rare at diagnosis.

Morphology

SMZL has its most characteristic morphology in the spleen.[53] In typical cases, the neoplastic lymphocytes centrifugally expand out from the margins of atrophic germinal centers (**Fig. 9**A), irregularly infiltrate the adjacent splenic red pulp, and exhibit dimorphic cytologic features (**Fig. 9**B). The neoplastic cells immediately adjacent to the germinal center are similar to mantle zone lymphocytes. These are surrounded by coronas of neoplastic cells that resemble normal splenic marginal zone lymphocytes (**Fig. 9**C). They are small to medium sized with partially dispersed chromatin, small or inconspicuous nucleoli, and abundant pale staining cytoplasm. Large lymphocytes with features similar to immunoblasts are often singly distributed near the border between the expanded white pulp and the adjacent red pulp.

Because a subset of patients with SMZL present with a prominent leukemic phase, bone marrow involvement, and an enlarged spleen (ie, splenic lymphoma with villous lymphocytes) (**Fig. 10**A), the bone marrow is often the site from which the diagnosis is attempted so that splenectomy can be avoided. Though both paratrabecular and intertrabecular nodules of SMZL occur, an intravascular distribution is highly characteristic of SMZL (**Fig. 10**B, C)[58] and, when present, can be used to suggest the diagnosis.

Phenotype

The cells of SMZL express CD19, CD20, CD22, and PAX-5 and show either kappa or lambda immunoglobulin light chain restriction. SMZL cells are occasionally positive for CD5, DBA.44, CD11c, and CD103.[59] Care must be taken in these instances to exclude MCL and hairy cell leukemia. However, typically the cells of this lymphoma type are negative for CD10, CD21, CD35, BCL6, CD103 Annexin A1, and CD5.

Genetics

The two most common anomalies in SMZL, del7q31-32 and trisomy 3, neither of which is exclusive for SMZL, occur in 40% and 15% of cases, respectively.[60]

NODAL MARGINAL ZONE B-CELL LYMPHOMA

Nodal marginal zone B cell lymphomas (NMZLs) are uncommon.[4,61] They occur with a median age of 60 to 65 years with a striking female predominance. The disease

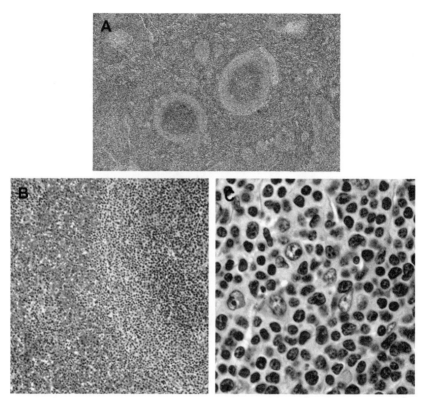

Fig. 9. Splenic marginal zone lymphoma involving spleen. (*A*) The splenic white pulp is preferentially involved. (*B*) The neoplastic cells involve the splenic B-cell follicles (*right*) and spill into the red pulp (*left*). (*C*) The dimorphic cytology is illustrated.

presents with painless, very slowly progressive, or waxing and waning lymph node enlargement. Although most reports suggest that 50% to 65% of patients with this lymphoma type have Ann Arbor stage I or II disease, some reports indicate advanced stage in up to 71% of patients, with bone marrow involvement in 32%. B symptoms are unusual. Because there is considerable morphologic and phenotypic overlap among nodal, splenic, and extranodal MALT-type marginal zone B-cell lymphomas, involvement of the spleen and of anatomic sites commonly affected by MALT lymphoma should be excluded by staging before a case is accepted as an NMZL.

Morphology

Three basic architectural patterns characterize NMZL. The abnormal cells can be distributed immediately adjacent to the lymph node sinusoids (perifollicular— **Fig. 11**).[62,63] They can circumferentially surround germinal centers (analogous to the distribution of SMZL) (**Fig. 11**).[61,64,65] They can expand the interfollicular areas. The neoplastic lymphocytes are usually medium sized with round to irregular nuclear contours, partially condensed chromatin, inconspicuous nucleoli, and voluminous clear cytoplasm with distinct cell membranes. NMZL contains variable numbers of large lymphocytes resembling immunoblasts or centroblasts, and

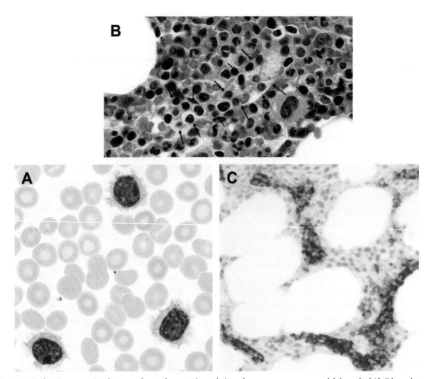

Fig. 10. Splenic marginal zone lymphoma involving bone marrow and blood. (A) Blood containing abnormal "villous lymphocytes." (B) Sinusoidal involvement is subtle in H and E stains and is highlighted here by the arrows. (C) Immunoperoxidase stains for CD20 illuminate the degree and intravascular distribution of the neoplastic B cells.

a subset of cases, particularly those involving the interfollicular areas, contains plasma cells.[65]

Phenotype

NMZL cells express CD19, CD20, CD22, and PAX-5 and show either kappa or lambda immunoglobulin light chain restriction. Light chain–restricted plasma cells are present in a minority of cases. In contrast to normal monocytoid B cells that do not express BCL2 or CD43, NMZL cells are BCL2 and /or CD43 positive in many cases.[32,66] Typically, the cells of this lymphoma type are negative for CD10, CD21, CD35, BCL6, and CD5.

Genetics

No nodal NMZL-specific chromosomal abnormalities have been detected. Trisomies 3 and 18 are the most common abnormalities.

LYMPHOPLASMACYTIC LYMPHOMA

LPL is an uncommon neoplasm of older adults with a slight male predominance.[67] Usually, LPL affects the bone marrow with less common involvement of spleen and lymph nodes and is associated with IgM paraproteinemia and manifestations of hyperviscosity or cryoglobulinemia (Waldenstrom macroglobulinemia–WM). Although most patients with WM have LPL, patients with IgM paraproteins in general can have

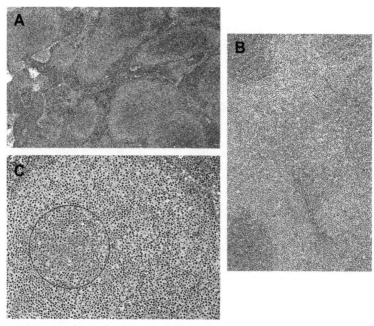

Fig. 11. Nodal marginal zone lymphoma. (*A*) Nodular pattern of involvement. (*B*) Perifollicular involvement. (*C*) The non-neoplastic germinal center (*within the circle*) is surrounded by the neoplastic marginal zone cells.

a variety of B-cell lymphoma types, and not all cases of LPL are associated with an IgM paraprotein.[68] Once cases of WM are excluded, LPL as a disease predominantly involving lymph nodes is rare.

Morphology

The neoplastic cells infiltrate the paracortex and hilum of the lymph node, often with sparing or dilatation of the subcapsular and marginal sinuses (**Fig. 12**A).[67,69–71] LPL cells span a spectrum from small lymphocytes with clumped chromatin, inconspicuous nucleoli, and sparse cytoplasm to plasma cells (**Fig. 12**B). Subsets of the tumor cells contain intranuclear (Dutcher bodies) or cytoplasmic (Russell bodies) immunoglobulin inclusions. Varying numbers of large transformed lymphocytes may be present. In LPL-involved bone marrows, the abnormal lymphoplasmacytic infiltrates can form any combination of paratrabecular or intertrabecular lymphoid aggregates or involve the bone marrow interstitium and are typically accompanied by frequent mast cells.

Phenotype

The neoplastic lymphocytes and plasmacytoid lymphocytes express CD19, CD20, CD79a, and PAX-5 and show either kappa or lambda immunoglobulin light chain restriction. They are typically negative for CD5 and CD10, but cases with expression of these markers have been well described.[59,71] The neoplastic plasma cells variably express CD138 and the same immunoglobulin light chain type as the neoplastic lymphocytes (**Fig. 12**C, D). Typically, LPL cells are positive for IgM, but they may express any immunoglobulin isotype.

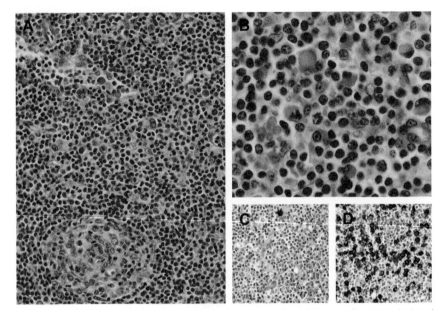

Fig. 12. Lymphoplasmacytic lymphoma. (*A*) A non-neoplastic germinal center is in the bottom of the field. The interfollicular areas (*top*) are expanded by the neoplastic cells, but the lymph node sinus (*top left*) is not effaced. (*B*) The neoplastic cells form a cytologic spectrum from small lymphocytes to plasma cells. Prominent intra- and extracellular eosinophilic immunoglobulin globules are present. Immunoperoxidase stains for kappa (*C*) and lambda (*D*) immunoglobulin light chains show lambda light chain restriction in the plasma cell component of this lymphoplasmacytic lymphoma.

Genetics

Although not completely specific for LPL, del(6)(q21) is the most common abnormality.[72]

This concludes the discussion of the indolent lymphomas of mature B cells, a clinically, morphologically, phenotypically, and genetically diverse group of lymphoid neoplasms. As discussed, careful consideration of the distinctive morphologic features coupled with immunophenotyping can lead to a confident diagnosis in most cases. In those that are diagnostically difficult, the distinctive genetic characteristics of these tumors can supplement morphology and phenotype.

REFERENCES

1. Muller-Hermelink HK, Montserrat E, Catovsky D, et al. Chronic lymphocytic leukemia/small lymphocytic lymphoma. In: Swerdlow S, Campo E, Harris NL, editors. WHO classification of tumours of haematopoietic and lymphoid tissues. Lyon: IARC Press; 2008. p. 180–2.
2. Ellison DJ, Nathwani BN, Cho SY, et al. Interfollicular small lymphocytic lymphoma: the diagnostic significance of pseudofollicles. Hum Pathol 1989;20(11):1108–18.
3. Ben-Ezra J, Burke JS, Swartz WG, et al. Small lymphocytic lymphoma: a clinicopathologic analysis of 268 cases. Blood 1989;73(2):579–87.
4. A clinical evaluation of the International Lymphoma Study Group classification of non-Hodgkin's lymphoma. The Non-Hodgkin's Lymphoma Classification Project. Blood 1997;89(11):3909–18.

5. Moynihan MJ, Bast MA, Chan WC, et al. Lymphomatous polyposis. A neoplasm of either follicular mantle or germinal center cell origin. Am J Surg Pathol 1996;20(4): 442–52.
6. Cohen PL, Kurtin PJ, Donovan KA, et al. Bone marrow and peripheral blood involvement in mantle cell lymphoma. Br J Haematol 1998;101(2):302–10.
7. Pittaluga S, Verhoef G, Criel A, et al. Prognostic significance of bone marrow trephine and peripheral blood smears in 55 patients with mantle cell lymphoma. Leuk Lymphoma 1996;21(1–2):115–25.
8. Majlis A, Pugh WC, Rodriguez MA, et al. Mantle cell lymphoma: correlation of clinical outcome and biologic features with three histologic variants. J Clin Oncol 1997;15(4):1664–71.
9. Swerdlow S, Campo E, Seto M, et al. Mantle cell lymphoma. In: Swerdlow S, Campo E, Harris NL, editors. WHO classification of tumours of haematopoietic and lymphoid tissues. Lyon: IARC Press; 2008. p. 229–32.
10. Kurtin PJ. Mantle cell lymphoma. Adv Anat Pathol 1998;5(6):376–98.
11. Bernard M, Gressin R, Lefrere F, et al. Blastic variant of mantle cell lymphoma: a rare but highly aggressive subtype. Leukemia 2001;15(11):1785–91.
12. Miranda RN, Briggs RC, Kinney MC, et al. Immunohistochemical detection of cyclin D1 using optimized conditions is highly specific for mantle cell lymphoma and hairy cell leukemia. Mod Pathol 2000;13(12):1308–14.
13. Rimokh R, Berger F, Delsol G, et al. Rearrangement and overexpression of the BCL-1/PRAD-1 gene in intermediate lymphocytic lymphomas and in t(11q13)-bearing leukemias. Blood 1993;81(11):3063–7.
14. Remstein ED, Kurtin PJ, Buno I, et al. Diagnostic utility of fluorescence in situ hybridization in mantle-cell lymphoma. Br J Haematol 2000;110(4):856–62.
15. Fu K, Weisenburger DD, Greiner TC, et al. Cyclin D1-negative mantle cell lymphoma: a clinicopathologic study based on gene expression profiling. Blood 2005;106(13):4315–21.
16. Wlodarska I, Dierickx D, Vanhentenrijk V, et al. Translocations targeting CCND2, CCND3, and MYCN do occur in t(11;14)-negative mantle cell lymphomas. Blood 2008;111(12):5683–90.
17. Orchard J, Garand R, Davis Z, et al. A subset of t(11;14) lymphoma with mantle cell features displays mutated IgVH genes and includes patients with good prognosis, nonnodal disease. Blood 2003;101(12):4975–81.
18. Harris NL, Swerdlow S, Jaffe ES, et al. Follicular lymphoma. In: Swerdlow S, Campo E, Harris NL, et al, editors. WHO classification of tumours of haematopoietic and lymphoid tissues. Lyon: IARC Press; 2008. p. 220–6.
19. Solal-Celigny P, Roy P, Colombat P, et al. Follicular lymphoma international prognostic index. Blood 2004;104(5):1258–65.
20. Nathwani BN, Winberg CD, Diamond LW, et al. Morphologic criteria for the differentiation of follicular lymphoma from florid reactive follicular hyperplasia: a study of 80 cases. Cancer 1981;48(8):1794–806.
21. Schmid U, Cogliatti SB, Diss TC, et al. Monocytoid/marginal zone B-cell differentiation in follicle centre cell lymphoma. Histopathology 1996;29(3):201–8.
22. Keith TA, Cousar JB, Glick AD, et al. Plasmacytic differentiation in follicular center cell (FCC) lymphomas. Am J Clin Pathol 1985;84(3):283–90.
23. Martin AR, Weisenburger DD, Chan WC, et al. Prognostic value of cellular proliferation and histologic grade in follicular lymphoma. Blood 1995;85(12):3671–8.
24. Kansal R, Ross CW, Singleton TP, et al. Histopathologic features of splenic small B-cell lymphomas. A study of 42 cases with a definitive diagnosis by the World Health Organization classification. Am J Clin Pathol 2003;120(3):335–47.

25. Sato Y, Ichimura K, Tanaka T, et al. Duodenal follicular lymphomas share common characteristics with mucosa-associated lymphoid tissue lymphomas. J Clin Pathol 2008;61(3):377–81.

26. Bergman R, Kurtin PJ, Gibson LE, et al. Clinicopathologic, immunophenotypic, and molecular characterization of primary cutaneous follicular B-cell lymphoma. Arch Dermatol 2001;137(4):432–9.

27. Hsi ED. Pathology of primary cutaneous B-cell lymphomas: diagnosis and classification. Clin Lymphoma 2004;5(2):89–97.

28. Willemze R, Swerdlow S, Harris NL, et al. Primary cutaneous follicle centre lymphoma. In: Swerdlow S, Campo E, Harris NL, editors. WHO classification of tumours of haematopoietic and lymphoid tissues. Lyon: IARC Press; 2008. p. 227–8.

29. Yang B, Tubbs RR, Finn W, et al. Clinicopathologic reassessment of primary cutaneous B-cell lymphomas with immunophenotypic and molecular genetic characterization. Am J Surg Pathol 2000;24(5):694–702.

30. Lorsbach RB, Shay-Seymore D, Moore J, et al. Clinicopathologic analysis of follicular lymphoma occurring in children. Blood 2002;99(6):1959–64.

31. Dogan A, Bagdi E, Munson P, et al. CD10 and BCL-6 expression in paraffin sections of normal lymphoid tissue and B-cell lymphomas. Am J Surg Pathol 2000;24(6):846–52.

32. Lai R, Arber DA, Chang KL, et al. Frequency of bcl-2 expression in non-Hodgkin's lymphoma: a study of 778 cases with comparison of marginal zone lymphoma and monocytoid B-cell hyperplasia. Mod Pathol 1998;11(9):864–9.

33. Cheung KJ, Shah SP, Steidl C, et al. Genome-wide profiling of follicular lymphoma by array comparative genomic hybridization reveals prognostically significant DNA copy number imbalances. Blood 2009;113(1):137–48.

34. Horsman DE, Okamoto I, Ludkovski O, et al. Follicular lymphoma lacking the t(14;18)(q32;q21): identification of two disease subtypes. Br J Haematol 2003; 120(3):424–33.

35. Jardin F, Gaulard P, Buchonnet G, et al. Follicular lymphoma without t(14;18) and with BCL-6 rearrangement: a lymphoma subtype with distinct pathological, molecular and clinical characteristics. Leukemia 2002;16(11):2309–17.

36. Davies AJ, Rosenwald A, Wright G, et al. Transformation of follicular lymphoma to diffuse large B-cell lymphoma proceeds by distinct oncogenic mechanisms. Br J Haematol 2007;136(2):286–93.

37. Isaacson PG, Chott A, Nakamura S, et al. Extranodal marginal zone lymphoma of mucosa-associated lymphoid tissue (MALT lymphoma). In: Swerdlow S, Campo E, Harris NL, editors. WHO classification of tumours of haematopoietic and lymphoid tissues. Lyon: IARC Press; 2008. p. 214–7.

38. Isaacson PG, Du MQ. MALT lymphoma: from morphology to molecules. Nat Rev Cancer 2004;4(8):644–53.

39. Zinzani PL, Magagnoli M, Galieni P, et al. Nongastrointestinal low-grade mucosa-associated lymphoid tissue lymphoma: analysis of 75 patients. J Clin Oncol 1999; 17(4):1254–8.

40. Zucca E, Conconi A, Pedrinis E, et al. Nongastric marginal zone B-cell lymphoma of mucosa-associated lymphoid tissue. Blood 2003;101(7):2489–95.

41. Isaacson PG, Spencer J, Finn T. Primary B-cell gastric lymphoma. Hum Pathol 1986;17(1):72–82.

42. Zucca E, Bertoni F, Roggero E, et al. The gastric marginal zone B-cell lymphoma of MALT type. Blood 2000;96(2):410–9.

43. Kurtin PJ, Myers JL, Adlakha H, et al. Pathologic and clinical features of primary pulmonary extranodal marginal zone B-cell lymphoma of MALT type. Am J Surg Pathol 2001;25(8):997–1008.

44. Thieblemont C, Berger F, Dumontet C, et al. Mucosa-associated lymphoid tissue lymphoma is a disseminated disease in one third of 158 patients analyzed. Blood 2000;95(3):802–6.

45. Remstein ED, James CD, Kurtin PJ. Incidence and subtype specificity of API2-MALT1 fusion translocations in extranodal, nodal, and splenic marginal zone lymphomas. Am J Pathol 2000;156(4):1183–8.

46. Dierlamm J, Baens M, Wlodarska I, et al. The apoptosis inhibitor gene API2 and a novel 18q gene, MLT, are recurrently rearranged in the t(11;18)(q21;q21)p6ssociated with mucosa-associated lymphoid tissue lymphomas. Blood 1999;93(11): 3601–9.

47. Willis TG, Jadayel DM, Du MQ, et al. Bcl10 is involved in t(1;14)(p22;q32) of MALT B cell lymphoma and mutated in multiple tumor types. Cell 1999;96(1): 35–45.

48. Vinatzer U, Gollinger M, Mullauer L, et al. Mucosa-associated lymphoid tissue lymphoma: novel translocations including rearrangements of ODZ2, JMJD2C, and CNN3. Clin Cancer Res 2008;14(20):6426–31.

49. Streubel B, Lamprecht A, Dierlamm J, et al. T(14;18)(q32;q21) involving IGH and MALT1 is a frequent chromosomal aberration in MALT lymphoma. Blood 2003; 101(6):2335–9.

50. Remstein ED, Dogan A, Einerson RR, et al. The incidence and anatomic site specificity of chromosomal translocations in primary extranodal marginal zone B-cell lymphoma of mucosa-associated lymphoid tissue (MALT lymphoma) in North America. Am J Surg Pathol 2006;30(12):1546–53.

51. Du MQ. MALT lymphoma: recent advances in aetiology and molecular genetics. J Clin Exp Hematop 2007;47(2):31–42.

52. Remstein ED, Kurtin PJ, James CD, et al. Mucosa-associated lymphoid tissue lymphomas with t(11;18)(q21;q21) and mucosa-associated lymphoid tissue lymphomas with aneuploidy develop along different pathogenetic pathways. Am J Pathol 2002;161(1):63–71.

53. Isaacson PG, Piris MA, Berger F, et al. Splenic B cell marginal zone lymphoma. In: Swerdlow S, Campo E, Harris NL, editors. WHO classification of tumours of haematopoietic and lymphoid tissues. Lyon: IARC Press; 2008. p. 185–7.

54. Chacon JI, Mollejo M, Munoz E, et al. Splenic marginal zone lymphoma: clinical characteristics and prognostic factors in a series of 60 patients. Blood 2002; 100(5):1648–54.

55. Hammer RD, Glick AD, Greer JP, et al. Splenic marginal zone lymphoma. A distinct B-cell neoplasm. Am J Surg Pathol 1996;20(5):613–26.

56. Mollejo M, Menarguez J, Lloret E, et al. Splenic marginal zone lymphoma: a distinctive type of low-grade B-cell lymphoma. A clinicopathological study of 13 cases. Am J Surg Pathol 1995;19(10):1146–57.

57. Isaacson PG, Matutes E, Burke M, et al. The histopathology of splenic lymphoma with villous lymphocytes. Blood 1994;84(11):3828–34.

58. Audouin J, Le Tourneau A, Molina T, et al. Patterns of bone marrow involvement in 58 patients presenting primary splenic marginal zone lymphoma with or without circulating villous lymphocytes. Br J Haematol 2003;122(3):404–12.

59. Morice WG, Kurtin PJ, Hodnefield JM, et al. Predictive value of blood and bone marrow flow cytometry in B-cell lymphoma classification: comparative analysis of flow cytometry and tissue biopsy in 252 patients. Mayo Clin Proc 2008;83(7):776–85.

60. Remstein ED, Law M, Mollejo M, et al. The prevalence of IG translocations and 7q32 deletions in splenic marginal zone lymphoma. Leukemia 2008;22(6):1268–72.
61. Campo E, Pileri S, Jaffe ES, et al. Nodal marginal zone lymphoma. In: Swerdlow S, Campo E, Harris NL, editors. WHO classification of tumours of haematopoietic and lymphoid tissues. Lyon: IARC Press; 2008. p. 218–9.
62. Cousar JB, McGinn DL, Glick AD, et al. Report of an unusual lymphoma arising from parafollicular B-lymphocytes (PBLs) or so-called "monocytoid" lymphocytes. Am J Clin Pathol 1987;87(1):121–8.
63. Sheibani K, Burke JS, Swartz WG, et al. Monocytoid B-cell lymphoma. Clinicopathologic study of 21 cases of a unique type of low-grade lymphoma. Cancer 1988;62(8):1531–8.
64. Camacho FI, Algara P, Mollejo M, et al. Nodal marginal zone lymphoma: a heterogeneous tumor: a comprehensive analysis of a series of 27 cases. Am J Surg Pathol 2003;27(6):762–71.
65. Campo E, Miquel R, Krenacs L, et al. Primary nodal marginal zone lymphomas of splenic and MALT type. Am J Surg Pathol 1999;23(1):59–68.
66. Lai R, Weiss LM, Chang KL, et al. Frequency of CD43 expression in non-Hodgkin lymphoma. A survey of 742 cases and further characterization of rare CD43+ follicular lymphomas. Am J Clin Pathol 1999;111(4):488–94.
67. Swerdlow S, Berger F, Harris NL, et al. Lymphoplasmacytic lymphoma. In: Swerdlow S, Campo E, Harris NL, editors. WHO classification of tumours of haematopoietic and lymphoid tissues. Lyon: IARC Press; 2008. p. 194–5.
68. Lin P, Hao S, Handy BC, et al. Lymphoid neoplasms associated with IgM paraprotein: a study of 382 patients. Am J Clin Pathol 2005;123(2):200–5.
69. Lennert K, Feller AC. Lymphoplasmacytic/lymphoplasmacytoid lymphoma (immunocytoma). In: Lennert K, Feller AC, editors. Histopathology of non-Hodgkin's lymphomas (based on the updated Kiel classification). New York: Springer-Verlag; 1992. p. 64–75.
70. Andriko JA, Swerdlow SH, Aguilera NI, et al. Is lymphoplasmacytic lymphoma/immunocytoma a distinct entity? A clinicopathologic study of 20 cases. Am J Surg Pathol 2001;25(6):742–51.
71. Remstein ED, Hanson CA, Kyle RA, et al. Despite apparent morphologic and immunophenotypic heterogeneity, Waldenstrom's macroglobulinemia is consistently composed of cells along a morphologic continuum of small lymphocytes, plasmacytoid lymphocytes, and plasma cells. Semin Oncol 2003;30(2):182–6.
72. Cook JR, Aguilera NI, Reshmi S, et al. Deletion 6q is not a characteristic marker of nodal lymphoplasmacytic lymphoma. Cancer Genet Cytogenet 2005;162(1):85–8.

Diffuse Large B-Cell Lymphomas and Burkitt Lymphoma

Laurence de Leval, MD, PhD[a],*, Robert Paul Hasserjian, MD[b]

KEYWORDS

- WHO 2008 classification • Diffuse large B-cell lymphoma
- Burkitt • Burkitt-like • High-grade • Pathology • Genetics
- Diagnosis

DIFFUSE LARGE B-CELL LYMPHOMAS

Diffuse large B-cell lymphomas (DLBCLs), defined as neoplasms of large transformed B cells (with nuclear diameter more than twice that of a normal lymphocyte), account for 30% to 40% of all adult non-Hodgkin lymphomas. Although an increasing number of subtypes and entities have been recognized by virtue of their distinctive immunophenotypic and/or clinical and pathologic features, the majority of cases fall into the category of DLBCL, not otherwise specified (DLBCL, NOS). DLBCL, NOS is the usual form of DLBCL and represents the diagnosis assigned after exclusion of more specific categories (**Box 1**).

Diffuse Large B-cell Lymphoma, Not Otherwise Specified

DLBCL, NOS usually affects adults with a median age at presentation in the seventh decade, but it also affects children and young adults. The disease may arise in any anatomic location and up to one-third of cases present in extranodal sites. DLBCL, NOS may occur de novo or as a transformation from an underlying small B-cell lymphoma.

Morphology

By order of decreasing frequency, the centroblastic, immunoblastic, and anaplastic variants are the most common morphologic variants (**Fig. 1**). Occasional tumors are made up of signet ring or spindled cells and may be confused with nonhematologic tumors. Given the poor reproducibility of cytologic classification and unresolved

Laurence de Leval is a senior research associate of the Belgian National Fund for Scientific Research.

[a] Department of Pathology, C.H.U. Sart Tilman, Institute of Pathology, B23, +1, B – 4000-Liège, Belgium

[b] Department of Pathology, Massachusetts General Hospital, 55 Fruit Street, Boston, MA 02114, USA

* Corresponding author.

E-mail address: l.deleval@ulg.ac.be (L. de Leval).

Hematol Oncol Clin N Am 23 (2009) 791–827
doi:10.1016/j.hoc.2009.04.004
0889-8588/09/$ – see front matter © 2009 Elsevier Inc. All rights reserved.

hemonc.theclinics.com

Box 1
Classification of diffuse large B-cell lymphomas and Burkitt lymphoma

Diffuse large B-cell lymphomas (DLBCLs)

Diffuse large B-cell lymphoma, not otherwise specified

    Morphologic variants: centroblastic, immunoblastic, anaplastic

    Molecular subgroups[a]

    Immunohistochemical subgroups[a]

Diffuse large B-cell lymphoma subtypes

    T-cell/histiocyte-rich large B-cell lymphoma

    Primary DLBCL of the central nervous system[a]

    Primary cutaneous DLBCL, leg type[a]

    Epstein Barr virus-positive DLBCL of the elderly[a]

Diffuse large B-cell lymphoma entities

    Primary mediastinal (thymic) large B-cell lymphoma

    Intravascular large B-cell lymphoma

    DLBCL associated with chronic inflammation (previously called pyothorax-associated lymphoma)

    Lymphomatoid granulomatosis

    Anaplastic lymphoma kinase–positive large B-cell lymphoma[b]

    Plasmablastic lymphoma[b]

    Large B-cell lymphoma arising in human herpesvirus-8–associated multicentric Castleman disease[a]

    Primary effusion lymphoma

Burkitt lymphoma (BL)

Borderline categories

    B-cell lymphoma, unclassifiable, with features intermediate between DLBCL and BL[a]

    B-cell lymphoma, unclassifiable, with features intermediate between DLBCL and classical Hodgkin lymphoma[a]

[a] designates recently recognized entities in the 2008 WHO Classification that were not listed in the 2001 Classification.
[b] listed as DLBCL variants in the 2001 Classification.
   Data from Swerdlow SH, Campo E, Harris NL, et al. WHO Classification of tumours of haematopoietic and lymphoid tissues. Lyon: IARC Press; 2008.

---

controversy regarding possible worse prognosis of immunoblastic tumors, there is no consensus on the usefulness of morphologic subtyping.[1,2]

    Bone marrow involvement in DLBCL, seen in about 15% of the cases, may appear either as a large-cell infiltrate or, slightly more commonly, as an infiltrate of predominantly small B cells ("discordant" marrow involvement); prognosis in the latter is not worse than that in cases without marrow involvement, but it may confer a higher risk of late relapses.[3,4]

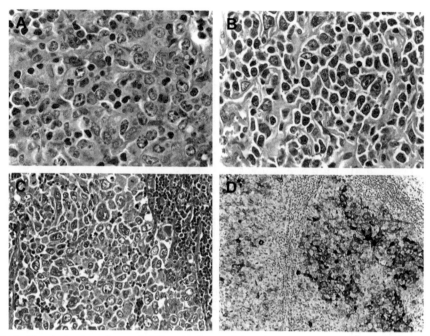

Fig. 1. Morphologic variants of diffuse large B-cell lymphoma. (*A*) The centroblastic variant of DLBCL is composed predominantly of centroblasts that have smooth nuclear contours and multiple nucleoli. (*B*) The immunoblastic variant of DLBCL is composed predominantly of immunoblasts that have round nuclei with a prominent central nucleolus. (*C*) The anaplastic variant of DLBCL typically displays sinusoidal infiltration by large pleomorphic cells that grow in cohesive sheets. (*D*) This lymphoma frequently expresses CD30.

Immunophenotype

DLBCLs express CD45 and pan-B cell antigens, such as CD19, CD20, CD45RA, CD79a, and the nuclear transcription factor PAX5, but they may lack one or more of these. Notably, treatment with rituximab can result in the loss of CD20 expression.[5] The tumor cells usually express a monotypic surface immunoglobulin (Ig), with or without cytoplasmic Ig, usually IgM. The proliferation fraction is typically high (median, 65%). Expression of CD30, characteristic of the anaplastic morphologic variant, may be seen occasionally in other morphologic types.

About 10% of de novo DLBCL cases express CD5 and are distinguished from blastoid mantle cell lymphoma by their negativity for cyclin D1. CD5-positive DLBCL tends to occur in older women, with a predilection for extranodal involvement, especially bone marrow and spleen; intravascular tumor cells are often present.[6] CD5 expression in DLBCL is associated with a shorter survival.[7]

Genetic features

DLBCLs have clonally rearranged *IG* genes with somatic mutations in the variable regions and hence are thought to derive from antigen-exposed B cells that have migrated to or passed through the germinal center (GC).[8]

No single genetic aberration typifies DLBCL. Many cases exhibit complex karyotypes, and genetic imbalances are found in up to two-thirds of the cases.[9] In addition to point mutations, gene amplifications, and deletions that are common to many types

Table 1
Recurrent genetic alterations in DLBCL, NOS

Target Gene or Chromosomal Region	Normal Gene Function	Frequency of Alteration	Functional Consequence of Alteration and Clinical Implications
Translocations			
BCL6 (3q27) translocation to *IG* or *non-IG* genes	Critical role in GC development, transcriptional repressor of genes involved in lymphocyte activation and differentiation, cell cycle control and inflammation[12]	25%–40%	Constitutive expression of BCL6 may (1) lead to maturation arrest and confer a proliferative advantage and (2) induce down-modulation and functional inactivation of the p53 tumor suppressor gene, allowing GC B cells to tolerate genomic alterations and promoting the persistence of malignant clones[13] Prognostic impact of *BCL6* gene rearrangements is controversial.[14,15]
BCL2 (18q21) translocation to *IGH*	Control of apoptosis	15%–20% of de novo DLBCL, most transformed follicular lymphomas	Overexpression of the BCL2 antiapoptotic protein leads to survival advantage. In contrast with the adverse prognostic significance of BCL2 overexpression,[16] detection of the *BCL2* translocation alone has no predictive value on survival.[17]
MYC (8q24) translocation to *IG* or *non-IG* genes	Control of proliferation and apoptosis	10%	MYC overexpression leads to increased cell proliferation. Associated with complex karyotypes and negative prognostic significance « Double hit » lymphomas (*MYC* rearrangement with BCL2 and/or BCL6 rearrangements) are extremely resistant to therapy, may show features partially overlapping those of BL, and are best categorized as unclassifiable B-cell lymphomas intermediate between DLBCL and BL.

Hypermutations		
FAS (10q24)	Proapoptotic receptor involved in the initiation of caspase-induced apoptosis	20%	Destabilization of trimeric FAS proapoptotic receptors
BCL6	GC development, transcriptional repressor	75%	Possible BCL6 deregulation[18]
Point mutations		
p53 (17p)	Cell cycle regulation	20%	Functional inactivation of p53 Clinical drug resistance and poor outcome[19]
Amplifications		
2p12-16 region	Candidate target genes include REL, a member of the NFkappaB family and BCL11A[9]	15%–20%	No direct correlation with NFkappaB activation[20] More common in extranodal tumors
BCL2 (18q21)	Control of apoptosis	25%	Overexpression of BCL2 antiapoptotic protein leads to survival advantage

of malignancies, chromosomal translocations and aberrant somatic hypermutation represent important mechanisms of oncogenesis in DLBCL. Recurrent translocations involving the *BCL6, BCL2,* and/or *MYC* genes occur in about 50% of cases[10] and induce deregulated expression of these proto-oncogenes by promoter substitution, usually as a result of their juxtaposition to *IG* genes. Somatic hypermutation activity not only affects "physiologic" target genes such as the *IG* variable regions but may also aberrantly target multiple other proto-oncogenes, including *MYC, PIM1, PAX5,* and *RhoH/TTF*.[11] Hypermutation appears to represent a powerful mechanism of transformation by facilitating translocations by the induction of DNA double-strand breaks.[11] **Table 1** summarizes the most frequent recurrent genetic aberrations found in DLBCL.

Gene expression profiling
Gene expression profiling studies have identified two distinct molecular DLBCL subgroups, namely, the GC B cell-like DLBCL (GCB DLBCL) harboring a gene expression profile similar to that of GC B cells, and the activated B cell-like DLBCL (ABC DLBCL), with a gene expression profile similar to that of in vitro mitogenically activated peripheral blood cells. A subset of cases cannot be categorized as either GCB or ABC (so-called "type 3" tumors).[21,22] The GCB and ABC subgroups of DLBCL differ in their oncogenic mechanisms and clinical outcome, validating the notion of pathogenetically distinct subgroups **(Table 2)**.[23] Both subgroups harbor mutated *IG* genes, but ongoing somatic hypermutation is only a feature of GCB tumors.[24] The t(14;18)(q32;q21) translocation and chromosomal amplifications of the *c-REL* locus at 2p occur predominantly

Table 2
Characteristics of the DLBCL molecular subgroups identified by gene expression profiling

Characteristics	Germinal Center B-cell (GCB) DLBCL	Activated B-cell (ABC) DLBCL
Overexpressed genes	CD10, BCL6, HGAL, LMO2	MUM1/IRF4, XBP1, CD44, FOXP1
Postulated cell of origin	Germinal center B cell	Postgerminal center B cell that is blocked during plasmacytic differentiation
Ongoing IG mutations	Yes	No
Genetic alterations and oncogenic mechanisms	t(14;18)(q32;q21): BCL2 translocation c-REL amplification at 2p Gains at 12q12 Deletion of PTEN tumor suppressor	t(3;X)(q27;X): BCL6 translocation PRDM1/BLIMP1 inactivation Trisomy 3, trisomy 18 Deletion 6q Constitutive NFkappaB activation Deletion of the INK4a/ARF tumor suppressor locus
Morphology	Centroblastic	Immunoblastic rich
Immunophenotype	CD10+ BCL6+/− MUM1+/− or CD10− BCL6+ MUM-1-	All other combinations
Outcome with CHOP-like chemotherapy	60% 5-year survival	35% 5-year survival
Outcome with chemotherapy plus rituximab	75% 5-year survival	50% 5-year survival

Abbreviation: CHOP, cyclophosphamide, doxorubicin, vincristine, prednisone.

if not exclusively in the GCB group,[22] whereas *BCL6* translocations are three times more common in ABC than in GCB DLBCLs.[25] Activation of the nuclear factor-kappa B (NFκB) signaling pathway, relying on the CARD11/MALT1/BCL10 signaling complex, is a feature of the ABC subgroup, and interference with this pathway selectively kills ABC-type DLBCL tumor cells.[26] Importantly, patients with GCB DLBCL have significantly better outcomes than those with ABC DLBCL, a difference that remains significant with chemotherapy regimens that include rituximab.[27] Analysis of the expression of a limited number of genes by real-time RT-PCR can also predict outcome in DLBCL and may be more amenable to routine diagnostic use.[28,29]

The ABC and GCB molecular signatures are reflected at the protein level by differential expression of antigens normally related to physiologic B-cell differentiation, including GC markers such as CD10 and BCL6 and post-GC markers such as multiple myeloma 1 (MUM1), VS38c, and CD44. An algorithm developed by Hans and colleagues,[30] based on the expression of CD10, BCL6, and MUM1 as assessed by immunohistochemistry, correlates with the gene expression profiling classification, although the concordance is imperfect. Immunohistochemistry is at best semiquantitative and suffers from intra- and interobserver variation.[31] Although several studies demonstrated the favorable predictive value of the GC-like immunophenotype,[30,32,33] others failed to show such correlation.[34,35] Moreover, it is unclear whether the addition of rituximab to chemotherapy may eliminate or attenuate the prognostic value of immunohistochemically defined GC and non-GC groups.[36]

Prognostic biomarkers
Numerous biomarkers (summarized in **Table 3**) have been studied with respect to their correlation with distinct clinical features and/or outcome in DLBCL (reviewed by de Leval and Harris and Lossos and Morgensztern[37,38]).[39–41] Most of the markers have been assessed by immunohistochemistry. The predictive value of some biomarkers validated in the prerituximab era appears to be lost with new rituximab-containing treatment protocols that have improved the prognosis significantly.[42]

T-Cell/Histiocyte-Rich Large B-cell Lymphoma
In the T-cell/histiocyte-rich variant of DLBCL (THRLBCL), there are few large neoplastic B cells scattered in a background of non-neoplastic T cells with or without histiocytes. THRLBCL usually presents in middle-aged or older male adults, often with advanced-stage disease and frequent involvement of spleen, liver, and bone marrow.

The pattern of involvement in lymph nodes is usually diffuse or may be vaguely nodular, but an associated follicular dendritic cell proliferation is lacking. In the spleen, a micronodular pattern involving the white pulp is typical (**Fig. 2**).[43] The neoplastic cells may resemble centroblasts, immunoblasts, lymphocyte-predominant Hodgkin cells, or classic Reed-Sternberg cells.[44] They express CD45 and B-cell antigens, are strongly positive for BCL6, variably express BCL2 and EMA, are negative for CD30 and CD15, and do not harbor Epstein Barr virus (EBV).[44,45] The reactive cells comprise CD68+ histiocytes and variable proportions of CD4+ and CD8+ mature T cells. In contrast to nodular lymphocyte-predominant Hodgkin lymphoma (NLPHL), small B cells are virtually absent, and T cells with a follicular helper T-cell phenotype (CD57+ and/or PD1+) are not numerous and do not form rosettes around the neoplastic B cells.[46,47] Because of the scarcity of neoplastic cells, THRLBCL may be mistaken as a reactive granulomatous process, especially in cases encountered in liver or pulmonary biopsies. Conversely, THRLBCL may develop an increasing density of neoplastic cells with progression or relapse and exhibit an appearance indistinguishable from DLBCL, NOS.

Table 3
Prognostic biomarkers in DLBCL, NOS

Molecular Marker	Biologic Function	High Expression Correlation with Outcome
HLA-II	Immune response	Favorable
Ki67	Proliferation	Unfavorable
p53	Cell cycle control	Unfavorable
BCL2	Inhibition of apoptosis	Unfavorable[a]
Survivin	Inhibition of apoptosis	Unfavorable
sCD44, CD44v6	Adhesion molecules, lymphocyte homing, and dissemination	Unfavorable
ICAM-1	Adhesion molecule, lymphocyte trafficking	Unfavorable
BCL6	Transcriptional repressor, GC marker	Favorable[a]
MUM1	Transcription factor, post-GC marker	Unfavorable
CD5	T-cell lineage antigen	Unfavorable
GC-like immunophenotype	Reflective of GCB molecular subtype	Favorable[a]
Non-GC–like immunophenotype	Reflective of ABC molecular subtype	Unfavorable[a]
FOXP-1	Transcription factor	Unfavorable
PKC-beta	Enhances B-cell proliferation and survival	Unfavorable
LMO2	GC marker	Favorable[b]

Abbreviations: ABC, activated B-cell; FOXP-1, forkhead box protein 1; GC, germinal center; GCB, germinal center B-cell; HLA, human leukocyte antigen; ICAM, intercellular adhesion molecule; MUM1, multiple myeloma 1; PKC-beta, protein kinase C-beta.
[a] Prognostic significance not confirmed for DLBCL patients treated with chemotherapy and anti-CD20 antibody therapy.
[b] Prognostic significance confirmed for DLBCL patients treated with chemotherapy and anti-CD20 antibody therapy.

By molecular profiling, most THRLBCL cases fall into a subset of DLBCL characterized by "host inflammatory response" genes.[48]

A possible relationship between THRLBCL and NLPHL is controversial. Both diseases contain neoplastic cells with similar morphologic and immunophenotypic features but differ with respect to their architecture and the nature of the reactive background. This distinction, however, is crucial, as THRLBCL and NLPHL have clearly distinct clinical courses. Some have suggested that NLPHL and THRLBCL form a biologic continuum,[49] but this concept is not supported by comparative genomic hybridization studies.[50] It is currently recommended that the diagnosis of THRLBCL be restricted to de novo cases and not be applied in patients with a history of NLPHL.

Although some studies have suggested that THRLBCL follows a more aggressive clinical course than DLBCL, NOS,[51] other reports indicate a similar prognosis.[52]

Primary Diffuse Large B-cell Lymphoma of the Central Nervous System

Primary DLBCL of the central nervous system (CNS) comprises all primary intracerebral (PCNSL) or intraocular (PIOL) DLBCL. These diagnoses require exclusion of

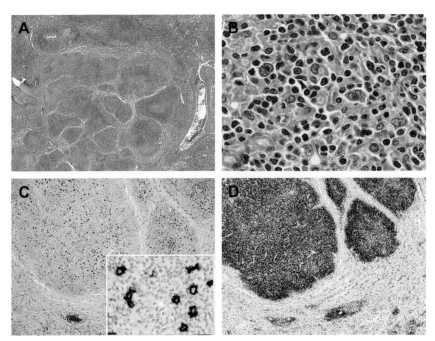

Fig. 2. T-cell/histiocyte-rich large B-cell lymphoma (THRLBCL). (*A*) THRLBCL involving the spleen as multiple cellular nodules. (*B*) There are few large neoplastic cells, scattered in a background of histiocytes and small lymphocytes. (*C*) CD20 highlights few large neoplastic cells and no small cells. (*D*) CD5 stains most of the background small lymphocytes.

a systemic primary lymphoma and do not apply to patients with immunodeficiency conditions. PCNSL accounts for 2% to 3% of all primary brain tumors and usually affects elderly individuals with a slight male predominance (for review, see Batchelor and Loeffler [53]). PCNSL can present as solitary (75%) or multiple (25%) masses in the brain parenchyma; approximately one-fifth of the patients go on to develop ocular lesions, and conversely, the majority of patients with PIOL ultimately develop brain lesions. Relapses typically remain confined to the CNS but may occasionally occur outside the CNS, especially in the testis or breast. The prognosis of PCNSL is poorer than that of DLBCL, NOS occurring outside the CNS.

Morphologically, the tumor cells usually infiltrate perivascular spaces and adjacent brain parenchyma (**Fig. 3**A, B). Treatment with steroids before biopsy can induce regression of the lesions and complicate the histologic interpretation. In addition to CD20, the tumor cells are positive for BCL6 in the majority of cases (60%–80%), and almost all cases are MUM1-positive, whereas CD10 expression is infrequent (see **Fig. 3**C, D).[54,55] At the molecular level, PCNSL carries a high load of somatic hypermutations in the *IG* variable region genes, with ongoing mutations in some cases. These features suggest the derivation of PCNSL from late GC B cells.[56]

Chromosomal translocations involving *BCL6* are frequent (17%–47% of cases), often involve non-*IG* partners, and are associated with poor outcome. Conversely, rearrangements of *BCL2* and *cMYC* are virtually never found in PCNSL.[57]

By gene expression profiling, the molecular signature of PCNSL includes both the GCB and the ABC subtypes; PCNSL shows a gene expression pattern that is distinct from non-CNS DLBCL, but the identified "CNS signature" might in fact reflect the

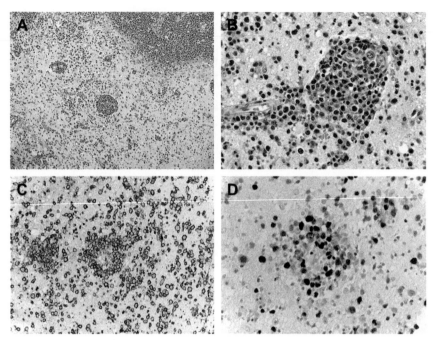

Fig. 3. Primary DLBCL of the CNS. (*A*) Primary DLBCL of the CNS involves the perivascular spaces and spreads into the adjacent brain parenchyma. (*B*) The lymphoma cells usually display centroblastic morphology, as in this case. (*C*) CD20 highlights the perivascular distribution of the tumor cells. (*D*) The lymphoma cells show nuclear expression of MUM-1.

non-neoplastic brain microenvironment. Activation of the interleukin (IL-4) pathway in endothelial cells may account for the angiotropism typically encountered in PCNSL.[58–60]

Primary Cutaneous Diffuse Large B-cell Lymphoma, Leg Type

This primary cutaneous DLBCL, accounting for about one-fifth of primary cutaneous B-cell lymphomas, is a tumor-forming nonepidermotropic neoplasm that preferentially affects the lower limb but may occur elsewhere. It usually affects elderly women. It is composed of large B cells with a striking round cell morphology. The tumor cells express CD20, BCL6, and MUM1 but are usually negative for CD10. BCL2 is overexpressed in most cases as a consequence of *BCL2* amplification.[61] The gene expression profile is that of the ABC DLBCL subgroup.[62] The disease frequently disseminates to noncutaneous sites and has an aggressive course.

Epstein Barr Virus-Positive Diffuse Large B-cell Lymphoma of the Elderly

This DLBCL subtype occurs in elderly patients (by definition, older than 50 years, with a median age in the eighth decade) without HIV infection and without any known immunodeficiency syndrome. Other EBV-related DLBCL entities (**Table 4**) and infectious mononucleosis should be excluded. This subtype of DLBCL is believed to be related to altered immune function caused by immune senescence.

The disease often involves extranodal sites (skin, tonsil, lung, stomach), with or without lymph node involvement. On histology, the tumor resembles a monomorphous

Table 4
EBV-positive large B-cell lymphoid proliferations

Type of Lymphoid Proliferation	Clinical Setting	Presentation
EBV+ DLBCL	Associated with primary immune disorders Associated with HIV infection Post-transplant-associated Iatrogenic immunodeficiency-associated (methotrexate, TNFα antagonists) With no known predisposing conditions, <50 years old	Nodal or extranodal
Plasmablastic lymphoma	HIV infection Less often: HIV-negative individuals	Extranodal (oral cavity or other), less commonly nodal
Primary effusion lymphoma[a]	HIV infection Less often: post-transplant, elderly Mediterranean individuals	Body cavity effusion Solid extracavitary
Lymphomatoid granulomatosis	Congenital immunodeficiency syndromes HIV infection Post-transplant	Lung, brain, skin; often multifocal involvement
DLBCL associated with chronic inflammation	Chronic pyothorax or chronic infection	Pleural-based mass, bone, or joint tumor
EBV+ DLBCL of the elderly	>50 years old, immune senescence	Extranodal
Germinotropic lymphoproliferative disorder[a/b]	Immunocompetent individuals	Germinal center of lymph nodes

Abbreviation: HHV8, human herpesvirus 8.
[a] These disorders are characterized by coinfection by EBV and HHV8.
[b] Exceedingly rare disorder.

large-cell lymphoma or a polymorphous large-cell infiltrate with a variable inflammatory background. Some cases may resemble THRLBCL (**Fig. 4**). Angiocentricity and extensive necrosis are frequent. Reed-Sternberg–like cells may be numerous, raising the differential diagnosis with classical Hodgkin lymphoma (cHL). The tumor cells express CD20 and CD79a, are positive for EBER, LMP-1, and EBV nuclear antigen (EBNA)-2, and variably express CD30, but are negative for CD15.[63–65] The prognosis is inferior to that of patients with EBV-negative DLBCLs; the presence of B symptoms and age more than 70 years are additional adverse prognostic factors.[64,66]

Primary Mediastinal (Thymic) Large B-cell Lymphoma

Primary mediastinal large B-cell lymphoma (PMLBCL) is a distinct DLBCL entity arising in the mediastinum from putative thymic B cells[67,68] and comprises 2% to 4% of all non-Hodgkin lymphomas.

PMLBCL: a distinct DLBCL entity
PMLBCL (**Table 5**) tends to occur in young patients (median age, about 35 years) and affects women more commonly than men. Patients present with an often bulky

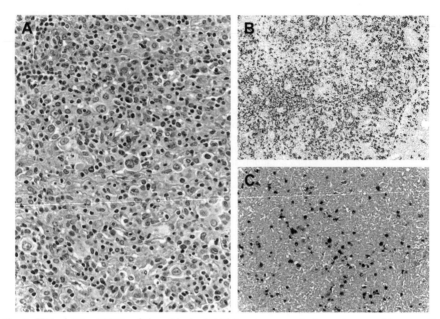

Fig. 4. EBV-positive DLBCL of the elderly. (*A*) This case presented as a tumor of large cells, some of which resemble Reed-Sternberg cells, in a background rich in histiocytes. (*B*) CD20 highlights numerous large B cells. (*C*) Many of the tumor cells are positive for EBER by in situ hybridization.

anterior mediastinal mass and symptoms related to impingement of local anatomic structures.[69,70] The disease is usually localized at presentation, but progression can be characterized by dissemination to other extranodal sites, including lung, liver, kidneys, adrenals, ovaries, brain, and the gastrointestinal tract.[70] Although PMLBCL was initially believed to carry an adverse prognosis, recent studies have shown an overall survival similar or superior to that of DLBCL, NOS.[71,72]

Histologically, PMLBCL is a diffuse proliferation of medium to large cells. Particular (but not entirely specific) morphologic features include the presence of fine compartmentalizing sclerosis, the presence of cells with abundant clear cytoplasm and/or multilobated nuclei, and the presence of large cells with Reed-Sternberg–like morphology (**Fig. 5**).[73] The tumor cells express the B-cell–associated antigens CD19, CD20, and CD79a but often lack surface Ig, despite expression of the IG-associated transcription factors BOB.1, Oct-2, and PU.1.[74] Most cases express BCL6, MUM1/IRF4, BCL2, and CD23, and a variable proportion of cases also express CD30; in contrast to cHL, the CD30 expression is usually weak and is present only on a subset of the tumor cells.[74-76] Expression of MAL, FIG1 (the product of the IL-4–induced gene 1), and tumor necrosis factor (TNF)-receptor–associated factor 1 (TRAF-1) is characteristic of PMLBCL, especially when combined with nuclear c-REL localization.[77-80]

The tumor cells contain hypermutated *IG* genes with no evidence of ongoing mutation.[81] PMLBCL only rarely exhibit *BCL2* or *BCL6* rearrangements.[82] The most frequent genetic abnormalities are gains in chromosomes 9p24 (including the *JAK2* locus) in up to 75% of cases and gain of *REL* on chromosome 2p in about 50% of cases.[83,84]

In gene expression profiling studies, a PMLBCL molecular signature distinct from that of DLBCL, NOS was delineated and is characterized by low levels of expression

Table 5
Distinguishing features between PMLBCL and DLBCL, NOS

	DLBCL, NOS	PMLBCL
Clinical features	Adults, M > F Stages I–II: 50% Bulky mass occasional	Young women Stages I–II >50% Bulky mass frequent
Morphology	Common to both: sheets of large cells Variable	Clear cells Sclerosis
Immunophenotype	Common to both: CD45+ CD20+ CD79a+PAX5+ BOB-2+ Oct-1+ sIg+	sIg- CD30 +/− CD23+ MAL+ TRAF-1+/c-REL+ (50%)
Genetics	Rearranged *BCL6*: 30% Rearranged *BCL2*: 20%	Gains at 2p15: *cREL, BCL11* (50%) Gains at 9p24: *JAK* (75%)

Molecular signature	GCB and ABC subtypes	PMLBCL signature
		Downregulation:
		  BCR signaling pathway
		Overexpression:
		  Extracellular matrix components
		  Cytokines/JAK/STAT

of multiple B-cell signaling components and coreceptors and high expression of cytokine pathway components, TNF family members, and extracellular matrix elements.[72,79]

PMLBCL: overlapping features with cHL

Although PMLBCL and cHL have several distinctive pathologic features, PMLBCL and nodular sclerosis HL exhibit strikingly similar clinical presentations (young women with an anterior mediastinal mass) and some overlap in pathologic, genetic, and molecular features (see **Fig. 5**B–D). The chromosome 2p and 9p aberrations characteristic of PMLBCL are also detectable in a subset of cHL.[85] Activation of the NFκB pathway, known to enhance the survival of Reed-Sternberg cells, is also a feature of PMLBCL[79,86] and may represent a survival pathway shared by both neoplasms. Altered JAK/STAT signaling, manifested by constitutive activation of STAT5 and STAT6, represents another alteration common to both PMLBCL and cHL and may cause defective suppression of cytokine signaling.[87–89] Aberrant tyrosine kinase activities and activation of the PI3K/AKT pathway were recently identified as a further shared pathogenic mechanism between PMLBCL and cHL.[90]

Mediastinal "gray zone" lymphomas

The identification of molecular links between PMLBCL and cHL supports the hypothesis that there may be some pathogenetic overlap between the two entitles and that these diseases may in fact represent the opposite ends of a continuum. Indeed, "gray zone" lymphomas, which represent a range of tumors having characteristics of both PMLBCL and cHL, either as composite neoplasms (synchronous or metachronous) or as more homogeneous neoplasms with transitional features, have been described.[91–96] A novel category designated "B-cell lymphoma, unclassifiable, with

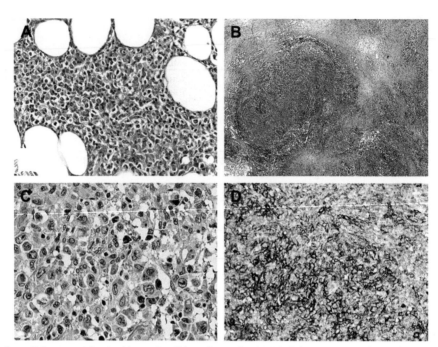

Fig. 5. Primary mediastinal large B-cell lymphoma (PMLBCL). (*A*) PMLBCL involving the mediastinal fat, composed of medium to large cells with abundant clear cytoplasm. (*B–D*) PMLBCL shows overlapping features with nodular sclerosis Hodgkin lymphoma. (*B*) PMLBCL characterized by abundant sclerosis imparting a vaguely nodular pattern. (*C*) PMBCL comprising cells with lobated nuclei and Reed-Sternberg–like morphology. (*D*) PMBCL often displays variable expression of CD30, in this case moderate to strong.

features intermediate between DLBCL and cHL" has been created to encompass such cases.

Intravascular Large B-cell Lymphoma

Intravascular large B-cell lymphoma (IVLBCL) is a rare subtype of DLBCL characterized by the selective growth of lymphoma cells within small blood vessels, with occasional limited infiltration of perivascular tissue, but without an obvious extravascular tumor mass or leukemia.[97]

The clinical presentation tends to vary according to the geographic region. Western patients present with symptoms related to organ involvement, most frequently the skin and the brain. Involvement of vascular sinuses of the bone marrow, liver, and spleen is frequent, whereas lymph nodes are usually spared.[98] IVLBCL in Asian patients is often associated with a hemophagocytic syndrome (HPS) with pancytopenia, hepatosplenomegaly, and bone marrow involvement, while lacking neurologic or cutaneous manifestations.[94] Both types predominantly affect elderly patients and present as disseminated and aggressive malignancies eventually resulting in multiorgan failure. There have been recent encouraging reports suggesting that the usually dismal prognosis of IVLBCL may be substantially improved by the addition of rituximab to conventional chemotherapy regimens.[95] Another subset of IVLBCL (the "cutaneous variant") has disease limited to the skin at presentation, affects mainly younger women, and has a much more favorable clinical behavior.[98]

The neoplastic cells in IVLBCL are large lymphoid cells expressing CD20, with coexpression of CD5 in up to one-third of the cases, and negative for EBV.[96] Expression of BCL6 and CD10 is infrequent, whereas MUM1/IRF4 is often positive. Many cases express BCL2, but the t(14;18) translocation is usually absent.[99] The selective localization of the tumor cells within vessels has been ascribed to defective expression of specific surface molecules, such as CD29 and CD54, that are necessary for transvascular migration.[100]

DLBCL Associated with Chronic Inflammation

This category comprises DLBCL occurring in the context of chronic inflammation and associated with EBV, of which pyothorax-associated lymphoma (PAL) is the prototypic form. This rare disease develops in the pleural cavity of patients with a history of longstanding (>10 years) pyothorax, usually resulting from artificial pneumothorax for treatment of tuberculosis. PAL is more common in Japan than in Western countries.[101,102] The disease affects elderly patients and shows a strong male predominance. Chronic inflammation may promote the growth of EBV-infected B cells and contribute to the development of PAL by creating a microenvironment that is less accessible to T-cell immune surveillance and by providing local production of cytokines such as IL-6, which acts as a growth factor on PAL cells.[103,104] PAL presents as a pleural-based tumor mass, often with direct invasion of the chest wall and lung. The clinical, pathologic, and genetic features of PAL are summarized in **Table 6**.[105,106]

Occasional cases of EBV-positive lymphomas complicating longstanding chronic suppuration in other extranodal sites (such as bone or joint lymphomas occurring in the setting of chronic osteomyelitis or in association with metallic implants and skin lymphomas in patients with chronic venous ulcers) are also considered part of the disease spectrum.[107,108]

Lymphomatoid Granulomatosis

Lymphomatoid granulomatosis (LYG) is a rare angiocentric and angiodestructive lymphoproliferative process involving the lungs. LYG represents an EBV-positive large B-cell proliferation associated with an exuberant T-cell reaction.[109]

LYG affects patients of all ages, most often between the fourth and sixth decades, with a slight male predominance. Patients typically present with multinodular bilateral lung involvement and respiratory symptoms. The CNS, kidneys, and skin are also commonly involved.[110] Lymphoid organs are usually spared. LYG often occurs in the setting of HIV infection or iatrogenetic immunosuppression due to organ transplant or autoimmune diseases (see **Table 4**).[111]

Histologically, LYG consists of a polymorphous cellular infiltrate including lymphocytes, histiocytes, plasma cells, and varying numbers of large atypical lymphoid cells, exhibiting an angioinvasive pattern with or without associated infarct-type necrosis. The neoplastic cells are positive for CD45 and CD20 and may weakly express CD30. The B cells express EBER as well as LMP-1 and EBNA-2.[109,112] The small lymphocytes consist mostly of CD4+ T cells. LYG encompasses a spectrum of histologic grades (from 1 to 3). Its clinical aggressiveness is related to the proportion of EBV-positive large B cells and necrosis, with grade 3 lesions resembling EBV-positive DLBCL.

Plasmablastic Lymphoma

Plasmablastic lymphoma (PBL) designates a group of tumors that morphologically resemble DLBCL but have an immunophenotypic profile of plasma cells. The

Table 6
Comparison of lymphomas presenting in body cavities

	DLBCL Associated with Chronic Inflammation	Primary Effusion Lymphoma
Clinical setting	Elderly men with chronic pyothorax Other chronic infections (osteomyelitis)	AIDS patients, profound immunodeficiency, previous history of or concomitant Kaposi sarcoma Post-transplant Elderly Mediterranean individuals (HHV8 endemic)
Epidemiology	More frequent in Japan Very rare in Western countries	1%–2% of AIDS-associated NHL
Presentation	Tumor mass	Effusion in a body cavity +/− tumor mass (extracavitary PEL)
Morphology	DLBCL with immunoblastic and angiocentric features, abundant necrosis	Large pleomorphic cells immunoblastic, plasmablastic, or anaplastic morphology
Viruses		
HHV8	−	+
EBV	EBER+, LMP1+/−, EBNA2+	EBER+, LMP1−, EBNA2−
Immunophenotype		
CD45	+	+
CD20	+/−	−
CD79a	+	−
Ig expression	+/−	−
CD10, BCL6	−	−
MUM1/IRF4	+	+
CD138	−/+	+
T-cell antigens	−/+ (CD2, CD3, CD4)	−
CD30	−/+	+
EMA	−	+
Genetic features		
IGH gene rearrangement	Monoclonal	Monoclonal
TCR gene rearrangement	Polyclonal	May be monoclonal
IG mutations	Yes, without ongoing mutations	Yes
Genetic alterations	p53 mutations (70%)	Gains in chromosomes 12 and X
Gene expression profile	Distinct from nodal DLBCLs, different expression of interferon response genes	Features of plasma cells and EBV-transformed lymphoblastoid cell lines
Cell of origin	Late GC/post-GC B cell	Post-GC B cell
Prognosis	Heterogeneous, 20%–35% 5-y survival	Poor, <6 month median survival

Abbreviations: EBNA, EBV nuclear antigen; EBV, Epstein-Barr virus; GC, germinal center; HHV8, human herpesvirus 8; LMP, latent membrane protein; +/−, usually positive, may be negative; −/+, usually negative, may be positive.

neoplastic cells of PBL have absent or weak expression of CD45 and B-cell–associated antigens and exhibit strong expression of the plasma-cell–associated antigens CD138 and MUM-1/IRF4, with or without monotypic expression of cytoplasmic Ig (usually IgG or IgA type). Since the original description as a rare variant of DLBCL occurring in the oral cavity in HIV-infected patients,[113] its spectrum has been expanded to include similar lesions in immunocompetent patients and in other extranodal sites, such as the anorectal region, nasopharynx, intestine, and lymph nodes.[114–116] PBL has a highly aggressive clinical behavior,[113] but improved survival outcomes have been reported in HIV-infected patients in the era of highly active antiretroviral therapy.

Histologically, PBL is usually a diffuse proliferation of immunoblastic cells, but a subset of tumors can show plasmacytic differentiation (**Fig. 6**). PBL usually exhibits a high proliferation rate with frequent apoptotic cells, and a starry-sky pattern may be present. Virtually all cases are positive for EBER but lack the EBV-associated proteins LMP1 and EBNA. HHV8 is consistently absent.

Table 7 summarizes the main clinical and pathologic features of PBL and its differential diagnosis with other neoplasms that exhibit plasmablastic features.[114,116–118]

Anaplastic Lymphoma Kinase–Positive Large B-cell Lymphoma

This very rare neoplasm is composed of large immunoblast-like cells with abundant cytoplasm and occasional plasmablastic differentiation that shows a prominent intrasinusoidal growth pattern within affected lymph nodes (**Fig. 7**A). Tumor cells bear chromosomal translocations affecting the anaplastic lymphoma kinase gene (*ALK*).[119] Most cases express clathrin-ALK fusion protein and show a membranous

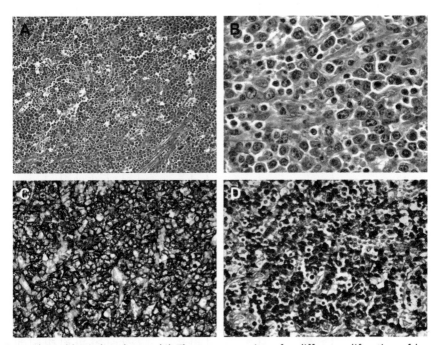

Fig. 6. Plasmablastic lymphoma. (*A*) The tumor consists of a diffuse proliferation of large cells (*B*) with immunoblastic/plasmablastic features. (*C*) The tumor cells show strong membranous positivity for CD138 (*D*) and are positive for EBER.

Table 7
Lymphomas with plasmablastic features

	Plasmablastic Lymphoma	Plasma Cell Neoplasms	Primary Effusion Lymphoma	Plasmablastic Lymphoma with Multicentric Castleman Disease	ALK + Diffuse Large B-cell Lymphoma
Clinical presentation	Oral cavity, other extranodal sites, less commonly lymph nodes	Bone marrow and/or extramedullary	Body cavity effusion Extracavitary solid PEL	Lymph nodes and spleen, diffuse lymphadenopathy	Lymph nodes, sinusoidal pattern
Association with HIV	Yes	No	Yes	Yes	No
Morphology	Immunoblastic and plasmablastic +/− plasma cells	Plasma cells +/− plasmablasts	Pleomorphic with immunoblastic +/− plasmablastic +/− anaplastic features	Plasmablastic	Immunoblastic and plasmablastic
Associated viruses					
EBV	+	−	+	−	−
HHV8	−	−	+	+	−
Immunophenotype					
CD45	−/+	−	+	+	−
CD20	−/+	−	−	+/−	−
CD79a	+/−	−	−	−	−
BCL6	−	−	−	−	−

MUM1/IRF4	+	+	+	+	+
CD138	+	+	+	–	+
cIg	+/– (IgG)	+/– (IgG > A > M > D)	–	IgM lambda	+/– (IgA)
CD30	+/–	–/+	+	–	–
EMA	+/–	–/+	+	–	+
ALK	–	–	–	–	+
Ig variable regions	Unmutated or mutated	Mutated	Mutated	Unmutated	NA
Cell of origin	Plasmablast (proliferating B cell that has switched its phenotype to the plasma cell gene expression profile)	Terminally differentiated B cell	Post-GC B cell	Naïve B cell	Post-GC B cell
Clinical course	Aggressive	Variable	Very aggressive	Very aggressive	Usually aggressive

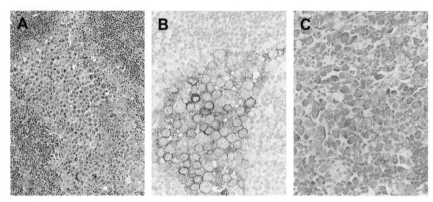

Fig. 7. Anaplastic lymphoma kinase–positive DLBCL. (*A*) The tumor is composed of large cells with immunoblastic and plasmablastic features and shows a sinusoidal growth pattern. (*B*) The lymphoma cells are positive for EMA. (*C*) ALK-1 stain reveals fine granular cytoplasmic localization of the ALK protein.

and granular cytoplasmic staining for ALK.[120] A few cases express the NPM-ALK fusion[121] and show a nuclear and diffuse cytoplasmic ALK staining. The tumor cells are negative for CD20, CD79a, and CD30 but are positive for EMA and CD138 and express cytoplasmic IgA (see **Fig. 7**B, C). A subset of cases may also express CD4 and CD57. The disease affects mostly adult males and is often disseminated at presentation, with a poor prognosis.

Primary Effusion Lymphoma

Primary effusion lymphoma (PEL) was originally identified in AIDS as a neoplasm of large pleomorphic B cells usually presenting as effusions in serous cavities (pleural, pericardial, or peritoneal). Generally, there are no tumor masses, but some cases may have concomitant or subsequent solid tissue involvement of adjacent structures. The tumor cells are characteristically infected by the human herpesvirus 8 (HHV8), which likely plays a major role in lymphomagenesis; most cases are also coinfected with EBV.[122,123] The clinicopathological and genetic features of PEL are summarized in **Table 6**.[124–127]

Rare HHV8-positive lymphomas may present as extranodal or less commonly nodal masses with no associated effusions. These "extracavity PELs" exhibit clinicopathologic features similar to those of PEL except for a somewhat more frequent expression of B-cell antigens and Ig.[117]

Large B-cell Lymphoma Arising in HHV8-Associated Multicentric Castleman Disease

This lymphoma is composed of monoclonal HHV8-positive, EBV-negative large B cells resembling plasmablasts that express cytoplasmic IgM lambda immunoglobulin in the setting of HHV8-associated multicentric Castleman disease. The majority of cases occur in HIV-infected patients. The disease involves lymph nodes and spleen, can evolve toward a leukemic phase, and has a short median survival.[128] The neoplastic cells are naïve, unmutated B cells that usually express CD20 but are negative for CD138.[129] Precursor lesions to this lymphoma can manifest as clusters or aggregates of large IgM lambda-positive, HHV8-positive B cells with a plasmablastic appearance in the mantle zones of lymph nodes involved by multicentric Castleman disease; this pattern of involvement has been called "microlymphoma."

BURKITT LYMPHOMA

Burkitt lymphoma (BL) is an aggressive B-cell lymphoma that mainly affects children and young adults. The tumor is composed of medium-sized, monomorphous lymphoid cells with a high mitotic rate and very high Ki67 proliferation index. A translocation between *MYC* and an *IG* gene is characteristic.

Clinical Features

BL has the highest doubling time of any tumor. Patients often present acutely and may present with oncologic emergencies such as spinal cord compression (**Fig. 8**A). There are 3 clinical variants of BL, which differ in their geographic distribution, epidemiology, and pathogenesis: endemic BL, sporadic BL, and immunodeficiency-associated BL (**Table 8**). Regardless of the clinical presentation, BL has a predilection for CNS involvement. BL may involve the peripheral blood in advanced disseminated disease and may rarely present as a purely leukemic form limited to the blood and bone marrow.[133] Such cases were previously classified as "L3" type of acute lymphoblastic leukemia (ALL), are otherwise identical to tissue-based BL, and are not considered to represent a variant of ALL in the World Health Organization (WHO) Classification.

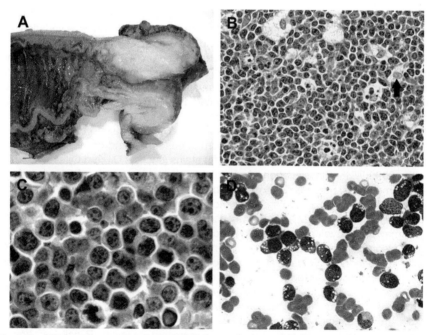

Fig. 8. Burkitt lymphoma morphology. (*A*) Gross photograph of a case of sporadic BL, presenting as an ileal mass causing intussusception. (*B*) Case of BL showing characteristic "starry-sky" appearance and monomorphous tumor cells with nuclear size approximating that of interspersed histiocytes (*arrow*). (*C*) On high power, this case of BL occurring in an HIV+ patient shows molding of cytoplasmic borders, moderately dispersed chromatin, and multiple small nucleoli as well as plasmacytoid features. (*D*) BL involving the bone marrow, with basophilic, vacuolated cytoplasm evident on a Wright-Giesma–stained aspirate smear.

			Immunodeficiency
Feature	**Endemic**	**Sporadic**	**Associated**
Age	Mainly children, peak age incidence 4–7 y	Children and young adults (median age, 30 y)	HIV+ adults and patients with congenital or iatrogenic immunodeficiency
Male: Female ratio	2: 1	2.5: 1	Males more commonly affected
Geographic distribution	Equatorial Africa and Papua, New Guinea	Worldwide	Worldwide
Sites of involvement	Commonly extranodal, jaw and facial bones in 50% of cases	Commonly extranodal, often ileocecal region	More frequently nodal or bone marrow involvement
EBV association	>90% of cases	15%–30% of cases	25%–40% of cases

Table 8
Features of the clinical variants of BL

Data from Refs.[130–132]

Morphology

BL is a diffuse lymphoma composed of medium-sized lymphocytes (defined by having a nucleus that is similar in diameter to a histiocyte nucleus) with little size variation. As BL exhibits a very high rate of both mitosis and apoptosis, frequent phagocytic histiocytes containing nuclear debris are interspersed throughout the tumor, imparting the characteristic (but nonspecific) "starry-sky" appearance on low magnification. Nonneoplastic small lymphocytes are usually sparse. The tumor cells have round nuclei with no or minimal irregularities, finely dispersed nuclear chromatin with multiple small nucleoli, and well-delineated cytoplasmic borders that are often angulated ("squared off") in relation to other cells (see **Fig. 8**B–C). On a Giemsa-stained tissue section or Wright-Giemsa stained smear, the cytoplasm is basophilic and on air-dried smears contains vacuoles that stain positively with fat stains (such as Oil Red O)(see **Fig. 8**D).

In the 2008 WHO Classification, no formal morphologic variants of BL are recognized. Some cases, particularly those associated with immunodeficiency, may exhibit plasmacytoid features, including eccentric scant basophilic cytoplasm and single central nucleoli (see **Fig. 8**C).[130] Some cases of BL (including most cases arising in adults) may have atypical morphology, such as increased nuclear irregularity, slight nuclear pleomorphism, and/or more prominent, single nucleoli; if these cases otherwise fit immunophenotypically and genetically with BL, they are classified as such and are no longer considered to comprise a discrete BL variant. Indeed, it was recently shown that these "atypical BL cases" have a molecular signature similar to classic BL.[134] Cases with marked variation in cytomorphology and/or large cell size, an unusual immunophenotype, and/or unusual genetic features should be excluded from the BL category altogether and often represent cases of B-cell lymphoma, unclassifiable, with features intermediate between DLBCL and BL (DLBCL/BL) (**Table 9**).

Immunophenotype

BL is positive for pan–B-cell markers (CD20, PAX5, and CD79a). The classic immunophenotype, present in almost all cases, is strong CD10 expression, expression of

Table 9
Morphologic, immunophenotypic, and genetic features used to distinguish Burkitt lymphoma from DLBCL/BL and DLBCL

Expected BL Finding	Relative Contraindication for a Diagnosis of BL	Absolute Contraindication for a Diagnosis of BL[a]
Uniform, medium-sized cells	Mild or moderate cellular pleomorphism	Blastic morphology[b] Large cell size or marked cellular pleomorphism[c]
CD10 strongly positive	CD10 negative	NA
BCL6 positive	BCL6 negative	NA
BCL2 negative	NA	BCL2 strongly positive[a]
Ki67	NA	<95% proliferation index[a]
MYC rearrangement with LG locus (usually LGH, but sometimes with kappa or lambda loci)	Absent or shown to be with a non-LG locus	NA
Simple karyotype	Complex karyotype (3 or more abnormalities in addition to 8q24)	NA
No BCL6 rearrangement	NA	BCL6 rearrangement present[a]
No BCL2 rearrangement	NA	BCL2 rearrangement present[a]

Abbreviation: NA, not applicable.
[a] Cases with any absolute contraindications should be diagnosed as DLBCL/BL, irrespective of the other features. Consideration should also be given to placing cases with two or more relative contraindications into the DLBCL/BL category.
[b] If TdT is positive and surface immunoglobulin is negative, consider a diagnosis of B-lymphoblastic leukemia. Otherwise, should be classified as DLBCL/BL.
[c] Cases that have the morphology of DLBCL should be classified as such irrespective of morphology, immunophenotype, or genetic features.

BCL6, and negativity for BCL2 (**Fig. 9A–C**).[135] BL also expresses CD43, TCL1, and CD38 but is negative for CD5, CD23, CD44, CD138, CD34, and TdT.[136] MUM1/IRF4 is expressed in some cases.[137] Ki67 reveals a proliferation fraction of near 100% (at least 95% of tumor cells)(see **Fig. 9D**). BL cells exhibit monotypic surface IgM kappa or lambda expression; rare cases may lack surface light chain expression, raising the differential diagnosis of lymphoblastic lymphoma, but unlike these are TdT negative.[131] Cases with plasmacytoid features may contain abundant cytoplasmic Ig.

The association with EBV varies among the clinical variants of BL and is shown in **Table 8**. BL cases presenting as leukemia are only rarely EBV positive.[131] More than half of BL cases arising in HIV-infected patients are EBV negative and tend to occur early in the course of disease when the CD4+ T-cell count is preserved;[138] this observation suggests that the development of BL requires a relatively intact immune system. Indeed, chronic B-cell stimulation due to recurrent infections by *P. falciparum* in regions endemic for malaria has been postulated to underlie the development of endemic BL.[139]

Genetic Features

Nearly all cases of BL have a translocation involving the MYC gene at the 8q24 locus. The translocation partner is most often the *IGH* region at 14q32, but less commonly, it can be the genes encoding lambda or kappa light chains (located at 22q11 or 2p12,

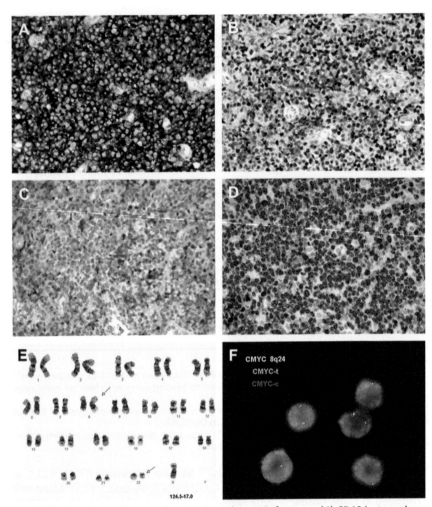

Fig. 9. Burkitt lymphoma immunophenotypic and genetic features. (A) CD10 is strongly positive. (B) BCL6 is positive. (C) BCL2 is negative in the tumor cells. (D) Ki67 shows a proliferation index of 100%. (E) Karyotype shows the variant t(8;22)(q24;q11) translocation between *MYC* and *IGL* genes. (F) Interphase FISH shows split of the *MYC* probe signal in two nuclei on the left, confirming a *MYC* rearrangement.

respectively) (see **Fig. 9E**). Recent data indicate that the *MYC-IGH* translocation arises due to aberrant activity of the activation-induced cytidine deaminase (AID) enzyme.[140] AID is normally involved in producing somatic hypermutations and class switching that underlie the generation of antibody diversity. Indeed, all clinical subtypes of BL show evidence of somatic hypermutation of the *IG* genes during lymphomagenesis, although without ongoing somatic mutation.[141] The *IGH* gene breakpoint in endemic BL is usually located within the joining region and may reflect aberrant somatic hypermutation activity, whereas abnormal *IGH* switch region recombination appears to cause the *MYC* translocation in sporadic BL; the *IGH* breakpoints in BL presenting as leukemia are variable.[131,141,142] Taken together, these data suggest that BL originates from a B cell that has undergone the GC reaction and in some cases has been stimulated by antigen; the precise stage of B-cell development at which the

IG-MYC translocation arises is uncertain. Both HIV-related and endemic BL (but not sporadic BL) also show evidence of antigen selection during somatic hypermutation, providing further evidence that these lymphomas may originate from an immune reaction gone awry.[141]

Rearrangement of *MYC* can be demonstrated by routine karyotyping or interphase fluorescent in situ hybridization (FISH) (see **Fig. 9**F). Due to the wide range of the *IGH* breakpoints in BL and the occurrence of other translocation partners such as light chain genes, PCR is generally not routinely used to detect *MYC* rearrangement. In BL, the *MYC* rearrangement is almost always with an *IG* gene partner, a feature that can be confirmed with dual-color FISH using probes to the *IG* gene loci. BL usually displays a simple karyotype,[143] and array-based comparative genomic hybridization shows relatively low genetic complexity compared with DLBCL.[134] Nevertheless, other genetic mutations in addition to the *IGH-MYC* rearrangement are likely to play a role in the pathogenesis of BL, including mutations of *p53*.[144] Rare cases that are otherwise characteristic for BL lack an *MYC* translocation; the percentage of these cases is variable in published studies, likely reflecting differing pathologic inclusion criteria.[145] These cases bear a molecular signature similar to other BL cases that have rearranged *MYC*, validating their classification as BL.[134,146]

Gene Expression Profiling

MYC is an oncogene that markedly enhances cell proliferation and affects cell cycle progression, apoptosis, and differentiation.[147] Recent studies have shown that BL exhibits a characteristic gene expression profile that is distinct from DLBCL. As expected, the BL molecular signature includes many *MYC* target genes, but differences in the expression of GC-related genes, MHC Class I genes, and NFκB target genes are also observed.[146] Interestingly, some cases with a molecular signature identical to classic BL cases would not be classified as BL by the current diagnostic criteria, because they had morphologic features of DLBCL or other "nonconforming" features. Although gene expression profiling is not a routine test at the present time, these studies suggest that our current diagnostic methods are imperfect in clearly defining biologically discrete groups of BL and DLBCL. Gene expression profiling may hold future promise in better dictating optimal therapy for patients with aggressive lymphomas.

Outcome and Prognostic Features

BL is not effectively treated by CHOP-like (cyclophosphamide, doxorubicin, vincristine, and prednisone) regimens that are used to treat DLBCL.[148] However, both adult and pediatric BL patients can be cured by intensive chemotherapeutic regimens that contain high-dose methotrexate, etoposide, and cytarabine.[149,150] BL also requires the administration of intrathecal chemotherapy, as it carries a high-risk of relapse in the CNS.

Most BL patients present with disseminated high-stage disease. The bone marrow is involved in 10% to 30% of cases and is less commonly involved in endemic BL than in the other types.[132,147] BL has a superior prognosis when it is limited stage and when it occurs in children rather than adults. In adults, elevated serum LDH level and older age are other risk factors.[151] In patients with a single site of disease and in children, the 5-year overall survival rate is up to or exceeding 90%.[152] Even in advanced stages and with leukemic presentation, the 5-year survival rate is at least 50%.[151,153,154]

B-CELL LYMPHOMA UNCLASSIFIABLE, WITH FEATURES INTERMEDIATE BETWEEN DIFFUSE LARGE B-CELL LYMPHOMA AND BURKITT LYMPHOMA

With the increased use of immunophenotyping panels and genetic studies, there is increased recognition of cases that share many features with BL but deviate with respect to one or more findings. Pathologists have handled these cases variously, most commonly diagnosing them as "high-grade lymphomas." There is poor reproducibility when pathologists attempt to assign such cases to BL or DLBCL categories, even when using the results of cytogenetic and immunophenotypic studies.[155] Underscoring this diagnostic "haziness," molecular profiling studies have shown that 17% to 34% of cases that had a molecular signature of BL were not classified as BL by hematopathologists; conversely, cases diagnosed as BL almost always displayed a BL molecular signature.[134,146] The molecular profiling study of Hummel and colleagues[134] also identified a group of cases displaying a molecular signature intermediate between BL and DLBCL.

Given the different therapies that are indicated, pathologists' hedging between BL and DLBCL frustrates clinicians and also affects the validity of clinical trials evaluating the effectiveness of therapies on discrete biologic disease entities. For these reasons, the WHO 2008 Classification established a new diagnostic category of B-cell lymphoma, unclassifiable, with features intermediate between DLBCL and BL (DLBCL/BL).[2] DLBCL/BL is unlikely to represent a single biologic disease entity but rather comprises a heterogeneous group of cases that have some features (morphologic, immunophenotypic, or genetic) resembling BL and others that resemble DLBCL.

Morphology

Morphologic features are useful in the distinction between BL and DLBCL, however, accurate assessment of cell size, cytoplasmic borders, and nuclear chromatin requires excellent fixation, thin sectioning, and high-quality staining of sections.[156] If there is moderate cellular pleomorphism that is considered to be unacceptable for BL but the cell size is smaller than would be expected for DLBCL, a case may be classified as BL/DLBCL if it has an immunophenotype resembling BL and has an *MYC* translocation. Similarly, cases that have the morphology of BL (medium-sized cells that are uniform or only mildly pleomorphic) may be placed into the DLBCL/BL category if they have immunophenotypic and/or genetic deviations from BL (**Fig. 10** and **Table 9**).

Immunophenotype

Although occasional BL cases may have some immunophenotypic deviations from the expected profile (such as negativity for BCL6, weak positivity for BCL2, or lack of CD10 expression), any such deviations should lead to investigation for genetic features of DLBCL/BL (see below). In particular, strong BCL2 staining and/or a Ki67 proliferation index of less than 90% are absolute contraindications for a diagnosis of BL, and such cases should be placed in the DLBCL/BL category even if they have BL morphology (see **Fig. 10**C). Strong BCL2 staining by immunohistochemistry is often, but not always, associated with a *BCL2* translocation and can also be associated with *BCL6* translocation.[155]

Genetic Features

DLBCL/BL may or may not contain an *MYC* rearrangement. When *MYC* rearrangement is absent, there should be other deviations from BL, such as atypical morphology and/or immunophenotype. When an *MYC* rearrangement is present in DLBCL/BL

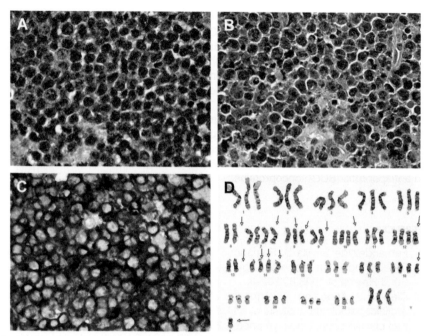

Fig. 10. B-cell lymphoma, unclassifiable, with features intermediate between DLBCL and Burkitt lymphoma (DLBCL/BL). (*A*) Case with morphology resembling BL but with concurrent *MYC* and *BCL2* rearrangements ("double-hit" lymphoma). (*B*) Case with a medium-cell size similar to BL but nuclear irregularity and pleomorphism unacceptable for BL. (*C*) Double-hit case with concurrent *MYC* and *BCL2* rearrangement and strong BCL2 staining. (*D*) Case with t(8;14) and complex karyotype, including extra copies of both der(8) and der(14) chromosomes. Such karyotypic complexity would be highly unusual for BL.

cases, it often has atypical features, including one or more of the following: (1) rearrangement with a non-*IG* partner (demonstrated by FISH, showing *IGH IGK*, and *IGL* loci); (2) a complex karyotype;[157] (3) concurrent rearrangements of *BCL2* and/or *BLC6* genes (so-called "double-hit" or "triple-hit" lymphoma cases) (see **Fig. 10D**). The double-hit lymphomas with both *MYC* and *BCL2* rearrangements comprise a large and relatively well-characterized subset of DLBCL/BL. These cases exhibit a spectrum of morphology and a wide range of Ki67 proliferation index, but all strongly express BCL2 and have a very poor prognosis with current therapies.[157,158] Most *MYC* and *BCL2* double-hit lymphomas have a complex karyotype with a t(14;18) abnormality in addition to the *MYC* 8q24 rearrangement. It should be emphasized that approximately 10% of all DLBCL cases DLBCL bear a *MYC* rearrangement,[159] and cases that are morphologically consistent with DLBCL but have a *MYC* rearrangement should not be placed in the DLBCL/BL category. DLBCL/BL with concurrent *MYC* and *BCL2* rearrangements can occur as high-grade transformation of a previous low-grade follicular lymphoma.[160] Such cases may exhibit complex *IGH-MYC-BCL2* rearrangements on karyotypic analysis.[161]

Gene Expression Profiling and Outcome

While gene expression profiling data are not available on DLBCL/BL as a group, some double-hit cases with both *MYC* and *BCL2* rearrangements have been shown to have a molecular signature similar to classic BL, other cases had a signature intermediate between BL and DLBCL.[146] Importantly, DLBCL with *MYC* translocation shares the molecular signature of DLBCL, not BL.[146] Cases with a molecular signature intermediate between BL and DLBCL may encompass many of the DLBCL/BL group, but this remains uncertain because the criteria for the DLBCL/BL group were developed after publication of these gene expression profiling studies.[134] It is anticipated that DLBCL/BL represents a biologically heterogeneous group that requires further genetic characterization.

The double-hit DLBCL/BL lymphomas are highly aggressive tumors that usually present at a high stage of disease and do poorly whether treated with intensive regimens used to treat BL or CHOP-like regimens.[156,162] The aggressive nature of these tumors likely reflects their simultaneous expression of both proproliferative (MYC) and antiapoptotic (BCL2) oncoproteins.

REFERENCES

1. Fernandez de Sevilla S, Romagosa V, Domingo-Claros A, et al. Diffuse large B-cell lymphoma: is morphologic subdivision useful in clinical management? Eur J Haematol 1998;60:202–8.
2. Diebold J, Anderson JR, Armitage JO, et al. Diffuse large B-cell lymphoma: a clinicopathologic analysis of 444 cases classified according to the updated Kiel classification. Leuk Lymphoma 2002;43(1):97–104.
3. Cabanillas F, Velasquez WS, Hagemeister FB, et al. Clinical, biologic, and histologic features of late relapses in diffuse large cell lymphoma. Blood 1992;79(4):1024–8.
4. Kremer M, Spitzer M, Mandl-Weber S, et al. Discordant bone marrow involvement in diffuse large B-cell lymphoma: comparative molecular analysis reveals a heterogeneous group of disorders. Lab Invest 2003;83(1):107–14.
5. Davis T, Czerwinski K, Levy R. Therapy of B-cell lymphoma with anti-CD20 antibodies can result in the loss of CD20 antigen expression. Clin Cancer Res 1999;5:611–5.
6. Yamaguchi M, Seto M, Okamoto M, et al. De novo CD5+ diffuse large B-cell lymphoma: a clinicopathologic study of 109 patients. Blood 2002;99:815–21.
7. Ennishi D, Takeuchi K, Yokoyama M, et al. CD5 expression is potentially predictive of poor outcome among biomarkers in patients with diffuse large B-cell lymphoma receiving rituximab plus CHOP therapy. Ann Oncol 2008;19(11):1921–6.
8. Kuppers R, Klein U, Hansmann ML, et al. Cellular origin of human B-cell lymphomas. N Engl J Med 1999;341(20):1520–9.
9. Bea S, Colomo L, Lopez-Guillermo A, et al. Clinicopathologic significance and prognostic value of chromosomal imbalances in diffuse large B-cell lymphomas. J Clin Oncol 2004;22(17):3498–506.
10. Chaganti RS, Nanjangud G, Schmidt H, et al. Recurring chromosomal abnormalities in non-Hodgkin's lymphoma: biologic and clinical significance. Semin Hematol 2000;37(4):396–411.
11. Pasqualucci L, Neumeister P, Goossens T, et al. Hypermutation of multiple protooncogenes in B-cell diffuse large-cell lymphomas. Nature 2001;412(6844):341–6.
12. Dent A, Vasanwala F, Toney L. Regulation of gene expression by the proto-oncogene BCL-6. Crit Rev Oncol Hematol 2002;41:1–9.
13. Phan RT, Dalla-Favera R. The BCL6 proto-oncogene suppresses p53 expression in germinal-centre B cells. Nature 2004;432(7017):635–9.

14. Bastard C, Deweindt C, Kerckaert JP, et al. LAZ3 rearrangements in non-Hodgkin's lymphoma: correlation with histology, immunophenotype, karyotype, and clinical outcome in 217 patients. Blood 1994;83(9):2423–7.

15. Barrans S, O'Connor S, Evans P, et al. Rearrangement of the BCL6 locus at 3q27 is an independent poor prognostic factor in nodal diffuse large B-cell lymphoma. Br J Haematol 2002;117:322–32.

16. Hermine O, Haioun C, Lepage E, et al. Prognostic significance of bcl-2 protein expression in aggressive non-Hodgkin's lymphoma. Groupe d'Etude des Lymphomes de l'Adulte (GELA). Blood 1996;87(1):265–72.

17. Gascoyne RD, Adomat SA, Krajewski S, et al. Prognostic significance of Bcl-2 protein expression and Bcl-2 gene rearrangement in diffuse aggressive non-Hodgkin's lymphoma. Blood 1997;90(1):244–51.

18. Pasqualucci L, Migliazza A, Basso K, et al. Mutations of the BCL6 proto-oncogene disrupt its negative autoregulation in diffuse large B-cell lymphoma. Blood 2003;101(8):2914–23.

19. Young KH, Leroy K, Moller MB, et al. Structural profiles of TP53 gene mutations predict clinical outcome in diffuse large B-cell lymphoma: an international collaborative study. Blood 2008;112(8):3088–98.

20. Houldsworth J, Olshen AB, Cattoretti G, et al. Relationship between REL amplification, REL function, and clinical and biologic features in diffuse large B-cell lymphomas. Blood 2004;103(5):1862–8.

21. Alizadeh AA, Eisen MB, Davis RE, et al. Distinct types of diffuse large B-cell lymphoma identified by gene expression profiling [In Process Citation]. Nature 2000;403(6769):503–11.

22. Rosenwald A, Wright G, Chan WC, et al. The use of molecular profiling to predict survival after chemotherapy for diffuse large-B-cell lymphoma. N Engl J Med 2002;346(25):1937–47.

23. Lenz G, Wright GW, Emre NC, et al. Molecular subtypes of diffuse large B-cell lymphoma arise by distinct genetic pathways. Proc Natl Acad Sci U S A 2008; 105(36):13520–5.

24. Lossos IS, Alizadeh AA, Eisen MB, et al. Ongoing immunoglobulin somatic mutation in germinal center B cell-like but not in activated B cell-like diffuse large cell lymphomas. Proc Natl Acad Sci U S A 2000;97(18):10209–13.

25. Iqbal J, Greiner TC, Patel K, et al. Distinctive patterns of BCL6 molecular alterations and their functional consequences in different subgroups of diffuse large B-cell lymphoma. Leukemia 2007;21(11):2332–43.

26. Ngo VN, Davis RE, Lamy L, et al. A loss-of-function RNA interference screen for molecular targets in cancer. Nature 2006;441(7089):106–10.

27. Lenz G, Wright G, Dave SS, et al. Stromal gene signatures in large-B-cell lymphomas. N Engl J Med 2008;359(22):2313–23.

28. Lossos IS, Czerwinski DK, Alizadeh AA, et al. Prediction of survival in diffuse large-B-cell lymphoma based on the expression of six genes. N Engl J Med 2004;350(18):1828–37.

29. Rimsza LM, Leblanc ML, Unger JM, et al. Gene expression predicts overall survival in paraffin-embedded tissues of diffuse large B-cell lymphoma treated with R-CHOP. Blood 2008;112(8):3425–33.

30. Hans CP, Weisenburger DD, Greiner TC, et al. Confirmation of the molecular classification of diffuse large B-cell lymphoma by immunohistochemistry using a tissue microarray. Blood 2004;103(1):275–82.

31. de Jong D, Rosenwald A, Chhanabhai M, et al. Immunohistochemical prognostic markers in diffuse large B-cell lymphoma: validation of tissue microarray

as a prerequisite for broad clinical applications–a study from the Lunenburg Lymphoma Biomarker Consortium. J Clin Oncol 2007;25(7):805–12.

32. Barrans SL, Carter I, Owen RG, et al. Germinal center phenotype and bcl-2 expression combined with the International Prognostic Index improves patient risk stratification in diffuse large B-cell lymphoma. Blood 2002;99(4):1136–43.

33. Chang CC, McClintock S, Cleveland RP, et al. Immunohistochemical expression patterns of germinal center and activation B-cell markers correlate with prognosis in diffuse large B-cell lymphoma. Am J Surg Pathol 2004;28(4): 464–70.

34. Colomo L, Lopez-Guillermo A, Perales M, et al. Clinical impact of the differentiation profile assessed by immunophenotyping in patients with diffuse large B-cell lymphoma. Blood 2003;101(1):78–84.

35. De Paepe P, Achten R, Verhoef G, et al. Large cleaved and immunoblastic lymphoma may represent two distinct clinicopathologic entities within the group of diffuse large B-cell lymphomas. J Clin Oncol 2005;23(28):7060–8.

36. Nyman H, Adde M, Karjalainen-Lindsberg ML, et al. Prognostic impact of immunohistochemically defined germinal center phenotype in diffuse large B-cell lymphoma patients treated with immunochemotherapy. Blood 2007;109(11):4930–5.

37. de Leval L, Harris NL. Variability in immunophenotype in diffuse large B-cell lymphoma and its clinical relevance. Histopathology 2003;43(6):509–28.

38. Lossos IS, Morgensztern D. Prognostic biomarkers in diffuse large B-cell lymphoma. J Clin Oncol 2006;24(6):995–1007.

39. Shipp MA, Ross KN, Tamayo P, et al. Diffuse large B-cell lymphoma outcome prediction by gene-expression profiling and supervised machine learning. Nat Med 2002;8(1):68–74.

40. Banham AH, Connors JM, Brown PJ, et al. Expression of the FOXP1 transcription factor is strongly associated with inferior survival in patients with diffuse large B-cell lymphoma. Clin Cancer Res 2005;11(3):1065–72.

41. Natkunam Y, Farinha P, Hsi ED, et al. LMO2 protein expression predicts survival in patients with diffuse large B-cell lymphoma treated with anthracycline-based chemotherapy with and without rituximab. J Clin Oncol 2008;26(3):447–54.

42. Coiffier B. Rituximab therapy in malignant lymphoma. Oncogene 2007;26(25): 3603–13.

43. Dogan A, Burke JS, Goteri G, et al. Micronodular T-cell/histiocyte-rich large B-cell lymphoma of the spleen: histology, immunophenotype, and differential diagnosis. Am J Surg Pathol 2003;27(7):903–11.

44. Lim MS, Beaty M, Sorbara L, et al. T-cell/histiocyte-rich large B-cell lymphoma: a heterogeneous entity with derivation from germinal center B cells. Am J Surg Pathol 2002;26(11):1458–66.

45. Achten R, Verhoef G, Vanuytsel L, et al. Histiocyte-rich, T-cell-rich B-cell lymphoma: a distinct diffuse large B-cell lymphoma subtype showing characteristic morphologic and immunophenotypic features. Histopathology 2002;40(1):31–45.

46. Rudiger T, Ott G, Ott MM, et al. Differential diagnosis between classic Hodgkin's lymphoma, T-cell-rich B-cell lymphoma, and paragranuloma by paraffin immunohistochemistry. Am J Surg Pathol 1998;22(10):1184–91.

47. Nam-Cha SH, Roncador G, Sanchez-Verde L, et al. PD-1, a follicular T-cell marker useful for recognizing nodular lymphocyte-predominant Hodgkin lymphoma. Am J Surg Pathol 2008;32(8):1252–7.

48. Monti S, Savage KJ, Kutok JL, et al. Molecular profiling of diffuse large B-cell lymphoma identifies robust subtypes including one characterized by host inflammatory response. Blood 2005;105(5):1851–61.

49. Rudiger T, Gascoyne RD, Jaffe ES, et al. Workshop on the relationship between nodular lymphocyte predominant Hodgkin's lymphoma and T cell/histiocyte-rich B cell lymphoma. Ann Oncol 2002;13(Suppl 1):44–51.
50. Franke S, Wlodarska I, Maes B, et al. Comparative genomic hybridization pattern distinguishes T-cell/histiocyte-rich B-cell lymphoma from nodular lymphocyte predominance Hodgkin's lymphoma. Am J Pathol 2002;161(5):1861–7.
51. Maes B, Anastasopoulou A, Kluin-Nelemans JC, et al. Among diffuse large B-cell lymphomas, T-cell-rich/histiocyte-rich BCL and CD30+ anaplastic B-cell subtypes exhibit distinct clinical features. Ann Oncol 2001;12(6):853–8.
52. Bouabdallah R, Mounier N, Guettier C, et al. T-cell/histiocyte-rich large B-cell lymphomas and classical diffuse large B-cell lymphomas have similar outcome after chemotherapy: a matched-control analysis. J Clin Oncol 2003;21(7):1271–7.
53. Batchelor T, Loeffler JS. Primary CNS lymphoma. J Clin Oncol 2006;24(8):1281–8.
54. Braaten KM, Betensky RA, de Leval L, et al. BCL-6 expression predicts improved survival in patients with primary central nervous system lymphoma. Clin Cancer Res 2003;9(3):1063–9.
55. Camilleri-Broet S, Criniere E, Broet P, et al. A uniform activated B-cell-like immunophenotype might explain the poor prognosis of primary central nervous system lymphomas: analysis of 83 cases. Blood 2006;107(1):190–6.
56. Montesinos-Rongen M, Siebert R, Deckert M. Primary lymphoma of the central nervous system: just DLBCL or not? Blood 2009;113(1):7–10.
57. Cady FM, O'Neill BP, Law ME, et al. Del(6)(q22) and BCL6 rearrangements in primary CNS lymphoma are indicators of an aggressive clinical course. J Clin Oncol 2008;26(29):4814–9.
58. Rubenstein JL, Fridlyand J, Shen A, et al. Gene expression and angiotropism in primary CNS lymphoma. Blood 2006;107(9):3716–23.
59. Montesinos-Rongen M, Brunn A, Bentink S, et al. Gene expression profiling suggests primary central nervous system lymphomas to be derived from a late germinal center B cell. Leukemia 2008;22(2):400–5.
60. Tun HW, Personett D, Baskerville KA, et al. Pathway analysis of primary central nervous system lymphoma. Blood 2008;111(6):3200–10.
61. Dijkman R, Tensen CP, Buettner M, et al. Primary cutaneous follicle center lymphoma and primary cutaneous large B-cell lymphoma, leg type, are both targeted by aberrant somatic hypermutation but demonstrate differential expression of AID. Blood 2006;107(12):4926–9.
62. Hoefnagel JJ, Dijkman R, Basso K, et al. Distinct types of primary cutaneous large B-cell lymphoma identified by gene expression profiling. Blood 2005;105(9):3671–8.
63. Oyama T, Ichimura K, Suzuki R, et al. Senile EBV+ B-cell lymphoproliferative disorders: a clinicopathologic study of 22 patients. Am J Surg Pathol 2003;27(1):16–26.
64. Oyama T, Yamamoto K, Asano N, et al. Age-related EBV-associated B-cell lymphoproliferative disorders constitute a distinct clinicopathologic group: a study of 96 patients. Clin Cancer Res 2007;13(17):5124–32.
65. Shimoyama Y, Oyama T, Asano N, et al. Senile Epstein-Barr virus-associated B-cell lymphoproliferative disorders: a mini review. J Clin Exp Hematop 2006;46(1):1–4.
66. Park S, Lee J, Ko YH, et al. The impact of Epstein-Barr virus status on clinical outcome in diffuse large B-cell lymphoma. Blood 2007;110(3):972–8.

67. Addis BJ, Isaacson PG. Large cell lymphoma of the mediastinum: a B-cell tumour of probable thymic origin. Histopathology 1986;10(4):379–90.

68. Isaacson P, Norton A, Addis B. The human thymus contains a novel population of B-lymphocytes. Lancet 1987;ii:1488–90.

69. Jacobson J, Aisenberg A, Lamarre L, et al. Mediastinal large cell lymphoma: an uncommon subset of adult lymphoma curable with combined modality therapy. Cancer 1988;62:1893–8.

70. Cazals-Hatem D, Lepage E, Brice P, et al. Primary mediastinal large B-cell lymphoma. A clinicopathologic study of 141 cases compared with 916 nonmediastinal large B-cell lymphomas, a GELA ("Groupe d'Etude des Lymphomes de l'Adulte") study. Am J Surg Pathol 1996;20(7):877–88.

71. Zinzani PL, Martelli M, Bendandi M, et al. Primary mediastinal large B-cell lymphoma with sclerosis: a clinical study of 89 patients treated with MACOP-B chemotherapy and radiation therapy. Haematologica 2001;86(2):187–91.

72. Rosenwald A, Wright G, Leroy K, et al. Molecular diagnosis of primary mediastinal B cell lymphoma identifies a clinically favorable subgroup of diffuse large B cell lymphoma related to Hodgkin lymphoma. J Exp Med 2003;198(6):851–62.

73. Lamarre L, Jacobson JO, Aisenberg AC, et al. Primary large cell lymphoma of the mediastinum. A histologic and immunophenotypic study of 29 cases. Am J Surg Pathol 1989;13(9):730–9.

74. Pileri SA, Gaidano G, Zinzani PL, et al. Primary mediastinal B-cell lymphoma: high frequency of BCL-6 mutations and consistent expression of the transcription factors OCT-2, BOB.1, and PU.1 in the absence of immunoglobulins. Am J Pathol 2003;162(1):243–53.

75. de Leval L, Ferry JA, Falini B, et al. Expression of bcl-6 and CD10 in primary mediastinal large B-cell lymphoma: evidence for derivation from germinal center B cells? Am J Surg Pathol 2001;25(10):1277–82.

76. Calaminici M, Piper K, Lee AM, et al. CD23 expression in mediastinal large B-cell lymphomas. Histopathology 2004;45(6):619–24.

77. Copie-Bergman C, Plonquet A, Alonso MA, et al. MAL expression in lymphoid cells: further evidence for MAL as a distinct molecular marker of primary mediastinal large B-cell lymphomas. Mod Pathol 2002;15(11):1172–80.

78. Copie-Bergman C, Boulland ML, Dehoulle C, et al. Interleukin 4-induced gene 1 is activated in primary mediastinal large B-cell lymphoma. Blood 2003;101(7):2756–61.

79. Savage KJ, Monti S, Kutok JL, et al. The molecular signature of mediastinal large B-cell lymphoma differs from that of other diffuse large B-cell lymphomas and shares features with classical Hodgkin's lymphoma. Blood 2003;102(12):3871–9.

80. Rodig SJ, Savage KJ, LaCasce AS, et al. Expression of TRAF1 and nuclear c-Rel distinguishes primary mediastinal large cell lymphoma from other types of diffuse large B-cell lymphoma. Am J Surg Pathol 2007;31(1):106–12.

81. Leithauser F, Bauerle M, Huynh MQ, et al. Isotype-switched immunoglobulin genes with a high load of somatic hypermutation and lack of ongoing mutational activity are prevalent in mediastinal B-cell lymphoma. Blood 2001;98(9):2762–70.

82. Tsang P, Cesarman E, Chadburn A, et al. Molecular characterization of primary mediastinal B cell lymphoma. Am J Pathol 1996;148(6):2017–25.

83. Joos S, Otano-Joos MI, Ziegler S, et al. Primary mediastinal (thymic) B-cell lymphoma is characterized by gains of chromosomal material including 9p and amplification of the REL gene. Blood 1996;87(4):1571–8.

84. Wessendorf S, Barth TF, Viardot A, et al. Further delineation of chromosomal consensus regions in primary mediastinal B-cell lymphomas: an analysis of 37 tumor samples using high-resolution genomic profiling (array-CGH). Leukemia 2007;21(12):2463–9.

85. Joos S, Granzow M, Holtgreve-Grez H, et al. Hodgkin's lymphoma cell lines are characterized by frequent aberrations on chromosomes 2p and 9p including REL and JAK2. Int J Cancer 2003;103(4):489–95.

86. Feuerhake F, Kutok JL, Monti S, et al. NF{kappa}B activity, function, and target-gene signatures in primary mediastinal large B-cell lymphoma and diffuse large B-cell lymphoma subtypes. Blood 2005;106(4):1392–9.

87. Guiter C, Dusanter-Fourt I, Copie-Bergman C, et al. Constitutive STAT6 activation in primary mediastinal large B-cell lymphoma. Blood 2004;104(2):543–9.

88. Melzner I, Bucur AJ, Bruderlein S, et al. Biallelic mutation of SOCS-1 impairs JAK2 degradation and sustains phospho-JAK2 action in the MedB-1 mediastinal lymphoma line. Blood 2005;105(6):2535–42.

89. Weniger MA, Melzner I, Menz CK, et al. Mutations of the tumor suppressor gene SOCS-1 in classical Hodgkin lymphoma are frequent and associated with nuclear phospho-STAT5 accumulation. Oncogene 2006;25(18):2679–84.

90. Renne C, Willenbrock K, Martin-Subero JI, et al. High expression of several tyrosine kinases and activation of the PI3K/AKT pathway in mediastinal large B cell lymphoma reveals further similarities to Hodgkin lymphoma. Leukemia 2007;21(4):780–7.

91. Rudiger T, Jaffe ES, Delsol G, et al. Workshop report on Hodgkin's disease and related diseases ('grey zone' lymphoma). Ann Oncol 1998;9(Suppl 5):S31–8.

92. Traverse-Glehen A, Pittaluga S, Gaulard P, et al. Mediastinal gray zone lymphoma: the missing link between classic Hodgkin's lymphoma and mediastinal large B-cell lymphoma. Am J Surg Pathol 2005;29(11):1411–21.

93. Calvo KR, Traverse-Glehen A, Pittaluga S, et al. Molecular profiling provides evidence of primary mediastinal large B-cell lymphoma as a distinct entity related to classic Hodgkin lymphoma: implications for mediastinal gray zone lymphomas as an intermediate form of B-cell lymphoma. Adv Anat Pathol 2004;11(5):227–38.

94. Murase T, Nakamura S, Kawauchi K, et al. An Asian variant of intravascular large B-cell lymphoma: clinical, pathological and cytogenetic approaches to diffuse large B-cell lymphoma associated with haemophagocytic syndrome. Br J Haematol 2000;111(3):826–34.

95. Ferreri AJ, Dognini GP, Bairey O, et al. The addition of rituximab to anthracycline-based chemotherapy significantly improves outcome in 'Western' patients with intravascular large B-cell lymphoma. Br J Haematol 2008;143(2):253–7.

96. Khalidi HS, Brynes RK, Browne P, et al. Intravascular large B-cell lymphoma: the CD5 antigen is expressed by a subset of cases. Mod Pathol 1998;11(10):983–8.

97. Ponzoni M, Ferreri AJ, Campo E, et al. Definition, diagnosis, and management of intravascular large B-cell lymphoma: proposals and perspectives from an international consensus meeting. J Clin Oncol 2007;25(21):3168–73.

98. Ferreri AJ, Campo E, Seymour JF, et al. Intravascular lymphoma: clinical presentation, natural history, management and prognostic factors in a series of 38 cases, with special emphasis on the 'cutaneous variant'. Br J Haematol 2004; 127(2):173–83.

99. Yegappan S, Coupland R, Arber DA, et al. Angiotropic lymphoma: an immunophenotypically and clinically heterogeneous lymphoma. Mod Pathol 2001; 14(11):1147–56.

100. Ponzoni M, Arrigoni G, Gould VE, et al. Lack of CD 29 (beta1 integrin) and CD 54 (ICAM-1) adhesion molecules in intravascular lymphomatosis. Hum Pathol 2000;31(2):220–6.
101. Nakatsuka S, Yao M, Hoshida Y, et al. Pyothorax-associated lymphoma: a review of 106 cases. J Clin Oncol 2002;20(20):4255–60.
102. Petitjean B, Jardin F, Joly B, et al. Pyothorax-associated lymphoma: a peculiar clinicopathologic entity derived from B cells at late stage of differentiation and with occasional aberrant dual B-and T-cell phenotype. Am J Surg Pathol 2002;26(6):724–32.
103. Kanno H, Aozasa K. Mechanism for the development of pyothorax-associated lymphoma. Pathol Int 1998;48(9):653–64.
104. Yamato H, Ohshima K, Suzumiya J, et al. Evidence for local immunosuppression and demonstration of c-myc amplification in pyothorax-associated lymphoma. Histopathology 2001;39(2):163–71.
105. Nishiu M, Tomita Y, Nakatsuka S, et al. Distinct pattern of gene expression in pyothorax-associated lymphoma (PAL), a lymphoma developing in long-standing inflammation. Cancer Sci 2004;95(10):828–34.
106. Takakuwa T, Tresnasari K, Rahadiani N, et al. Cell origin of pyothorax-associated lymphoma: a lymphoma strongly associated with Epstein-Barr virus infection. Leukemia 2008;22(3):620–7.
107. Copie-Bergman C, Niedobitek G, Mangham DC, et al. Epstein-Barr virus in B-cell lymphomas associated with chronic suppurative inflammation. J Pathol 1997;183(3):287–92.
108. Cheuk W, Chan AC, Chan JK, et al. Metallic implant-associated lymphoma: a distinct subgroup of large B-cell lymphoma related to pyothorax-associated lymphoma? Am J Surg Pathol 2005;29(6):832–6.
109. Guinee D Jr, Jaffe E, Kingma D, et al. Pulmonary lymphomatoid granulomatosis. Evidence for a proliferation of Epstein-Barr virus infected B-lymphocytes with a prominent T-cell component and vasculitis. Am J Surg Pathol 1994;18(8): 753–64.
110. Beaty MW, Toro J, Sorbara L, et al. Cutaneous lymphomatoid granulomatosis: correlation of clinical and biologic features. Am J Surg Pathol 2001;25(9): 1111–20.
111. Saxena A, Dyker KM, Angel S, et al. Posttransplant diffuse large B-cell lymphoma of "lymphomatoid granulomatosis" type. Virchows Arch 2002; 441(6):622–8.
112. Myers JL, Kurtin PJ, Katzenstein AL, et al. Lymphomatoid granulomatosis. Evidence of immunophenotypic diversity and relationship to Epstein-Barr virus infection. Am J Surg Pathol 1995;19(11):1300–12.
113. Delecluse HJ, Anagnostopoulos I, Dallenbach F, et al. Plasmablastic lymphomas of the oral cavity: a new entity associated with the human immuno-deficiency virus infection. Blood 1997;89(4):1413–20.
114. Colomo L, Loong F, Rives S, et al. Diffuse large B-cell lymphomas with plasma-blastic differentiation represent a heterogeneous group of disease entities. Am J Surg Pathol 2004;28(6):736–47.
115. Teruya-Feldstein J, Chiao E, Filippa DA, et al. CD20-negative large-cell lymphoma with plasmablastic features: a clinically heterogeneous spectrum in both HIV-positive and -negative patients. Ann Oncol 2004;15(11):1673–9.
116. Dong HY, Scadden DT, de Leval L, et al. Plasmablastic lymphoma in HIV-posi-tive patients: an aggressive Epstein-Barr Virus-associated extramedullary plas-macytic neoplasm. Am J Surg Pathol 2005;29(12):1633–41.

117. Chadburn A, Hyjek E, Mathew S, et al. KSHV-positive solid lymphomas represent an extra-cavitary variant of primary effusion lymphoma. Am J Surg Pathol 2004;28(11):1401–16.

118. Vega F, Chang CC, Medeiros LJ, et al. Plasmablastic lymphomas and plasmablastic plasma cell myelomas have nearly identical immunophenotypic profiles. Mod Pathol 2005;18(6):806–15.

119. Delsol G, Lamant L, Mariame B, et al. A new subtype of large B-cell lymphoma expressing the ALK kinase and lacking the 2; 5 translocation. Blood 1997;89(5): 1483–90.

120. Gascoyne RD, Lamant L, Martin-Subero JI, et al. ALK-positive diffuse large B-cell lymphoma is associated with Clathrin-ALK rearrangements: report of 6 cases. Blood 2003;102(7):2568–73.

121. Onciu M, Behm FG, Downing JR, et al. ALK-positive plasmablastic B-cell lymphoma with expression of the NPM-ALK fusion transcript: report of 2 cases. Blood 2003;102(7):2642–4.

122. Cesarman E, Chang Y, Moore PS, et al. Kaposi's sarcoma-associated herpesvirus-like DNA sequences in AIDS-related body-cavity-based lymphomas. N Engl J Med 1995;332(18):1186–91.

123. Horenstein MG, Nador RG, Chadburn A, et al. Epstein-Barr virus latent gene expression in primary effusion lymphomas containing Kaposi's sarcoma-associated herpesvirus/human herpesvirus-8. Blood 1997;90(3):1186–91.

124. Gaidano G, Gloghini A, Gattei V, et al. Association of Kaposi's sarcoma-associated herpesvirus-positive primary effusion lymphoma with expression of the CD138/syndecan-1 antigen. Blood 1997;90(12):4894–900.

125. Jenner RG, Maillard K, Cattini N, et al. Kaposi's sarcoma-associated herpesvirus-infected primary effusion lymphoma has a plasma cell gene expression profile. Proc Natl Acad Sci U S A 2003;100(18):10399–404.

126. Klein U, Gloghini A, Gaidano G, et al. Gene expression profile analysis of AIDS-related primary effusion lymphoma (PEL) suggests a plasmablastic derivation and identifies PEL-specific transcripts. Blood 2003;101(10): 4115–21.

127. Boulanger E, Gerard L, Gabarre J, et al. Prognostic factors and outcome of human herpesvirus 8-associated primary effusion lymphoma in patients with AIDS. J Clin Oncol 2005;23(19):4372–80.

128. Oksenhendler E, Boulanger E, Galicier L, et al. High incidence of Kaposi sarcoma-associated herpesvirus-related non-Hodgkin lymphoma in patients with HIV infection and multicentric Castleman disease. Blood 2002;99(7): 2331–6.

129. Dupin N, Diss TL, Kellam P, et al. HHV-8 is associated with a plasmablastic variant of Castleman disease that is linked to HHV-8-positive plasmablastic lymphoma. Blood 2000;95(4):1406–12.

130. Raphael M, Gentilhomme O, Tulliez M, et al. Histopathologic features of high-grade non-Hodgkin's lymphomas in acquired immunodeficiency syndrome. The French Study Group of Pathology for Human Immunodeficiency Virus-Associated Tumors. Arch Pathol Lab Med 1991;115(1):15–20.

131. Burmeister T, Schwartz S, Horst HA, et al. Molecular heterogeneity of sporadic adult Burkitt-type leukemia/lymphoma as revealed by PCR and cytogenetics: correlation with morphology, immunology and clinical features. Leukemia 2005;19(8):1391–8.

132. Hecht JL, Aster JC. Molecular biology of Burkitt's lymphoma. J Clin Oncol 2000; 18(21):3707–21.

133. Magrath IT, Janus C, Edwards BK, et al. An effective therapy for both undifferentiated (including Burkitt's) lymphomas and lymphoblastic lymphomas in children and young adults. Blood 1984;63(5):1102–11.

134. Hummel M, Bentink S, Berger H, et al. A biologic definition of Burkitt's lymphoma from transcriptional and genomic profiling. N Engl J Med 2006;354(23): 2419–30.

135. Dogan A, Bagdi E, Munson P, et al. CD10 and bcl-6 expression in paraffin sections of normal lymphoid tissue and B-cell lymphomas. Am J Surg Pathol 2000;24:846–52.

136. Rodig SJ, Vergilio JA, Shahsafaei A, et al. Characteristic expression patterns of TCL1, CD38, and CD44 identify aggressive lymphomas harboring a MYC translocation. Am J Surg Pathol 2008;32(1):113–22.

137. Chuang SS, Ye H, Du MQ, et al. Histopathology and immunohistochemistry in distinguishing Burkitt lymphoma from diffuse large B-cell lymphoma with very high proliferation index and with or without a starry-sky pattern: a comparative study with EBER and FISH. Am J Clin Pathol 2007;128(4):558–64.

138. Lim ST, Karim R, Tulpule A, et al. Prognostic factors in HIV-related diffuse large-cell lymphoma: before versus after highly active antiretroviral therapy. J Clin Oncol 2005;23(33):8477–82.

139. Rochford R, Cannon MJ, Moormann AM. Endemic Burkitt's lymphoma: a polymicrobial disease? Nat Rev Microbiol 2005;3(2):182–7.

140. Robbiani DF, Bothmer A, Callen E, et al. AID is required for the chromosomal breaks in c-myc that lead to c-myc/IgH translocations. Cell 2008;135(6): 1028–38.

141. Bellan C, Lazzi S, Hummel M, et al. Immunoglobulin gene analysis reveals 2 distinct cells of origin for EBV-positive and EBV-negative Burkitt lymphomas. Blood 2005;106(3):1031–6.

142. Shiramizu B, Barriga F, Neequaye J, et al. Patterns of chromosomal breakpoint locations in Burkitt's lymphoma: relevance to geography and Epstein-Barr virus association. Blood 1991;77(7):1516–26.

143. Boerma EG, Siebert R, Kluin PM, et al. Translocations involving 8q24 in Burkitt lymphoma and other malignant lymphomas: a historical review of cytogenetics in the light of today's knowledge. Leukemia 2009;23(2):225–34.

144. Gaidano G, Dalla-Favera R. Molecular pathogenesis of AIDS-related lymphomas. Adv Cancer Res 1995;67:113–53.

145. Leucci E, Cocco M, Onnis A, et al. MYC translocation-negative classical Burkitt lymphoma cases: an alternative pathogenetic mechanism involving miRNA deregulation. J Pathol 2008;216(4):440–50.

146. Dave SS, Fu K, Wright GW, et al. Molecular diagnosis of Burkitt's lymphoma. N Engl J Med 2006;354(23):2431–42.

147. Blum KA, Lozanski G, Byrd JC. Adult Burkitt leukemia and lymphoma. Blood 2004;104(10):3009–20.

148. Nomura Y, Karube K, Suzuki R, et al. High-grade mature B-cell lymphoma with Burkitt-like morphology: results of a clinicopathological study of 72 Japanese patients. Cancer Sci 2008;99(2):246–52.

149. Magrath I, Adde M, Shad A, et al. Adults and children with small non-cleaved-cell lymphoma have a similar excellent outcome when treated with the same chemotherapy regimen. J Clin Oncol 1996;14(3):925–34.

150. Mead GM, Sydes MR, Walewski J, et al. An international evaluation of CODOX-M and CODOX-M alternating with IVAC in adult Burkitt's lymphoma: results of United Kingdom Lymphoma Group LY06 study. Ann Oncol 2002;13(8):1264–74.

151. Divine M, Casassus P, Koscielny S, et al. Burkitt lymphoma in adults: a prospective study of 72 patients treated with an adapted pediatric LMB protocol. Ann Oncol 2005;16(12):1928–35.
152. Cairo MS, Sposto R, Perkins SL, et al. Burkitt's and Burkitt-like lymphoma in children and adolescents: a review of the Children's Cancer Group experience. Br J Haematol 2003;120(4):660–70.
153. Soussain C, Patte C, Ostronoff M, et al. Small noncleaved cell lymphoma and leukemia in adults. A retrospective study of 65 adults treated with the LMB pediatric protocols. Blood 1995;85(3):664–74.
154. Patte C, Auperin A, Gerrard M, et al. Results of the randomized international FAB/LMB96 trial for intermediate risk B-cell non-Hodgkin lymphoma in children and adolescents: it is possible to reduce treatment for the early responding patients. Blood 2007;109(7):2773–80.
155. Haralambieva E, Boerma EJ, van Imhoff GW, et al. Clinical, immunophenotypic, and genetic analysis of adult lymphomas with morphologic features of Burkitt lymphoma. Am J Surg Pathol 2005;29(8):1086–94.
156. McClure RF, Remstein ED, Macon WR, et al. Adult B-cell lymphomas with Burkitt-like morphology are phenotypically and genotypically heterogeneous with aggressive clinical behavior. Am J Surg Pathol 2005;29(12):1652–60.
157. Le Gouill S, Talmant P, Touzeau C, et al. The clinical presentation and prognosis of diffuse large B-cell lymphoma with t(14;18) and 8q24/c-MYC rearrangement. Haematologica 2007;92(10):1335–42.
158. Kanungo A, Medeiros LJ, Abruzzo LV, et al. Lymphoid neoplasms associated with concurrent t(14;18) and 8q24/c-MYC translocation generally have a poor prognosis. Mod Pathol 2006;19(1):25–33.
159. van Imhoff GW, Boerma EJ, van der Holt B, et al. Prognostic impact of germinal center-associated proteins and chromosomal breakpoints in poor-risk diffuse large B-cell lymphoma. J Clin Oncol 2006;24(25):4135–42.
160. Leoncini L, Delsol G, Gascoyne RD, et al. Aggressive B-cell lymphomas: a review based on the workshop of the XI Meeting of the European Association for Haematopathology. Histopathology 2005;46(3):241–55.
161. Knezevich S, Ludkovski O, Salski C, et al. Concurrent translocation of BCL2 and MYC with a single immunoglobulin locus in high-grade B-cell lymphomas. Leukemia 2005;19(4):659–63.
162. Macpherson N, Lesack D, Klasa R, et al. Small noncleaved, non-Burkitt's (Burkitt-Like) lymphoma: cytogenetics predict outcome and reflect clinical presentation. J Clin Oncol 1999;17(5):1558–67.

Peripheral T-Cell Lymphomas

William R. Macon, MD[a,b,c,*]

KEYWORDS

- Peripheral T-cell lymphoma • Angioimmunoblastic
- Anaplastic large cell • Hepatosplenic
- Enteropathy-associated • Mycosis fungoides • HTLV-1

Peripheral T-cell lymphomas (PTCLs) are malignancies of immunologically mature T-cells that have completed T-cell differentiation, generally in the thymus ("central" organ of T-cell differentiation), and have circulated to the "peripheral" lymphoid tissues (lymph nodes, spleen, gastrointestinal tract, skin, and so forth) where the tumors arise. Like normal human T-cells, most of the PTCLs express T-cell receptor (TCR) $\alpha\beta$ protein chains, with a minor subset expressing TCR $\gamma\delta$ protein chains. Unlike normal human T-cells, PTCLs often demonstrate phenotypic aberrancy,[1] such as loss of pan T-cell antigens, or have clonal TCR gene rearrangements.[2] Because natural killer (NK) cells and T cells have a common progenitor cell and some overlapping immunologic properties, NK-cell lymphomas are considered together with PTCLs in the World Health Organization (WHO) classification of malignant lymphomas.[3]

PTCLs are uncommon because they comprise only 5% to 10% of all non-Hodgkin lymphomas in North America and Western Europe and approximately twice that in Asia.[4] PTCLs can be grouped according to those that present primarily in lymph nodes or in extranodal/cutaneous sites or have leukemic and lymphomatous components (**Box 1**). The various PTCL entities in the WHO classification discussed herein follow that convention.

ANGIOIMMUNOBLASTIC T-CELL LYMPHOMA

Angioimmunoblastic T-cell lymphomas (AITCLs) present mainly in middle-aged to elderly adults who have generalized lymphadenopathy, often accompanied by hepatosplenomegaly and skin rash.[5] Patients often experience B-symptoms (fever, weight

This work was supported in part by the Iowa/Mayo SPORE (P50 CA97274).

[a] Mayo College of Medicine, 200 First Street SW, Rochester, MN 55905, USA

[b] Division of Anatomic Pathology, Department of Laboratory Medicine and Pathology, Mayo Clinic, 200 First Street SW, Rochester, MN 55905, USA

[c] Division of Hematopathology, Department of Laboratory Medicine and Pathology, Mayo Clinic, 200 First Street SW, Rochester, MN 55905, USA

* Mayo Clinic, 200 First Street SW, Rochester, MN 55905.

E-mail address: macon.william@mayo.edu

Hematol Oncol Clin N Am 23 (2009) 829–842
doi:10.1016/j.hoc.2009.04.007
0889-8588/09/$ – see front matter © 2009 Elsevier Inc. All rights reserved.

Box 1
Classification of peripheral T-cell and NK-cell lymphomas

Nodal

Angioimmunoblastic T-cell lymphoma

Anaplastic large cell lymphoma

Peripheral T-cell lymphoma, unspecified

Extranodal/cutaneous

Hepatosplenic T-cell lymphoma

Enteropathy-associated T-cell lymphoma

Extranodal NK/T-cell lymphoma, nasal type

Mycosis fungoides

Primary cutaneous peripheral T-cell lymphomas

    Primary cutaneous CD4+ small/medium T-cell lymphoma

    Primary cutaneous γδ T-cell lymphoma

    Primary cutaneous CD8+ aggressive epidermotropic cytotoxic T-cell lymphoma

Primary cutaneous anaplastic large cell lymphoma

Subcutaneous panniculitis-like T-cell lymphoma

Leukemic and lymphomatous components

Adult T-cell leukemia/lymphoma

---

loss, and night sweats) and may have polyclonal hypergammaglobulinemia and auto-immune hemolytic anemia. AITCL is an aggressive malignancy with a 5-year overall survival (OS) of approximately 32%.[4] Lymphoproliferations with features consistent with those described for angioimmunoblastic lymphadenopathy with dysproteinemia or for immunoblastic lymphadenopathy are considered AITCL from the onset.[5]

AITCLs partially or completely efface the lymph node architecture and often extend beyond the capsule into perinodal soft tissue (**Fig. 1**A). Clusters of neoplastic T-cell immunoblasts with "clear" cytoplasm have a perivascular distribution and are associated with a polymorphic reactive cell background of small lymphocytes, plasma cells, eosinophils, and histiocytes (see **Fig. 1**A inset). Proliferated blood vessels resemble high endothelial venules and often have a branching or "arborizing" pattern. An irregular meshwork of proliferated follicular dendritic cell (FDC) processes typically surrounds the vessels.

The T-cell immunoblasts usually comprise only 5% to 30% of the cells in the infiltrate and have phenotypic attributes of follicular T-helper cells, including expression of CD4, CD10, CXCL13, and PD-1 (CD279)[6–8] (see **Fig. 1**B, C). Furthermore, gene expression profiling has established a molecular link between AITCL and follicular T-helper cells.[9]

Other characteristics of AITCL include T-cell antigen loss, CD21 staining of the FDC meshworks (see **Fig. 1**D), and an increased number of Epstein-Barr virus (EBV)-positive B-cell immunoblasts, as detected by in situ hybridization using probes for EBV-encoded RNA.[5] Clonal TCR gene rearrangements are detected in 75% or more of AITCLs, and a smaller number of these cases have clonal immunoglobulin gene

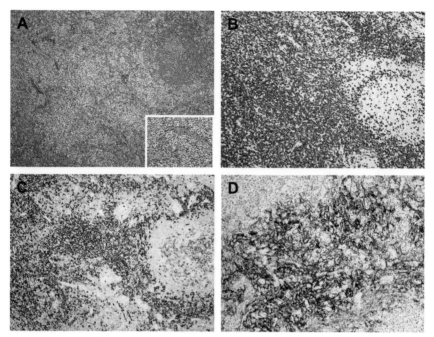

Fig. 1. Angioimmunoblastic T-cell lymphoma. (*A*) Stain of a lymph node showing distorted architecture with proliferation of clear cells and high endothelial cell venules (hematoxylin-eosin, medium power). Inset shows mixed infiltrate and clear cell cytology (hematoxylin-eosin, high power). (*B*) CD3 stain. (*C*) CD10 stain. (*D*) CD21 stain shows expanded and distorted FDC meshworks. (*Courtesy of* Dragan Jevremovic, MD, Rochester, MN.)

rearrangements.[5] Trisomy 3, trisomy 8, and an additional X chromosome are the most frequent cytogenetic abnormalities.[5]

Serial lymph node biopsies in patients with AITCL show that some of the lymphomas have histologic progression in total number of tumor cells with time, whereas a smaller number of cases may subsequently develop EBV+ diffuse large B-cell lymphomas or classical Hodgkin lymphomas.[10]

ANAPLASTIC LARGE CELL LYMPHOMA

Systemic anaplastic large cell lymphoma (ALCL) has a bimodal age distribution with a large peak in childhood and young adults and a small peak in older adults.[11] There is a male predominance in younger patients and a slight female predominance in older patients. Most patients present with lymphadenopathy and/or extranodal masses and B symptoms. Systemic ALCL is a moderately aggressive disease, and prognosis is closely associated with anaplastic lymphoma kinase (ALK) protein expression. ALK+ ALCLs have a 5-year OS of approximately 70%, whereas ALK− ALCLs have a 5-year OS of approximately 49%.[4] ALCLs have been reported adjacent to breast implants.[12,13] These cases are often seroma-associated and appear to have an indolent clinical course.[12]

The neoplastic cells are pleomorphic large cells that may appear cohesive and may completely efface the nodal architecture or be confined to the sinuses (**Fig. 2**A). The "hallmark" tumor cell is large with irregular nuclear contours, a prominent nucleolus,

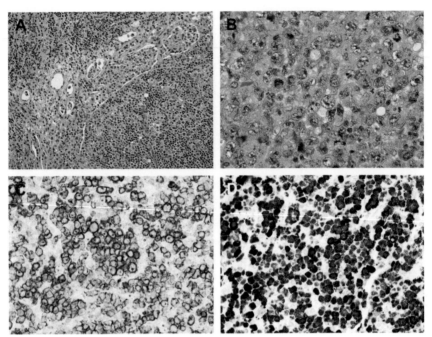

Fig. 2. ALCL. (*A*) Stain of a lymph node showing intrasinusoidal infiltrate of large atypical cells (hematoxylin-eosin, medium power). (*B*) Hallmark cells with kidney bean-shaped nuclei and high mitotic activity. (*C*) CD30 stain. (*D*) ALK-1 (nuclear and cytoplasmic positivity). (*Courtesy of* Dragan Jevremovic, MD, Rochester, MN.)

and abundant eosinophilic cytoplasm in which there may be a perinuclear clear region (see **Fig. 2**B). Some may have horseshoe- or doughnut-shaped nuclei or are multinucleate. Histologic patterns include the common variant (70% of cases) with pleomorphic or monomorphic cytology among the tumor cells, lymphohistiocytic variant (10%), small-cell variant (5% to 10%), and Hodgkin-like variant (3%).[14–17]

By definition, the tumor cells are CD30+ (see **Fig. 2**C). Most (70%–80%) have a T-cell phenotype, but absence of multiple T-cell antigens is frequently seen. A small number (10%–20%) completely lack T-cell and B-cell antigen expression and are regarded as having a null phenotype. CD30+ large-cell lymphomas that exclusively express B-cell antigens are classified among diffuse large B-cell lymphomas. Approximately 70% to 80% of ALCLs are ALK+ with most of these demonstrating cytoplasmic and nuclear staining (see **Fig. 2**D). Other ALK+ ALCLs have cytoplasmic staining only. No significant differences in survival have been seen between patients whose tumors have different ALK staining patterns.

A nonrandom t(2;5)(p23;q35) chromosomal abnormality is present in approximately 60% of ALCLs, which translocates a novel *ALK* gene (chromosome 2p23) next to the nucleolar organizing gene nucleophosmin (*NPM*) (chromosome 5q35) producing expression of a fusion protein recognized by cytoplasmic and nuclear staining by the ALK1 antibody.[14] Several variant 2p23 translocations have been described in approximately 20% of ALK+ ALCLs, which translocate the *ALK* gene to chromosome partners other than *NPM*.[18] These variant translocations are associated with cytoplasmic-only ALK staining. *ALK* translocations are seen mostly in young patients and in primary nodal cases.

Most (86%) ALCLs have clonal TCR gene rearrangements, and few (10%) have concomitant immunoglobulin gene rearrangements.[19] Gene expression profiling can distinguish ALK+ from ALK- systemic ALCLs, suggesting that they are two different entities.[20] Tumor cells are EBV− in most ALCLs.[19]

PERIPHERAL T-CELL LYMPHOMA, UNSPECIFIED

PTCL, unspecified is the most common type of PTCL and is a waste basket category for PTCLs that do not fit any of the defined disease entities in the WHO classification. However, specific entities may arise from this broad group of PTCLs. Patients with PTCL, unspecified are generally adults who present with generalized lymphadenopathy and B symptoms. This tends to be an aggressive group of tumors that have a 5-year OS of approximately 32%.[4]

Morphologic features are variable, but most cases have a diffuse growth pattern that effaces the nodal architecture. Tumor cells vary in size, often have clear cytoplasm, and may be multinucleate, resembling Reed-Sternberg cells (**Fig. 3**A). Histologic variants recognized by the WHO classification, but which do not merit segregating as specific diseases, include lymphoepithelioid (Lennert) lymphoma, T-zone lymphoma, and follicular T-cell lymphoma.[21] Lymphoepithelioid lymphoma effaces the tissue architecture and consists mostly of small tumor cells located between evenly dispersed clusters of epithelioid histiocytes (see **Fig. 3**B). T-zone lymphoma has a perifollicular growth pattern of small tumor cells that spare lymphoid follicles (see **Fig. 3**C). Follicular T-cell lymphoma is composed of intrafollicular

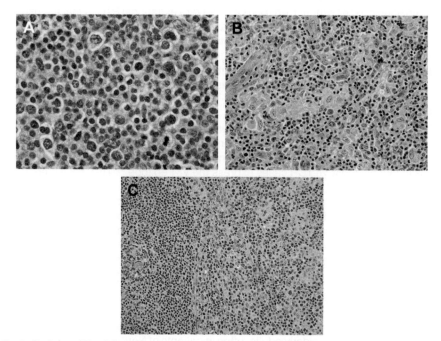

Fig. 3. Peripheral T-cell lymphoma, unspecified type (morphologic variants). (*A*) Stain of the pleomorphic variant (hematoxylin-eosin, high power). (*B*) Stain of the lymphoepithelioid (Lennert) variant (hematoxylin-eosin, medium power). (*C*) Stain of the T-zone variant (*right*) next to germinal center (*left*) (hematoxylin-eosin, high power). (*Courtesy of* Dragan Jevremovic, MD, Rochester, MN.)

aggregates of irregular T cells with clear cytoplasm that may mimic follicular or marginal zone lymphomas.[22]

Aberrant T-cell phenotypes are often encountered. Most nodal cases have αβ TCRs, but a few have γδ TCRs.[23] Occasional nodal PTCL, unspecified expresses a cytotoxic (TIA-1+, granzyme B+, and/or perforin+) T-cell phenotype, and these tumors may behave more aggressively than their noncytotoxic counterparts.[24] Most PTCLs, unspecified have clonal TCR gene rearrangements. EBV can be detected in a significant number of PTCLs, unspecified, and its presence in nodes involved by this lymphoma in elderly patients has been associated with a worse OS.[25]

Pathogenetic chromosomal abnormalities for PTCL, unspecified have been unrecognized for the most part.[26] However, some clinicopathologic entities may emerge based on recently identified recurrent cytogenetic abnormalities. For instance, a small number of cases with features of follicular T-cell lymphoma have a t(5;9)(q33;q32) that fuses *ITK* and *SYK*, which results in a fusion protein with constitutive activation of the SYK tyrosine kinase.[27] Additionally, 2 PTCLs, unspecified with t(6;14)(p25;q11.2), in which the interferon regulatory factor-4 (*IRF4*) locus is fused with the TCR-α (*TCRA*) locus, have been described, and both involved the skin and bone marrow and had a cytotoxic phenotype.[28]

Finally, gene expression profiling has not shown a single molecular profile for PTCL, unspecified, but has provided some insights into pathogenesis and identity of new potential therapeutic targets.[29,30]

HEPATOSPLENIC T-CELL LYMPHOMA

Hepatosplenic T-cell lymphomas (HSTCLs) are rare extranodal PTCLs that are usually diagnosed in patients who present with massive hepatosplenomegaly, no lymphadenopathy, B symptoms, moderate anemia, and marked thrombocytopenia. The subtype with δγ TCRs is generally seen in young adult males,[31] and the subtype with αβ TCRs seems to occur more frequently in females.[32] This tumor may also occur as a posttransplant lymphoproliferative disorder or in patients with Crohn disease treated with azathioprine and infliximab.[33,34] HSTCL is aggressive and has a 5-year OS of only 7%.[4]

The tumor cells are typically small to intermediate in size and preferentially infiltrate splenic sinuses, hepatic sinusoids, and bone marrow sinuses (**Fig. 4**). The neoplastic cells generally lack CD4, CD5, and CD7 and express either γδ TCRs (majority) or αβ TCRs (minority). Most γδ TCR cases express the Vδ1 epitope.[35] They have a nonactivated cytotoxic (TIA-1+ and granzyme B−/perforin−) T-cell phenotype and often show aberrant coincident expression of multiple killer immunoglobulin-like receptor isoforms.[36] Clonal TCR gene rearrangements are present in most cases. EBV is detectable in the tumor cells of very few cases. Isochromosome 7q is seen in many HSTCLs, but is not specific for this disease.[37] Trisomy 8 and loss of a sex chromosome are also frequently found. Gene expression profiling shows single clustering of HSγδTCLs, but a scattered distribution for other γδ PTCLs.[38]

ENTEROPATHY-ASSOCIATED T-CELL LYMPHOMA

Enteropathy-associated T-cell lymphomas (EATCLs) are rare extranodal PTCLs that occur in middle-aged to elderly adults, often in patients of Northern European descent with a history of celiac disease.[39] Patients present most often because of abdominal pain and weight loss. There may be signs of acute obstruction or perforation. Diarrhea may be present. The lymphomas are most often in the jejunum, but other gastrointestinal sites can be involved infrequently. The lesions may be multifocal small ulcers

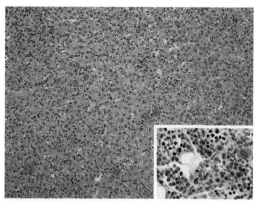

Fig. 4. HSTCL. Stain showing liver parenchyma with intrasinusoidal infiltrate of medium-sized atypical cells (hematoxylin-eosin, medium power). Inset shows intrasinusoidal infiltrate within the bone marrow. (*Courtesy of* Dragan Jevremovic, MD, Rochester, MN.)

("ulcerative jejunitis") or large masses. The lymphoma is aggressive and has a 5-year OS of approximately 20%.[4]

Two histologic subgroups have been identified that correlate with clinical and immunophenotypic features.[40] EATCLs with pleomorphic large tumor cells are usually associated with a history of celiac disease, have morphologic features of malabsorption, and tend to be CD56− (80% of cases) (**Fig. 5**). EATCLs with monomorphic small to medium size tumor cells often occur without a history of celiac disease, may lack morphologic features of malabsorption, and tend to be CD56+ (20%). Tumor cells, believed to arise from intraepithelial T cells, have a cytotoxic T-cell phenotype and often have lost T-cell antigens. Clonal TCR gene rearrangements can be detected in most cases. EBV is present in tumor cells in few EATCLs. Gains of chromosome 9q33-q34 are seen in up to 70% of EATCLs and are rarely detected in other PTCLs.[41]

EXTRANODAL NK/T-CELL LYMPHOMA, NASAL TYPE

Extranodal NK/T-cell lymphomas (NK/TCLs) almost always present in extranodal sites, particularly in the upper aerodigestive tract (nasal cavity, nasopharynx, and

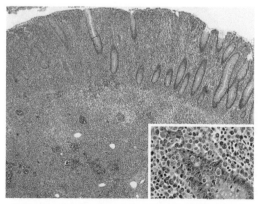

Fig. 5. EATCL. Stain of the ulcerated mass composed of atypical lymphocytes invading the bowel wall. Inset shows atypical intraepithelial lymphocytes (hematoxylin-eosin, medium power). (*Courtesy of* Dragan Jevremovic, MD, Rochester, MN.)

palate).[42] It has previously been termed "polymorphic reticulosis" and "lethal midline granuloma." NK/TCLs are most prevalent in adults in East Asia, Mexico, and Central and South America; they are uncommon in the Unites States, Canada, and Western Europe. Patients may have B symptoms and often present with nasal obstruction, epistaxis, or midfacial destructive lesions. The tumor may extend into the paranasal sinuses and orbit. It may disseminate to or arise at other sites, particularly skin, gastrointestinal tract, and testis. Primary nodal NK/TCLs are rare.[43] These lymphomas are aggressive and have a 5-year OS of approximately 42%.[4]

The characteristic morphologic features for NK/TCLs are angiocentric, angioinvasive, and angiodestructive infiltrates of cytologically atypical lymphocytes of varying size (**Fig. 6**). Necrosis is generally present and may be extensive. Most NK/TCLs appear to be lymphomas of true NK cells based on their phenotype (CD2+, surface CD3−, CD56+, TCRαβ− and TCRγδ−, and expression of cytotoxic granule-associated proteins) and on their lack of clonal TCR receptor gene rearrangements. A small number of NK/TCLs arise from T cells (CD2+, surface CD3±, CD56±, TCRαβ+ or TCRγδ+, and expression of cytotoxic granule-associated proteins), which demonstrate clonal TCR gene rearrangements. EBV+ tumor cells are found in the vast majority of NK/TCLs (see **Fig. 6** inset). No recurring chromosomal translocations have been reported.

MYCOSIS FUNGOIDES

Mycosis fungoides (MF) is rare, but it is the most common form of cutaneous T-cell lymphoma and is derived from CD4+ T cells of skin-associated lymphoid tissue.[44] It is an indolent disease with a protracted course that occurs most often in middle-aged to elderly adults. Two-thirds of cases are in males. The skin lesions of MF tend to be on the trunk and include erythematous patches, thickened plaques, nodular tumors, and generalized erythroderma. Patches and plaques may persist for years and eventually become more generalized and progress to tumors. Extracutaneous dissemination to lymph nodes and visceral organs is a late manifestation. Patients with Sézary syndrome (SS) have generalized erythroderma, lymphadenopathy, and peripheral blood involvement. Survival is dependent on stage, and patients with limited patch/plaque disease have survival equal to age-matched controls. The

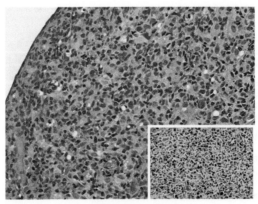

Fig. 6. Extranodal NK/TCL, nasal type: stain of the nasal polyp showing diffuse infiltrate by medium to large size atypical lymphocytes (hematoxylin-eosin, medium power). Inset shows in situ hybridization for Epstein-Barr virus. (*Courtesy of* Dragan Jevremovic, MD, Rochester, MN.)

10-year disease-specific survival for tumor stage is approximately 42%, and this drops to 20% with histologically proven lymph-node involvement.

Plaque-stage lesions are characterized by a dense, band-like, superficial dermal infiltrate of atypical, hyperchromatic cerebriform lymphocytes that extend into the epidermis (epidermotropism) (**Fig. 7**A). Pautrier microabscesses, intraepidermal collections of cerebriform lymphocytes, may be seen. Patch and early plaque stage lesions may be nondiagnostic because the lymphocytes are less dense and have less cytologic atypia. The most reliable histologic features of early MF are the presence of medium to large (nuclear diameters approximately equal to those of basal keratinocytes) cerebriform cells in the epidermis or in dermal clusters.[45] Epidermotropism as single cells lined up among basal keratinocytes at the epidermal-dermal junction, absence of significant papillary dermal fibrosis, and absence of significant numbers of blast-like cells are other useful histologic features of early MF.[45] Tumor-stage MF is generally concentrated in the upper dermis, but epidermotropism is often lost. Large cell transformation may occur in tumor-stage MF.[46] Cutaneous infiltrates in SS are often nondiagnostic because of the mild degree of lymphoid infiltrates and lack of epidermotropism. The diagnosis of SS can usually be made by examination of the peripheral blood for circulating tumor cells and by demonstration of restricted TCR Vβ chain use by flow cytometry.[47]

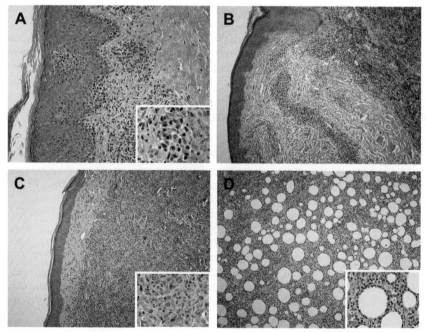

Fig. 7. Cutaneous T-cell lymphomas. (*A*) MF. Superficial dermal (lichenoid) and intraepidermal infiltrate of atypical small to medium size lymphocytes with irregular nuclear contours (cerebriform). (*B*) Primary cutaneous CD4+ small/medium T-cell lymphoma. Deep dermal infiltrate of atypical cells surrounding adnexal structures. (*C*) Primary cutaneous ALCL. Dermal infiltrate of large atypical cells with abundant cytoplasm. (*D*) Subcutaneous panniculitis-like T-cell lymphoma. Infiltrate of atypical lymphocytes in the subcutaneous tissue rimming individual adipocytes. (*Courtesy of* Dragan Jevremovic, MD, Rochester, MN.)

The tumor cells in most MF are CD4+ T cells that lack CD7. Aberrant T-cell phenotypes are not usually apparent until late plaque or tumor stages. Loss of CD26 is characteristic of the tumor cells in SS. Clonal TCR gene rearrangements can be detected in 80% to 90% of MF cases. Characteristic cytogenetic abnormalities have not been identified.

PRIMARY CUTANEOUS PERIPHERAL T-CELL LYMPHOMAS

The term cutaneous T-cell lymphomas should not be used synonymously with MF because of the recognition of a variety of primary cutaneous PTCLs that have no relationship with MF.

Primary cutaneous CD4+ small/medium T-cell lymphoma usually presents as a solitary plaque or nodule in the head and neck region or upper trunk.[44,48] Pleomorphic small to medium-sized CD4+ T cells form dense dermal infiltrates with little proclivity for epidermotropism (see **Fig. 7**B). This is an indolent disease with approximately 80% 5-year survival.

Primary cutaneous $\gamma\delta$ T-cell lymphoma usually presents as patches/plaques or deep dermal or subcutaneous nodules on the extremities of middle-aged patients.[44] Medium to large $\gamma\delta$ T cells that express CD56 and are negative for CD4, CD5, and CD8 infiltrate the dermis, sometimes with subcutaneous (resembling subcutaneous panniculitis-like T-cell lymphoma) or epidermal involvement. This is an aggressive disease with a median survival of 10 to 15 months.

Primary cutaneous CD8+ aggressive epidermotropic cytotoxic T-cell lymphoma is characterized by rapidly developing localized or disseminated papules or nodules that are often ulcerated.[44] Pleomorphic CD8+ cytotoxic (TIA-1+, granzyme B+, and perforin+) T cells infiltrate the superficial dermis and produce pagetoid epidermal involvement. This is an aggressive disease with median survival of approximately 32 months.

PRIMARY CUTANEOUS ANAPLASTIC LARGE CELL LYMPHOMA

Primary cutaneous anaplastic large cell lymphoma (C-ALCL) shares overlapping features with lymphomatoid papulosis (LyP) and with borderline lesions, all of which are included among the primary cutaneous CD30+ T-cell lymphoproliferative disorders in the WHO classification.[44] C-ALCL usually presents in adults as solitary or localized nodules that may undergo partial necrosis and resolution, but it does not spontaneously regress like LyP. C-ALCL has a 5-year OS of approximately 90%.[4]

The tumor cells involve the dermis extensively, may infiltrate subcutaneous tissue, and have little epidermotropism (see **Fig. 7**C). The neoplastic cells have similar cytologic features as those in systemic ALCL (see **Fig. 7**C inset). Greater than 75% of the atypical large cells are CD30+, and they are ALK−. C-ALCLs generally have clonal TCR gene rearrangements. They lack translocations involving ALK, but approximately one-half of C-ALCLs have IRF4 (6p25) translocations to yet-to-be-determined partner genes.[28]

SUBCUTANEOUS PANNICULITIS-LIKE T-CELL LYMPHOMA

Subcutaneous panniculitis-like T-cell lymphomas (SPTCLs) present as multiple nontender erythematous subcutaneous nodules of varying size on the extremities and/or trunk of younger adults who have B symptoms.[44,49] Dissemination to extracutaneous sites is unusual. Patients with SPTCLs have a 5-year OS of approximately 64%.[4]

Development of aggressive disease often correlates with the onset of a hemophago-cytic syndrome.

Pleomorphic tumor cells of varying size with hyperchromatic nuclei have a lobular panniculitis-like pattern of infiltration that is usually confined to the subcutis (see **Fig. 7**D). Tumor cells frequently rim the margins of fat spaces (see **Fig. 7**D inset). Karyorrhexis and fat necrosis are always present to some extent. Angioinvasion may occur, but angiodestruction is not a feature. The neoplastic cells are always cytotoxic (TIA-1+, granzyme B+, and perforin+) $\alpha\beta$ T cells that are usually CD8+. Aberrant T-cell phenotypes are commonly displayed. Clonal TCR gene rearrange-ments are present in most cases. SPTCLs are EBV−.

ADULT T-CELL LEUKEMIA/LYMPHOMA

Adult T-cell leukemia/lymphoma (ATLL) is a human T-lymphotropic virus 1 (HTLV-1)–associated malignancy that occurs in adults most frequently where the virus is endemic (southwestern Japan, central Africa, and the Caribbean basin).[50] There are 4 major presentations: acute, lymphomatous, chronic, and smoldering. The acute subtype is most common (60% of cases) and is associated with severe peripheral blood lymphocytosis, hypercalcemia, lytic bone lesions, hepatosplenomegaly, elevated serum lactate dehydrogenase, and a rapidly progressive course with a 6-month median survival. The lymphomatous subtype (20% of cases) is associated with generalized lymphadenopathy without leukemia and a median survival of approx-imately 1 year. The chronic subtype (15% of cases) may have a low level absolute lymphocytosis in the peripheral blood associated with an exfoliative skin rash and a median survival greater than 2 years. The smoldering subtype (5% of cases) has a normal peripheral blood lymphocyte count and a small number of circulating tumor cells and skin rashes. There is no lymphadenopathy, hepatosplenomegaly, or hyper-calcemia. Median survival for this type of ATLL is more than 2 years, but less than 10 years.

Circulating tumor cells are medium to large with multilobated nuclei (called "flower" or "cloverleaf" cells). Lymphomatous infiltrates are diffuse and are composed of pleo-morphic cells of varying size that efface the nodal architecture. Bone marrow speci-mens are generally involved by ATLL, but often to a lesser extent than would be expected for the degree of peripheral blood involvement. Cutaneous infiltrates are dermal, but may be epidermotropic with formation of Pautrier microabscesses similar to MF. The neoplastic cells are CD4+, CD7−, and CD25+ T cells that express FoxP3, phenotypic characteristics of regulatory T cells (Treg) responsible for suppressing T-cell effector function.[51] TCR gene rearrangements can be detected, and clonal inte-gration of HTLV-1 genome can be demonstrated.

ACKNOWLEDGMENT

The author greatly appreciates the contribution of the photomicrographs and figure legends by Dr. Dragan Jevremovic from the Division of Hematopathology, Department of Laboratory Medicine and Pathology, Mayo Clinic, Rochester, MN.

REFERENCES

1. Jamal S, Picker LJ, Aquino DB, et al. Immunophenotypic analysis of peripheral T-cell neoplasms. A multiparameter flow cytometric approach. Am J Clin Pathol 2001;116:512–26.

2. Brüggemann M, White H, Gaulard P, et al. Powerful strategy for polymerase chain reaction-based clonality assessment in T-cell malignancies. Report of the BIOMED-2 Concerted Action BHM4 CT98-3936. Leukemia 2007;21:215–21.
3. Jaffe ES, Harris NL, Stein H, et al. Introduction and overview of the classification of the lymphoid neolplasms. In: Swerdlow SH, Campo E, Harris NL, et al, editors. WHO classification of tumours of haematopoietic and lymphoid tissues. Lyon: IARC; 2008. p. 158–66.
4. Armitage J, Vose J, Weisenburger D. International peripheral T-cell and natural killer/T-cell lymphoma study: pathology findings and clinical outcomes. J Clin Oncol 2008;26:4124–30.
5. Dogan A, Attygalle AD, Kyriakou C. Angioimmunoblastic T-cell lymphoma. Br J Haematol 2003;121:681–91.
6. Attygalle A, Al-Jehani R, Diss TC, et al. Neoplastic T-cells in angioimmunoblastic T-cell lymphoma express CD10. Blood 2002;99:627–33.
7. Grogg KL, Attygalle AD, Macon WR, et al. Angioimmunoblastic T-cell lymphoma: a neoplasm of germinal-center T-helper cells? Blood 2005;106:1501–2.
8. Dorfman DM, Brown JA, Shahsafaei A, et al. Programmed death-1 (PD-1) is a marker of germinal center-associated T cells and angioimmunoblastic T-cell lymphoma. Am J Surg Pathol 2006;30:802–10.
9. de Leval L, Rickman DS, Thielen C, et al. The gene expression profile of nodal peripheral T-cell lymphoma demonstrates a molecular link between angioimmunoblastic T-cell lymphoma (AITL) and follicular helper T (T_{FH}) cells. Blood 2007;109:4952–63.
10. Attygalle AD, Kyriakou C, Dupuis J, et al. Histologic evolution of angioimmunoblastic T-cell lymphoma in consecutive biopsies: clinical correlation and insights into natural history and disease progression. Am J Surg Pathol 2007;31:1077–88.
11. Medeiros LJ, Elenitoba-Johnson KS. Anaplastic large cell lymphoma. Am J Clin Pathol 2007;127:707–22.
12. Roden AC, Macon WR, Keeney GL, et al. Seroma-associated primary anaplastic large-cell lymphoma adjacent to breast implants: an indolent T-cell lymphoproliferative disorder. Mod Pathol 2008;21:455–63.
13. de Jong D, Vasmel WLE, de Boer JP, et al. Anaplastic large-cell lymphoma in women with breast implants. JAMA 2008;300:2030–5.
14. Benharroch D, Meguerian-Bedoyan Z, Lamant L, et al. ALK-positive lymphoma: a single disease with a broad spectrum of morphology. Blood 1998;91:2076–84.
15. Pileri S, Falini B, Delsol G, et al. Lymphohistiocytic T-cell lymphoma (anaplastic large cell lymphoma CD30+/Ki-1+ with a high content of reactive histiocytes). Histopatholology 1990;16:383–91.
16. Kinney MC, Collins RD, Greer JP, et al. A small cell-predominant variant of primary Ki-1 (CD30)+ T-cell lymphoma. Am J Surg Pathol 1993;17:859–68.
17. Vassallo J, Lamant L, Brugieres L, et al. ALK-positive anaplastic large cell lymphoma mimicking nodular sclerosis Hodgkin's lymphoma: report of 10 cases. Am J Surg Pathol 2006;30:223–9.
18. Pulford K, Lamant L, Espinos E, et al. The emerging normal and disease-related roles of anaplastic lymphoma kinase. Cell Mol Life Sci 2004;61:2939–53.
19. Tan BT, Seo K, Warnke RA, et al. The frequency of immunoglobulin heavy chain gene and T-cell receptor γ-chain gene rearrangements and Epstein-Barr virus in ALK+ and ALK⁻ anaplastic large cell lymphoma and other peripheral T-cell lymphomas. J Mol Diagn 2008;10:502–12.
20. Lamant L, de Reyniès A, Duplantier MM, et al. Gene-expression profiling of systemic anaplastic large-cell lymphoma reveals differences based on ALK status and two distinct morphologic ALK+ subtypes. Blood 2007;109:2156–64.

21. Pileri SA, Weisenburger DD, Sng I, et al. Peripheral T-cell lymphoma, not otherwise specified. In: Swerdlow SH, Campo E, Harris NL, et al, editors. WHO classification of tumours of haematopoietic and lymphoid tissues. Lyon: IARC; 2008. p. 306–8.
22. de Leval L, Savilo E, Longtine J, et al. Peripheral T-cell lymphoma with follicular involvement and a CD4+/bcl-6+ phenotype. Am J Surg Pathol 2001;25: 395–400.
23. Saito T, Matsuno Y, Tanosaki R, et al. Gamma delta T-cell neoplasms: a clinicopathological study of 11 cases. Ann Oncol 2002;13:1792–8.
24. Asano N, Suzuki R, Kagami Y, et al. Clinicopathologic and prognostic significance of cytotoxic molecule expression in nodal peripheral T-cell lymphoma, unspecified. Am J Surg Pathol 2005;29:1284–93.
25. Dupuis J, Emile JF, Mounier N, et al. Prognostic significance of Epstein-Barr virus in nodal peripheral T-cell lymphoma, unspecified: a Groupe d'Etude des Lymphomes de l'Adulte (GELA) study. Blood 2006;108:4163–9.
26. Nelson M, Horsman DE, Weisenburger DD, et al. Cytogenetic abnormalities and clinical correlations in peripheral T-cell lymphoma. Br J Haematol 2008;141:461–9.
27. Streubel B, Vinatzer U, Willheim M, et al. Novel t(5;9)(q33;q22) fuses ITK to SYK in unspecified peripheral T-cell lymphoma. Leukemia 2006;20:313–8.
28. Feldman AL, Law M, Remstein ED, et al. Recurrent translocations involving the IRF4 oncogene locus in peripheral T-cell lymphomas. Leukemia 2009;23:574–80.
29. Ballester B, Ramuz O, Gisselbrecht C, et al. Gene expression profiling identifies molecular subgroups among nodal peripheral T-cell lymphomas. Oncogene 2006;25(10):1560–70.
30. Piccaluga PP, Agostinelli C, Califano A, et al. Gene expression analysis of peripheral T cell lymphoma, unspecified, reveals distinct profiles and new potential therapeutic targets. J Clin Oncol 2007;117:823–34.
31. Belhadj K, Reyes F, Farcet JP, et al. Hepatosplenic γδ T-cell lymphoma is a rare clinicopathologic entity with poor outcome: report of a series of 21 patients. Blood 2003;102:4261–9.
32. Macon WR, Levy NB, Kurtin PJ, et al. Hepatosplenic αβ T-cell lymphomas: a report of 14 cases and comparison with hepatosplenic γδ T-cell lymphomas. Am J Surg Pathol 2001;25:285–96.
33. Swerdlow SH. T-cell and NK-cell posttransplantation lymphoproliferative disorders. Am J Clin Pathol 2007;127:887–95.
34. Mackey AC, Green L, Liang LC, et al. Hepatosplenic T cell lymphoma associated with infliximab use in young patients treated for inflammatory bowel disease. J Pediatr Gastroenterol Nutr 2007;44:265–7.
35. Przybylski GK, Wu H, Macon WR, et al. Hepatosplenic and subcutaneous panniculitis-like γ/δ T cell lymphomas are derived from different Vγ subsets of γ/δ T lymphocytes. J Mol Diagn 2000;2:11–9.
36. Morice WG, Macon WR, Dogan A, et al. NK-cell-associated receptor expression in hepatosplenic T-cell lymphoma, insights into pathogenesis. Leukemia 2006;20: 883–6.
37. Feldman AL, Law M, Grogg KL, et al. Incidence of TCR and TCL1 translocations and isochromosome 7q in peripheral T-cell lymphomas using fluorescence in situ hybridization. Am J Clin Pathol 2008;130:178–85.
38. Miyazaki K, Yamaguchi M, Imai H, et al. Gene expression profiling of peripheral T-cell lymphoma including γδ T-cell lymphoma. Blood 2009;113:1071–4.
39. Zettl A, deLeeuw R, Haralambieva E, et al. Enteropathy-type T-cell lymphoma. Am J Clin Pathol 2007;127:701–6.

40. deLeeuw RJ, Zettl A, Klinker E, et al. Whole-genome analysis and HLA genotyping of enteropathy-type T-cell lymphoma reveals 2 distinct lymphoma subtypes. Gastroenterology 2007;132:1902–11.

41. Zettl A, Ott G, Makulik A, et al. Chromosomal gains at 9q characterize enteropathy-type T-cell lymphoma. Am J Pathol 2002;161:1635–45.

42. Hasserjian RP, Harris NL. NK-cell lymphomas and leukemias. A spectrum of tumors with variable manifestations and immunophenotype. Am J Clin Pathol 2007;127:860–8.

43. Takahashi E, Asano N, Li C, et al. Nodal T/NK-cell lymphoma of nasal type: a clinicopathologic study of six cases. Histopathology 2008;52:585–96.

44. Kinney MC, Jones D. Cutaneous T-cell and NK-cell lymphomas. The WHO-EORTC classification and the increasing recognition of specialized tumor types. Am J Clin Pathol 2007;127:670–86.

45. Santucci M, Biggeri A, Feller AC, et al. Efficacy of histologic criteria for diagnosing early mycosis fungoides. An EORTC Cutaneous Lymphoma Study Group investigation. Am J Surg Pathol 2002;24:40–50.

46. Salhany KE, Cousar JB, Greer JP, et al. Transformation of cutaneous T cell lymphoma to large cell lymphoma: a clinicopathologic and immunologic study. Am J Pathol 1988;132:265–77.

47. Morice WG, Kimlinger T, Katzmann JA, et al. Flow cytometric assessment of TCR-V_β expression in the evaluation of peripheral blood involvement by T-cell lymphoproliferative disorders. A comparison with conventional T-cell immunophenotyping and molecular genetic techniques. Am J Clin Pathol 2004;121:373–83.

48. Grogg KL, Jung S, Erickson LA, et al. Primary cutaneous CD4-positive small/medium-sized pleomorphic T-cell lymphoma: a clonal T-cell lymphoproliferative disorder with indolent behavior. Mod Pathol 2008;21:708–15.

49. Willemze R, Jansen PM, Cerroni L, et al. Subcutaneous panniculitis-like T-cell lymphoma: definition, classification, and prognostic factors: an EORTC Cutaneous Lymphoma Group Study of 83 cases. Blood 2008;111:838–45.

50. Matutes E. Adult T-cell leukaemia/lymphoma. J Clin Pathol 2007;60:1373–7.

51. Karube K, Ohshima K, Tsuchiya T, et al. Expression of FoxP3, a key molecule in CD4+CD25+ regulatory T-cells, in adult T-cell leukaemia/lymphoma cells. Br J Haematol 2004;126:81–4.

The Leukemias of Mature Lymphocytes

Eric D. Hsi, MD

KEYWORDS

- Leukemia • Chronic lymphocytic leukemia • Flow cytometry
- Interphase fluorescence in situ hybridization

The leukemias of mature B cells and T cells are a limited set of diseases in which blood and bone marrow are the primary sites of involvement. Although any B-cell lymphoproliferative disorder can eventually enter a leukemic phase, this article is limited to B-cell chronic lymphocytic leukemia (CLL), B-prolymphocytic leukemia (PLL), hairy cell leukemia (HCL), and HCL variant (HCLv). Burkitt leukemia/lymphoma and the so-called splenic lymphoma with villous lymphocytes (SLVL or splenic marginal zone lymphoma [SMZL]) are dealt with elsewhere. Likewise, we focus on T-cell lymphoproliferative processes that are primarily leukemic, including T-large granular lymphocyte leukemia, T-cell PLL, and adult T-cell leukemia/lymphoma (ATLL).

CHRONIC LYMPHOCYTIC LEUKEMIA
Introduction

CLL is the most common leukemia in the Western world. The age-adjusted estimated annual incidence in the United States is approximately 3.8/100,000.[1] The median age at diagnosis is approximately 65 years with a 2:1 male-to-female ratio.[1] CLL is an indolent leukemia with a disease course that can often span more than 15 years. In fact, many patients may die with their disease rather than from it. Effective therapies do exist, particularly when used early in the disease course, that can induce remissions. However, relapses inevitably occur. Thus, CLL is currently considered incurable in the vast majority of cases, and new therapies are needed.

Clinical Features

Patients present with lymphocytosis greater than $5.0 \times 10^9/l$ by definition.[2] However, it is recognized that patients with monoclonal B cells at lower levels exist and may be considered to have "monoclonal B-cell lymphocytosis" (MBL), which is discussed later. Some CLL patients may be discovered incidentally and are asymptomatic, whereas others may have symptoms relating to organ involvement (splenomegaly, hepatomegaly) or lymphadenopathy. Anemia and other cytopenias are often present due to immune hemolysis related to the leukemia or simple bone marrow replacement

Section of Hematopathology, Department of Clinical Pathology, Cleveland Clinic, L-11, 9500 Euclid Avenue, Cleveland, OH 44195, USA
E-mail address: hsie@ccf.org

Hematol Oncol Clin N Am 23 (2009) 843–871
doi:10.1016/j.hoc.2009.04.006
0889-8588/09/$ – see front matter © 2009 Elsevier Inc. All rights reserved.

by leukemic infiltrates. CLL may progress with increasing numbers of prolymphocytes in the blood, or patients may experience transformation to a large-cell lymphoma (Richter's syndrome), heralded by a sudden change in symptoms or rapid localized lymph node enlargement. Staging systems such as the modified Rai or Binet staging systems are used to predict prognosis in CLL patients (**Table 1**).[2–4] Although these systems are useful in stratifying patients, predicting outcome in intermediate stage patients is still difficult, and biologic predictors are needed.

Morphologic Features

The peripheral blood smear of patients with CLL is characterized by a variable lymphocytosis that may uncommonly reach more than $500 \times 10^9/l$. The lymphocytes are typically small and round with a condensed nuclear chromatin that is often mottled due to areas of extreme condensation alternating with lighter areas, imparting a "soccer ball" or "cracked" chromatin pattern (**Fig. 1**). The cytoplasm is usually scanty. Depending on the quality of blood smear, it may be difficult to distinguish a CLL cell from a normal mature lymphocyte. Variation from the typical form is acceptable within the spectrum of CLL, and some cases may have substantial numbers (>10%) of cells demonstrating nuclear irregularity and/or moderate amounts of pale blue cytoplasm (**Fig. 2**). Some studies have associated such variant morphology with worse outcome.[5,6] Prolymphocytes may be present in varying proportions. These cells are approximately 1.5 to 2.5 times larger than the typical CLL cells with slightly open chromatin and a central nucleolus. Cases in which prolymphocytes comprise greater than 10% but less than 55% of the lymphocytes have been termed "mixed cell" CLL or CLL/PL in the original French-American-British classification scheme[7] but this terminology has been omitted from the World Health Organization (WHO) classification.[8] Increased numbers of prolymphocytes have been associated with a poor prognosis (greater than $5 \times 10^9/l$)[9] and certain genetic abnormalities such as TP53 abnormalities and trisomy 12.[9–11]

The bone marrow may show variable involvement. Four major patterns are recognized: nodular, interstitial, mixed, and diffuse. The nodules tend to be nonparatrabecular. The cells are similar in appearance to those seen in lymph

Table 1
Staging systems for CLL

Staging System	Stage	Clinical Features	Median Survival (y)
Rai (modified)			
Low risk	0	Lymphocytosis[a]	14.5
Intermediate risk	I	Lymphocytosis, lymphadenopathy	7.5
	II	Lymphocytosis, hepatomegaly, and/or splenomegaly	
High risk	III	Lymphocytosis, anemia	2.5
	IV	Lymphocytosis, thrombocytopenia	
Binet	A	Normal Hgb, Plt, <3 areas	14
	B	Normal Hgb, Plt, ≥3 areas	5
	C	Anemia (<10 g/dL) and/or thrombocytopenia (<1 × 10⁹/l)	2.5

Areas, lymph nodes of the head/neck including Waldeyer's ring, lymph nodes of the axillae (bilateral counted as 1 area), lymph nodes of the groin (bilateral also counted as 1 area), splenomegaly, hepatomegaly.
[a] Greater than $5 \times 10^9/L$.

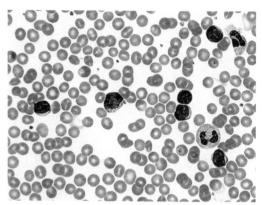

Fig. 1. Peripheral blood smear of a case of CLL demonstrating a lymphocytosis. The lymphocytes are small with condensed chromatin, imparting a "soccer ball" pattern and scant cytoplasm (Wright stain).

node—small and round with condensed chromatin. Proliferation centers (small collections of prolymphocytes in tissue section) can be seen. In the interstitial pattern, the lymphocytes infiltrate around preserved fat spaces, admixed with varying amounts of residual hematopoietic elements. The diffuse pattern, in which there is complete loss of the normal fat pattern with areas totally replaced by sheets of leukemia cells, has been associated with a poor prognosis and more advanced disease (**Fig. 3**).[12–14]

Transformation to PLL is defined by greater than 55% prolymphocytes and is usually characterized by worsening symptoms, loss of response to therapy, and poor prognosis.[15] Richter's syndrome (transformation to an aggressive NHL) occurs in approximately 5% of patients.[16] The transformation usually takes the form of a diffuse aggressive lymphoma such as diffuse large B-cell lymphoma, and survival is short.[17] In most, but not all, cases, the diffuse aggressive B-cell lymphoma is related to the CLL clone.[16,18] Unusual transformations/second malignancies, such as Hodgkin lymphoma, acute lymphoblastic leukemia (ALL), and multiple myeloma, have been reported.[19,20] Of note, Reed-Sternberg (RS) cells in some RS-like cells have been

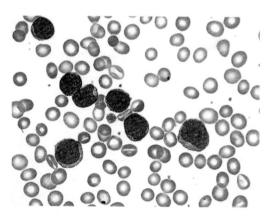

Fig. 2. CLL with variant morphology with irregular nuclei and occasional prolymphocyte in the lower right (Wright stain). Although unusual, cells with irregular nuclear contours can be seen in CLL.

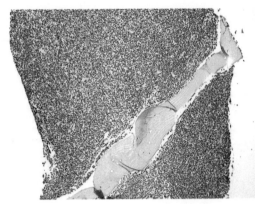

Fig. 3. Bone marrow biopsy of patient with CLL demonstrating a diffuse pattern (hematoxylin-eosin).

shown in some cases to be Epstein-Barr virus (EBV) positive and clonally related to the CLL.[21–23]

Immunophenotype

Multiparameter flow cytometric immunophenotyping is helpful in confirming the diagnosis of CLL and should be done in all cases. The typical immunophenotype has been well characterized. CLL cells express CD5, CD19, CD20, CD22, CD23, and restricted surface immunoglobulin light chain. The expression of CD20 and immunoglobulin is usually dim. Heavy chain expression is usually of the IgM and IgD type. FMC7 and CD79b are absent or only dimly expressed.[24,25] Deviation from this typical immunophenotype occurs, and scoring systems have been proposed to help quantify the likelihood that the diagnosis is CLL (**Table 2**).[25]

Table 2
Proposed scoring system for CLL

Score	CLL	Other B-cell Leukemias	B-NHL
		Number of Cases (%)	
5	209 (52)	0	0
4	139 (35)	0	1 (0.5)
3	39 (10)	1 (1)	7 (4)
2	11 (3)	8 (10)	43 (23)
1	1 (0.2)	25 (33)	75 (39)
0	1 (0.2)	43 (56)	63 (33)

Point system: surface Ig (weak, 1; moderate/strong, 0)
CD5 (positive, 1; negative, 0)
CD23 (positive, 1; negative, 0)
FMC7 (negative, 1; positive, 0)
CD22 (weak/negative, 1; moderate/strong, 0)
   Data from Matutes E, Owusu-Ankomah K, Morilla R, et al. The immunological profile of B-cell disorders and proposal of a scoring system for the diagnosis of CLL. Leukemia 1994; 8(10):1640–5.

One caveat to the presence of restricted light chain expression is the existence of rare cases of biclonal CLL in which a kappa CLL clone and a lambda CLL clone are seen. Cases might seem polytypic but have the other immunophenotypic features of CLL and, on molecular analysis, show biclonal rearrangement patterns. CD5 coexpression helps distinguish these cases from polyclonal B-cell lymphocytosis (see later section).

Two additional markers have been shown to be important in the prognosis of CLL. CD38 is a marker that, initially, was thought to correlate well with *IGH* variable region (*IGH V*) mutational status.[26] The correlation has subsequently been proven to be imperfect, but it has been shown in numerous studies that CD38 expression is a poor prognostic indicator in CLL.[27] Several studies have also shown it to be independent of other clinical parameters.[27–29] The most commonly used cutoff for defining positivity for CD38 is 30% CD38+ leukemic cells. The intracellular nonreceptor tyrosine kinase ZAP-70 has been recently shown to correlate fairly well with *IGH V* mutational status and can also be assessed by flow cytometry or immunohistochemistry.[30] Expression in greater than 20% of CLL cells is associated with germline *IGH V* genes and a poor prognosis.[31,32]

Although initially evaluated for their ability to predict *IGH V* mutational status, these markers are now best thought of as prognostic markers independent of mutational status, and recent studies suggest that, of the two markers, ZAP-70 provides the most valuable information when *IGH* mutational status is known.[33] Methodological variability exists, and standardization of the assay must be accomplished before broad application outside of clinical trials, or treatment stratification based on this assay can be contemplated.[34,35]

Molecular Genetics

Interphase fluorescence in situ hybridization (FISH) studies have revealed many common genetic abnormalities that also have clinical importance (**Table 3**).[36] Deletion of 13q is the most common abnormality and is associated with typical morphology and good prognosis. Trisomy 12 is associated with atypical morphology and intermediate prognosis. Deletion of 11q and deletion of 17p involving TP53 are relatively uncommon but associated with short survival compared with cases without these

Table 3
Frequency of chromosomal abnormalities[a]

Aberration	Percentage of Cases
13q deletion	55
11q deletion	18
Trisomy 12	16
17p deletion	7
6q deletion	6
Trisomy 8q	5
t(14q32)	4
Trisomy 3q	3
Normal	18

[a] Defined by FISH, some cases may have more than one abnormality.
Data from Dohner H, Stilgenbauer S, Benner A, et al. Genomic alterations and survival in chronic lymphocytic leukemia. N Engl J Med 2000; 343:1910–6.

abnormalities. In particular, 17p deletion is associated with resistance to therapy and may warrant alternate therapies.

IGH V mutational status has been shown to be an independent predictor of outcome in CLL.[26,37] IGH V mutational status can be characterized as unmutated based on greater than or equal to 98% homology to the germline sequence. Patients whose CLL cells have unmutated IGH V generally have a poorer prognosis than patients whose CLL cells have mutated IGH V genes. An exception to the prognostic significance of IGH V mutational status occurs when the VH3-21 family is used. This has been shown to be a poor prognostic factor regardless of mutational status.[38,39] ZAP-70 was identified as one molecule that was important in distinguishing mutated (ZAP-70 negative) versus nonmutated CLL (ZAP positive) and was associated with shorter time to treatment from diagnosis.[40,41] As noted above, ZAP-70 expression has subsequently been shown to be a prognostic indicator in CLL.

Differential Diagnosis

The differential diagnosis of CLL includes other B-cell leukemias and peripheralized lymphoma, particularly mantle cell lymphoma (MCL), marginal zone lymphoma, and follicular lymphoma (FL). Given the phenotypic and morphologic similarities, leukemic MCL is an important consideration. Morphologically, MCL cells may show slight nuclear irregularities and occasional intermediately sized cells. Flow cytometry is extremely helpful. Although both CLL and MCL express CD5, CD23 is expressed in most cases of CLL and is absent in MCL. Other useful features include bright CD20 and surface Ig expression in MCL and expression of CD79b and FMC7. The t(11;14)(q13;q32) involving IGH and CCND1 can confirm a diagnosis of leukemic MCL, with the caveat that some cases of myeloma may also have this translocation. However, plasma cell leukemia would not coexpress CD20 and CD5. **Table 4** shows the phenotypic and genetic features of the various B-cell lymphoproliferative disorders. Peripheralized FL may also have individual cells that resemble CLL cells but always has at least occasional, and often many, cells with deep nuclear clefts. Expression of CD10 and lack of CD5 is the rule in FL. Presence of a t(14;18)(q32;q21) is strong evidence against CLL and favors FL. SMZL will typically have occasional cells that have abundant cytoplasm and/or cytoplasmic villous projections. The immunophenotype is that of an immunoglobulin light chain–restricted, CD5-negative, lymphoproliferative disorder. Rare cases of MZL may express CD5.[42] Some cases of CLL do show atypical features such as irregular nuclei or mild deviation from the normal immunophenotype.[6] However, elimination of other serious considerations using combined morphology, flow cytometry, and, when needed, molecular studies allows a confident diagnosis in most cases.

Occasional cases of T-cell PLL can mimic CLL, but careful attention to the morphologic features (small nucleoli) and flow cytometric immunophenotype makes distinction straightforward. Likewise, some cells of ALL (ALL with a French-American-British L-1 morphologic subtype) might have small cells resembling CLL, but close attention to morphologic details, such as chromatin pattern and immunophenotyping, allows easy distinction from CLL.

Persistent polyclonal B-cell lymphocytosis might be mistaken for a B-cell leukemia. This disorder presents most commonly in female smokers with a modest lymphocytosis composed of polyclonal B cells, which may rarely coexpress CD5.[43] Deeply clefted lymphocytes are present, which makes confusion with CLL less likely than with other entities such as leukemic FL. In fact, BCL2/IGH translocations have been detected in these cases but are also polyclonal.[44] Immunophenotyping, as the name implies, shows polytypic B cells.

Table 4
Immunophenotype and molecular genetic features of B-cell chronic lymphoproliferative disorders

	CD5	CD10	CD20	CD23	CD79b	FMC7	CD103	sIg	t (14;18)	t (11;14)
CLL	+	−	+(dim)	+	−/+(dim)	−/+(dim)	−	±(dim)	−	−
MCL	+	−	+	−	+	+	−	+	−	+
MZL	−	−	+	−/+	+	+	−	+	−	−
HCL	−	−/+	+	−	+	+	+	+	−	−
FCL	−	+	+	−/+	+	+	−	±	+	−

Prognosis/Therapy

As noted above, the prognosis varies depending on the stage and biologic marker studies. Still the disease course is measured in years to decades. A conservative approach to therapy is often taken (watch and wait), withholding treatment until the patient becomes symptomatic. Current approved therapies are generally aimed at symptomatic disease and are not curative. Recently, nucleoside analogs such as fludarabine in combination with anti-CD20 (rituximab) have become prominent in first-line therapies.

With regard to the several prognostic factors noted here, routine use should be limited to clinical trials. However, there is agreement regarding the extremely aggressive behavior of CLL and lack of response to standard therapies with 17p deletion by FISH. Such patients should be considered for alternate therapies in the context of clinical trials.[35]

B-PROLYMPHOCYTIC LEUKEMIA

Introduction

PLL is defined as a B-cell leukemia that is composed of greater than 55% prolymphocytes in the peripheral blood.[7,45] PLL can arise from preexisting CLL (prolymphocytic transformation of CLL), in which case, this should be noted in the diagnosis. We consider the de novo form in this section. De novo PLL is a rare disorder. Our concept of PLL is evolving, because cases of leukemia with greater than 55% prolymphocytes appear to be a heterogeneous group of diseases encompassing transformed CLL, nucleolated variants of MCL, and de novo PLL.[46–48]

Clinical Features

Patients are usually older (median age, 70) with a male predominance. Patients present with splenomegaly and a high leukocyte count (often >100 × 10^9/l) and usually lack significant lymphadenopathy.[49,50] Cytopenias are common, usually due to marrow replacement.

Morphologic Features

The peripheral blood smear shows numerous (>55%) prolymphocytes, characterized by intermediate size, slightly dispersed chromatin, and a prominent central nucleolus. The cytoplasm is pale blue and moderate to abundant in amount. The nuclear contours are classically round, but indentations can be seen (**Fig. 4**). The bone marrow often shows extensive involvement with intermediately sized cells containing small nucleoli. The spleen may show white pulp involvement with or without red-pulp involvement. Again, the cells are round, intermediate in size, and show small central nucleoli in tissue section.

Immunophenotype

The reported immunophenotype of PLL is variable, likely because previous reports have included several entities (listed earlier). PLL expresses CD19, CD20 (bright), CD79b, FMC7, and sIg. CD5 may be expressed in some cases; however, prior data concerning CD5 expression may be inaccurate due to differences in inclusion criteria. Expression of cyclin D1 strongly suggests a nucleolated, typically blastoid variant of MCL and essentially excludes PLL.

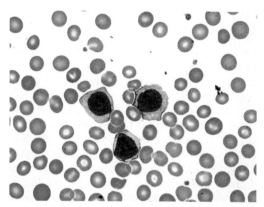

Fig. 4. B-PLL. Intermediately sized prolymphocytes are present with prominent central nucleoli (Wright stain).

Molecular Genetics

Rearranged immunoglobulin genes are present. Given the confusion in the precise definition related to MCL, the molecular genetic features of PLL are not yet precisely defined. The t(11;l4)(q13;q32) resulting in an *IGH/CCND1* fusion is present in a minority (20% of some series) of previously reported PLL. However, these cases are best considered a variant of MCL.[46] Other nonspecific abnormalities reported in PLL include TP53 abnormalities (deletion or mutation in 75% of cases) and deletions of 13q14 (55% of cases) and 11q23 (39% of cases).[51,52]

Differential Diagnosis

The differential diagnosis of a leukemia composed of prolymphocytes includes transformed CLL, MCL variant, T-PLL, and variant HCL. History of CLL allows one to reasonably diagnose a case of B-cell leukemia with greater than 55% prolymphocytes as prolymphocytic transformation of CLL. Presence of t(11;14)(q13;q32) allows one to confirm a diagnosis of MCL. T-PLL cells may resemble B-cell PLL cells morphologically because of the presence of nucleoli, although the T-PLL cells tend to have more nuclear irregularities, and the chromatin may be more condensed. Immunophenotyping easily identifies a T-cell process in T-PLL. HCLv may have small nucleoli but still have some cytoplasmic features of HCL that are not seen in PLL. The presence of CD103 and generally lower white count are seen in HCLv. Once these are excluded, PLL is the most likely diagnosis.

Prognosis/Therapy

PLL is usually an aggressive disease, although a subset of cases will not follow a rapidly progressive course that does not appear to be predictable. Older age, anemia, and presence of TP53 abnormalities may indicate more aggressive disease.[53]

Therapy has not been uniform for this uncommon disease and has varied from low-grade alkylator-based therapy to more aggressive anthracycline-containing regimens. More recently, nucleoside analogs such as cladribine and monoclonal antibody therapy with agents such as alemtuzumab have been successfully used.[53–56]

MONOCLONAL B-CELL LYMPHOCYTOSIS

With sensitive flow cytometric approaches, it has recently been found that a small proportion of people have minute B-cell clones with the phenotype of CLL. The finding of monoclonal B cells at a level below that required or CLL has been termed MBL. The criteria for MBL include demonstration of light chain restriction by flow cytometry, less than 5×10^9/L B cells, lack of known lymphoproliferative disease or autoimmune disease, and normal physical examination.[57] The incidence of MBL varies depending on the population studied but varies from 0.14% in blood donors, to 3.5% in outpatient donors without history of lymphoproliferative disease, to 13.5% in first-degree relatives with familial CLL.[57] Phenotypic studies have shown that most, but not all, MBLs have the phenotype of CLL. The significance of these "incidental" findings is as yet unknown but raises questions about the biology of CLL and risk factors for its development. Given that the incidence of CLL is orders of magnitude lower, clearly not all patients with MBL progress to CLL. A recent study found that patients with MBL and lymphocytosis progressed to CLL at the rate of 1.1%/y but that only a small fraction of patients with MBL (7%) required treatment for CLL and even fewer died of CLL.[58] Interestingly, the CLL phenotype MBL demonstrated 13q14 deletion at a similar frequency as that of full-blown CLL but showed increased incidence of *IGH V* mutated status (a favorable prognostic feature of CLL) compared with full-blown CLL.[58]

HAIRY CELL LEUKEMIA
Introduction

HCL is an uncommon mature B-cell leukemia composed of cells with cytoplasmic projections when examined on Wright stained smear. It represents 2% of lymphoid leukemias.[59]

Clinical Features

HCL presents in middle-aged to elderly patients (median age, 50 years) with a 4:1 male/female predominance. Patients present typically with cytopenias including monocytopenia and splenomegaly.[59,60] Infectious complications also occur, particularly with bacterial organisms. Monocytopenia has been suggested as a contributing factor.[61]

Morphology

On peripheral blood smear, HCL cells have a characteristic appearance. The chromatin is slightly less condensed than a mature non-neoplastic lymphocyte with a reticulated pattern. The cytoplasm is moderate in amount and stains pale gray blue. It has a "textured" or "lacy" quality to it. Fine cytoplasmic projections can be seen around the circumference of the cell (**Fig. 5**). The bone marrow aspirate may be hemodiluted, because reticulin fibrosis is usually present and accounts for frequent "dry taps" in HCL patients. Trephine biopsy is, therefore, very important. The infiltrate can be nodular, interstitial, or paratrabecular. The collections of lymphocytes may have a "fried egg" appearance, imparted due to the moderate amounts of cytoplasm, which results in the nuclei being spaced apart from one another. Nuclei are usually round to oval, but the cells may also have a spindled quality (**Fig. 6**).[62] Involvement may be subtle, and immunostains for B-cell markers such as CD20 or DBA.44 can highlight the cells, often showing many more cells than suspected on hematoxylin and eosin stained sections. Careful examination of a CD20 stained section may show the cytoplasmic projections. Mast cells are increased in the bone marrow of HCL patients and may be seen on aspirate smear and in tissue section.[63] In the spleen, HCL involves the

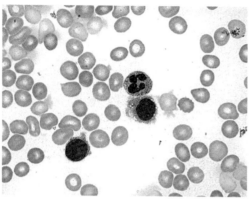

Fig. 5. Hairy cell leukemia. Small cells with round to bean-shaped nuclei with reticulated chromatin pattern and abundant "lacy" cytoplasm. Some cells may have ragged circumferential cytoplasmic borders imparting a "hairy" appearance (Wright stain).

red pulp preferentially. This is in contrast to the white pulp involvement seen in other low-grade B-cell lymphoproliferative disorders. Blood lakes are seen. These are non-endothelial lined spaces filled with erythrocytes and surrounded by leukemia cells.[64] A tartrate-resistant acid phosphatase stain is strongly positive in HCL cells but is not required for diagnosis in the era of multiparameter flow cytometry.

Immunophenotype

Flow cytometric analysis shows that the cells express CD19, CD11c, CD20, CD22, CD25, CD103, FMC7, and monotypic immunoglobulin light chains. Strong coexpression of CD11c, CD22, CD25, and CD103 is quite characteristic of this leukemia.[65–67] The latter marker is fairly sensitive and specific. It is present in approximately 95% of cases of HCL and uncommonly present in other B-cell chronic lymphoproliferative disorders.[67] Cyclin D1 can be overexpressed both at the messenger RNA and protein level (detectable by immunohistochemistry) in a minority of HCL cases.[68,69] Newer markers such as CD123 and annexin A1 (ANXA1) are expressed in HCL and appear to be useful in the diagnosis of HCL, as other B-cell lymphoproliferative disorders

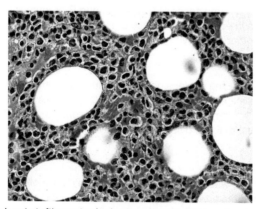

Fig. 6. Hairy cell leukemia infiltrate in the bone marrow trephine showing lymphocytes with round to indented nuclei and cytoplasmic clear halos (hematoxylin-eosin).

are negative for these makers.[70,71] CD10 can be seen in approximately 10% of cases.[72]

Molecular Genetics

There is no specific karyotypic abnormality; however, classical G-banded cytogenetic and comparative genomic hybridization studies show that gain of 5q13–31 and loss of 7q32 occur in a minority of cases and that the region at 7q32 is the same area also deleted in some cases of SMZL.[73,74] High-density gene mapping array studies have shown that HCL has a relatively stable genome. Loss of heterozygosity without copy number changes (suggesting uniparental disomy [UPD]) was found in approximately one-third of cases. Varying sites were seen, and 1p32 was commonly involved. Whether UPD plays a pathogenic role is unknown.[75] IGH mutational analysis shows that HCL cells have somatically hypermutated IGH genes with relatively low intraclonal heterogeneity, a feature of postgerminal center B cells.[76,77] Indeed, expression array studies have shown HCL cells to be related to postgerminal center memory B cells and that they differ from memory cells in the expression of chemokine and adhesion molecules.[78] As mentioned, although cyclin D1 is overexpressed in some cases, the t(11;14)(q13;q32) seen in MCL is absent.

Differential Diagnosis

The characteristic morphologic and immunophenotypic features usually allow easy separation from other B-cell lymphoproliferative disorders, such as CLL, PLL, and leukemic phase of FLs or MCLs. The main diagnostic considerations are SMZL and HCLv. Morphologically, HCL cells have characteristic nuclear features and cytoplasmic projections around the circumference of the cell, whereas SMZL cells usually have their cytoplasmic projections only around part of the cells, often at opposite ends of the cells. The cells in SMZL are often more heterogeneous appearing, with some containing nucleoli and others more closely resembling CLL cells. HCLv cells have a more condensed chromatin pattern than typical HCL cells and also have a small visible nucleolus. Immunophenotypically, the expression of bright CD11c, CD22, CD25, and CD103 is quite characteristic of HCL. Lack of CD25 is seen in HCLv. SMZL usually lacks these markers but may express them in a minority of cases. For example, CD103 can be expressed in approximately 15% of cases. When dealing with lymphocytes with villous/hairy projections, CD123 appears useful in distinguishing HCL (positive) from HCLv and SMZL (negative).[70] This latter marker is not specific, since it can be seen in some cases of CLL, AML, and B precursor ALL. ANXA1 is also reported to be seen in essentially all cases of HCL and is quite specific (approaching 100%) among the other B-cell lymphoproliferative disorders.[71]

Prognosis/Therapy

With recent therapies using nucleoside analogs such as pentostatin or cladribine, the prognosis of HCL is excellent, with a high complete response rate and excellent long-term survival.[59,60,79,80] Immunostaining of trephine biopsies using B-cell markers has identified the minimal residual disease that was associated with relapse.[80]

HAIRY CELL VARIANT

A variant form of HCL was first described by Cawley and colleagues[81] in 1980 and subsequently termed the prolymphocytic variant of HCL. It is quite uncommon, representing 0.4% of chronic lymphoproliferative disorders and an estimated 10% of HCL.[82] It differs from HCL in several clinical, morphologic, and immunophenotypic features. Thus, although the name suggests that this is related to HCL, it is still debatable whether such cases might actually represent a distinct entity or variant of another B-cell lymphoproliferative disorder. The following description reflects features currently accepted.

Clinical Features

The median age at onset is 71 years, older than that with typical HCL, and there is only a slight male predominance (1.6). Splenomegaly and cytopenias are common, as in typical HCL, but monocytopenia is not. There is usually a leukocytosis instead of leukopenia.[83]

Morphology

Morphologically, the cells resemble typical HCL cells in blood but have a more condensed chromatin pattern and a nucleolus. The cytoplasmic projections are less prominent than typical HCL. Bone marrow infiltration appears similar in pattern to typical HCL, with an interstitial pattern commonly seen. Some cases may show a "fried egg" appearance. In the spleen, as in typical HCL, there is a predilection for red-pulp involvement, and this can be a useful diagnostic feature. Unlike typical HCL, HCLv cells are negative for tartrate-resistant acid phosphatase.

Immunophenotype

Immunophenotyping shows some similarities to typical HCL. HCLv cells express CD19, CD20, CD22, and CD11c. CD103 is expressed in the majority of cases (60%) but CD25, CD123, and ANXA1 are absent.[71,82,84]

Molecular Genetics

No specific abnormalities have been described.

Differential Diagnosis

The main differential diagnosis is between typical HCL and SLVL. Besides the classical morphologic features described earlier, flow cytometric immunophenotyping can be very helpful. The former expresses the typical hairy cell markers such as CD11c, CD25, CD103, CD123, and ANXA1, whereas the variant form usually lacks CD25, CD123, and ANXA1. SLVL cells also lack CD103 (in most cases). CD123 and ANXA1 are also absent in SLVL. A series of cases of rare "splenic red-pulp lymphoma with numerous basophilic villous lymphocytes" has been described with clinical, pathologic, and phenotypic features similar to those of HCLv.[85] The relationship of this to HCLv is uncertain and remains to be explored; however, one morphologic difference may be the typical presence of nucleoli in HCLv, which was uncommon in splenic red-pulp lymphoma.

Prognosis/Therapy

Recognition of HCLv is of clinical importance because of the lack of response to standard HCL therapy. Splenectomy has been suggested as an alternative therapy in these patients.[82]

T-CELL GRANULAR LYMPHOCYTIC LEUKEMIA

T-cell granular lymphocytic leukemia (T-LGL) is an indolent T-cell leukemia that occurs most commonly in patients with a median age of 55 years. It was first recognized as a syndrome of increased large granular lymphocytes and chronic neutropenia.[86] Its neoplastic nature was confirmed by demonstrating clonal cytogenetic abnormalities, and careful clinicopathologic characterization defined its morphologic and immuno-phenotypic features.[87,88] Diagnostic criteria traditionally have been clonal T-LGL lymphocytosis greater than $2 \times 10^9/L$ for more than 6 months. However, some patients may have much lower lymphocyte levels, and, in practice, some patients may require therapy before the requisite 6 months.

Clinical Features

Patients vary widely in age, but the median age at diagnosis is 60 years.[89] The sex distribution is equal. Approximately two-thirds of patients are symptomatic, usually due to cytopenias such as neutropenia. "B" symptoms are seen in about one-third of patients. Organomegaly can be present in a minority of patients. Autoimmune disorders such as rheumatoid arthritis are commonly present, and T-LGL patients usually have associated cytopenias, which are often the major causes of morbidity for patients. Other described clinical associations include bone marrow failure syndromes, such as paroxysmal nocturnal hemoglobinuria, aplastic anemia, myelodysplasia, and red cell aplasia, suggesting an important role for immune dysregulation as part of the pathogenesis of this disease.[90]

Morphology

In the peripheral blood, one sees large granular lymphocytes that may be only modestly increased in number. These cells have abundant pale cytoplasm with azurophilic cytotoxic granules (**Fig. 7**). Since the normal number of LGLs is low (less than 520/μl), this can be easily overlooked.[91] Thus, the diagnosis is often difficult to make without special studies, such as flow cytometry or T-cell receptor gene rearrangement studies, due to the low level of circulating leukemia cells. Moreover, some degree of degranulation may occur during sample storage or transportation, resulting in cases with a typical immunophenotype that lack the characteristic morphology.

As in the blood, bone marrow involvement can be subtle. Bone marrow cellularity is usually increased, although normocellularity or hypocellularity can be seen.[92,93] A left shift in granulocytic cells is common, perhaps as a compensatory mechanism in patients with neutropenia, along with a relative increase in erythroid elements.[92,93] Megakaryocytes are normal. A subtle intravascular/intrasinusoidal pattern is also present, best seen with the aid of immunostains. A linear array of intrasinusoidal

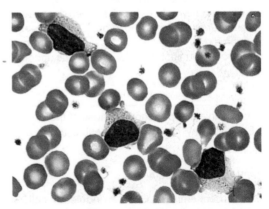

Fig. 7. T-LGL in blood. Mature lymphocytes with abundant cytoplasm containing cytotoxic granules (Wright stain).

lymphocytes is present in two-thirds of cases and is a relatively specific finding.[93] Interstitial clustering of eight or more CD8+ or TIA1 + T cells or six or more Granzyme B+ cells is characteristic of LGL and not seen in other reactive conditions (**Fig. 8**).

Immunophenotype

The most common immunophenotype is a CD3+/CD8+ $\alpha\beta$ T cell that also expresses CD16, CD57, and cytotoxic proteins such as TIA-1 and Granzyme B. With the availability of antibodies that have specificity to many of the TCR-Vβ families, a new modality that is useful in the diagnosis of T-LGL is flow cytometry for specific Vβ families, as a rapid and specific way to document skewed T-cell repertoire and thus T-cell clonality.[94,95] Lima and colleagues[95] showed an 81% sensitivity and 100% specificity when 60% of the total CD4+ or CD8+[bright] cells used a single Vβ family. Using a commercially available kit consisting of 24 Vβ family antibodies in a multicolor format to decrease the number of tubes used in the assay, good performance has been demonstrated in variety of T-cell leukemias, which may obviate the need for molecular studies.[96] However, because of incomplete T-cell repertoire coverage, a negative result must be further investigated with molecular studies. Such a flow cytometric assay also has the advantage of determining the particular Vβ family used by the leukemia for potential immunologic studies and may be a useful way to monitor therapy.[97] Restricted expression of a single isoform of killer inhibitory receptor (KIR) molecules can be detected in LGL leukemia and may serve as a clonality surrogate.[98] Rare cases of LGL have a $\gamma\delta$ phenotype but do not appear to differ substantially for the $\alpha\beta$ type.[99]

Molecular Genetics

T-cell receptor gene rearrangement studies should demonstrate monoclonal rearranged antigen receptor genes. This has become a very important diagnostic tool to confirm the diagnosis and differentiate reactive conditions, such as autoimmune disease or viral infection. In clinically borderline cases, it should be noted that monoclonal T-cell populations can be seen, particularly in elderly patients.[100] No specific chromosomal abnormalities have been identified.

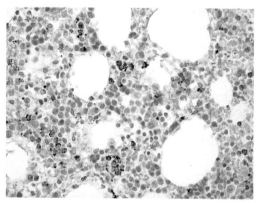

Fig. 8. T-LGL. A bone marrow trephine stained with granzyme B shows numerous cytotoxic T cells with focal clustering.

Differential Diagnosis

The differential diagnosis of T-LGL includes reactive nonclonal LGL expansions secondary to viral infection, skin disorders, and idiopathic thrombocytopenic purpura. These are often transient with relatively modest increases in LGLs. Clonality studies are usually negative. Features supporting the diagnosis of LGL rather than reactive processes are clinical features such as persistent cytopenias and persistence of a T-cell clone over time.

Prognosis

The course of LGL is generally indolent. In a multicenter series of 151 patients followed for a mean time of 29 months, most patients had nonprogressive disease.[101] However, some patients suffered more aggressive disease, and death within 4 years was seen in 19 patients.[101] Factors associated with poor outcome included fever at diagnosis and low percentage of LGLs in blood.[101] In another relatively large series, Dohdapka reported that 31% of patients required no therapy.[102] Median survival was 161 months.[102] Indicators of poor outcome included low neutrophil count and "B" symptoms/infection.[102] As more patients are studied and uniform diagnostic criteria are used, more reliable prognostic indicators will be defined. Treatment may include cyclosporine or methotrexate with or without corticosteroids.[89]

CHRONIC NATURAL KILLER CELL LYMPHOCYTOSIS

Rare cases of indolent natural killer (NK) cell lymphocytosis exist, characterized by persistent NK lymphocytosis, usually greater than 2×10^9/L. The uncommon indolent NK-cell variant of T-LGL lacks CD3 but expresses CD16 and CD56.[88,91,103,104]

Clinical Features

NK lymphocytosis occurs in adults with a median age of 60 years and may be associated with autoimmune diseases or viral infection. Patients present with cytopenias, usually neutropenia or anemia, whereas lymphadenopathy or organomegaly are uncommon. Rare patients had vasculitis or nephrotic syndrome.[103,104]

Morphology

Circulating granular lymphocytes are seen, similar to T-LGL leukemia. Bone marrow biopsy shows a subtle interstitial or sinusoidal infiltrate but generally requires immunohistochemistry to be clearly identified.

Immunophenotype

Flow cytometry demonstrates an NK-cell phenotype. The cells express CD16 and CD56 and lack surface CD3. CD2 and CD7 may be decreased, whereas CD5 may be abnormally expressed. A restricted pattern or absence of KIRs is indicative of an abnormal NK-cell population.[105]

Molecular Genetics

Being NK cells, antigen receptors are in the germline configuration. EBV genome is not present. Cytogenetic abnormalities may occur and are associated with worse prognosis.[106]

Differential Diagnosis

This disease should be distinguished from aggressive NK-cell leukemia, which, although of a similar immunophenotype, presents in younger patients with organomegaly and B-symptoms, and lacks an association with rheumatoid arthritis.[91,107]

Prognosis

This is an indolent disease that may progress with morbidity due to cytopenias and increasing lymphocytosis.

T-PROLYMPHOCYTIC LEUKEMIA
Introduction

T-prolymphocytic leukemia (T-PLL) is an uncommon T-cell lymphoproliferative disorder of mature, post-thymic T cells characterized by occurrence in older adults (median age, 69 years), with a male predominance. It represents approximately 2% of small lymphoid leukemias in adults.[108] Some confusion regarding this disease has been present in the past due to inconsistent terminology such as T-chronic lymphocytic leukemia (T-CLL). This may have lead to confusion with B-CLL and T-LGL. The current WHO classification does not recognize "T-CLL" as an entity, and most cases of T-CLL (once other leukemic T-cell processes such as Sézary syndrome, adult T-cell leukemia lymphoma, and T-LGL) are examples of the small-cell variant of T-PLL.[109,110] Some confusion also exists, because the name "prolymphocytic leukemia" to some may (erroneously) imply a morphologic similarity with B-PLL.

Clinical Features

Patients present with hepatosplenomegaly, lymphadenopathy, skin lesions, and marked leukocytosis (more than $100 \times 10^9/l$ in 75% of cases).[108] Cytopenias such as anemia and thrombocytopenia are common. The clinical course is generally aggressive; however, an indolent phase has been recognized.[111]

Morphology

The morphologic spectrum of T-PLL is variable.[112] The leukemic cells often are small to intermediate in size with slight to marked nuclear irregularities. The chromatin is condensed, and nucleoli are present but usually not as prominent as those seen in B-PLL. Nuclear contours are sound to irregular, and the irregularities can be quite marked. The cytoplasm is usually lightly basophilic and agranular, and cytoplasmic blebs can be found in some cases (**Fig. 9**). A minority of cases (approximately 20%) can be composed of small cells that may mimic typical B-CLL (so-called small-cell variant of T-PLL).

Bone marrow involvement is often extensive and present in an interstitial and diffuse pattern. Cutaneous involvement can be present in approximately 25% to 30% of patients and most commonly manifests as indurated erythema. Histologically, the pattern of infiltration is usually perivascular and periadnexal. Epidermotropism is not a feature.[113] This pattern is not specific, and knowledge of the complete clinical picture is required for one to make a diagnosis of cutaneous involvement by T-PLL rather than primary cutaneous T-cell lymphoma. Splenic involvement is characterized by red- and white-pulp involvement, whereas paracortical involvement may be seen in lymph node.[114] Hepatic involvement is frequent, and infiltration of sinusoids is seen.

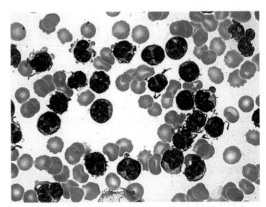

Fig. 9. T-PLL. This blood smear shows a marked lymphocytosis of atypical lymphocytes with mature chromatin, irregular nuclei, and small nucleoli. Cytoplasmic blebs or "knobs" are present (Wright stain).

Immunophenotype

Flow cytometric immunophenotypic is required to confirm the T-cell lineage of this leukemia. The common immunophenotype is CD2+, CD3+, CD4+, CD5+, CD7+, CD8-, CD19-, CD20-, CD26+, TdT-, and CD1a-. Although most cases (60%) are CD4+, a minority (25%) coexpress CD4 and CD8, and occasional cases are CD4-/CD8+ (15%).[108] TCL-1 expression is present in more than 70% of cases of T-PLL and, although expressed in other lymphoid malignancies such as B-cell lymphoma and CLL, appears to be specific for this entity when considering other T-cell leukemic processes that might enter the differential diagnosis, including T-LGL and Sézary syndrome (SS).[115]

Molecular Genetics

Cytogenetic analysis of T-PLL has shown frequent abnormalities of 14q32.1. Inv14(q11;q32.1) or 1(14;14)(q11;q32.1) is found in the majority (70%) of cases.[116]

Recent work has identified TCL1 as the oncogene at 14q32.1 of particular pathogenetic importance in T-PLL. Interestingly, the TCL1 homolog MTCP1, located at Xq28, is also involved in translocation with the TCR α/δ locus at 14q11. Transgenic mice overexpressing these genes develop leukemias, thus demonstrating the importance of these gene products in leukemogenesis.[117–119] The mechanism by which TCL1 overexpression promotes leukemia appears to relate to its function as a cofactor for AKT activation, resulting in nuclear localization of AKT and enhanced cell proliferation and survival.[120–122]

Differential Diagnosis

The differential diagnosis of T-PLL includes other B-cell leukemias, ALL, T-LGL, ATLL, and SS. B-cell leukemias can be excluded by basic immunophenotyping, which shows expression of pan B-cell antigens and lack of T-cell antigens. ALLs can also be excluded by morphologic examination demonstrating the fine chromatin of blasts that is not seen in T-PLL. Phenotyping would also differentiate precursor lymphoblastic processes, since these express such early precursor markers as CD1a, TdT, and the CD34. TdT would be absent in post-thymic T cells. ATLL can be excluded by typical clinical presentation, ethnic/geographic considerations, and presence of

HTLV-1, which is characteristic of ATLL. SS can be excluded by history of mycosis fungoides and clinical features such as erythroderma. Finally, as mentioned, expression of TCL1 in the specific setting of a mature T-cell leukemia appears to be fairly specific for T-PLL.[115]

Prognosis

The disease course is usually aggressive with short survival (less than one year).[108] In 1998, an indolent presentation was recognized; however, even these patients will convert to a more aggressive course typical of T-PLL with short survival.[111] A few reports of indolent T-cell PLL are appearing with complex karyotypes.[123,124] Recently, it has been shown that high levels of TCL1 and T-cell receptor expression are adverse prognostic factors.[125] Therapy with alemtuzumab has resulted in complete responses in a high proportion of cases and may improve the outlook for many patients.[126,127]

MYCOSIS FUNGOIDES AND SEZARY SYNDROME
Introduction

SS is generally regarded as the leukemic form of epidermotropic cutaneous T-cell lymphoma (mycosis fungoides). It is defined as the presence of erythroderma, generalized lymphadenopathy, and clonally related neoplastic T cells in the blood, skin, and lymph nodes. In addition, an absolute Sézary cell count of greater than 1000 cells/μl, CD4:CD8 ratio greater than 10, or loss of 1 or more T-cell antigens have been added as laboratory criteria.

Clinical Features

SS is characterized by erythroderma, palmoplantar keratoderma, partial alopecia, lymphadenopathy, and pruritus.

Morphology

The morphologic identification of Sézary cells is somewhat subjective, with Sézary-like cells being seen frequently in some patients with benign dermatoses and also in patients with clinical features of SS who lack detectable T-cell clones in the blood.[128,129] Atypical lymphocytes can be seen in the blood and take the form of lymphocytes with cleaved "cerebriform" nuclei of large (typical Sézary cells,) or small (so-called Lutzner cells) size (**Fig. 10**).

Immunophenotype

Flow cytometric immunophenotyping is used to detect Sézary cells in blood. The cells are mature T cells that express CD4+. Several phenotypic abnormalities can be seen. CD3 antigen density is often altered compared with normal T cells. Deletion of CD7 is common but can be found in some reactive conditions.[130–132] Uncommonly, loss of other T-cell antigens, such as CD5 or CD2, may be seen. CD26, dipeptidyl aminopeptidase IV, is absent in the great majority of cases of SS, and lack of this marker is a diagnostic feature useful in identifying Sézary cells in blood samples.[133,134] Sézary cells express the KIR CD158k and appear to be a useful marker for the diagnosis of SS.[135] T-cell clonality can be inferred from restricted use of T-cell receptor Vβ.[96] This approach has also been used to follow patients with SS on treatment with phototherapy.[97,136] Use of all of these markers will maximize one's ability to detect Sézary cells.[137]

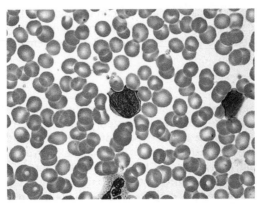

Fig.10. Sézary syndrome. A blood smear shows atypical lymphocytes with "creased," cerebriform nuclei (Wright stain).

Molecular Genetics

Gene rearrangement studies in the blood will demonstrate a monoclonal T-cell population related to clones present in the skin. Array-based studies show that genomic instability appears to be a feature of SS, and some recurrent gains and losses are being identified. Genes involved appear to include *cMYC*, *cMYC*-regulating proteins, mediators of *MYC*-induced apoptosis, and interleukin-2 (IL-2) signaling pathway components.[138]

Differential Diagnosis

The differential diagnosis includes other T-cell leukemias. The clinical picture will allow identification of a T-cell leukemic process as SS, since the patients will have a cutaneous T-cell lymphoma with erythroderma and adenopathy. Such a history will be absent in other processes such as T-PLL and LGLs. ATLL may have skin involvement, but the cells are much more lobulated than those in typical are SS. The phenotype as listed here, particularly the lack of CD26 and expression of CD158k, will strongly support SS.

Prognosis

SS is an aggressive disease with overall survival at 5 years of 10% to 20%.[139]

ADULT T-CELL LEUKEMIA/LYMPHOMA

ATLL is an HTLV-1–driven lymphoproliferative disorder. It occurs at high frequency in areas where HTLV-1 infection is endemic, such as Southwestern Japan and the Caribbean basin. Several clinical variants are described, including smoldering, chronic, lymphomatous, and acute variants. Circulating neoplastic cells are not present in the lymphomatous variant and are present at only a low level in the chronic and smoldering variants.[140] Since this article features mature lymphoid leukemias, we focus on the acute variant, the most common variant and one with a leukemic phase.

Clinical Features

Patients with the acute form of ATLL present with lymphadenopathy, organomegaly, and skin rash. They have constitutional symptoms, and laboratory examination shows leukocytosis with circulating neoplastic cells, eosinophilia, hypercalcemia, and elevated LDH.

Morphology

Peripheral blood examination reveals numerous atypical medium to large sized cells with polylobated nuclei and basophilic cytoplasm. These cells have been termed "flower" cells (**Fig. 11**). Bone marrow infiltration is usually patchy. Prominent osteo-clastic activity can be seen.

Immunophenotype

The neoplastic cells express pan T-cell antigens, including CD2, CD3, CD5, but usually lack CD7. Most cases are CD4+/CD8-, but other combinations including lack of both CD4 and CD8 are present. CD25+ (IL-2 receptor alpha) is expressed in almost all cases. CD4+/CD25+ expression is similar to that in regulatory T cells (Tregs) and expression of other Treg markers, such as FOXP3 and CTLA-4, has been shown in at least a subset of cases. Whether ATLL cells function as Tregs is still the subject of investigation.[141,142]

Genetics

T-cell receptor gene rearrangement studies are clonally rearranged. HTLV-1 genome is also clonally integrated. Different patterns of integration (complete, defective, and multiband) occur by Southern blot analysis and have been associated with disease type.[143]

Differential Diagnosis

The differential diagnosis includes other T-cell leukemias and leukemic phase of lymphoma. With regard to LGL and T-PLL, the morphologic features of ATLL help point one away from such diagnoses. SS cells typically do not have the extreme nuclear lobulation seen in ATLL. Demonstration of HTLV-1 viral genome confirms the diagnosis of ATLL and effectively excludes other T-cell leukemias.

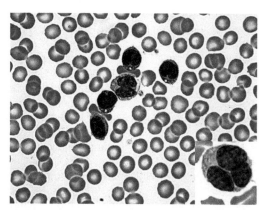

Fig. 11. ATLL. A blood smear shows circulating atypical lobulated lymphocytes or so-called flower cells (Wright stain).

REFERENCES

1. Dores GM, Anderson WF, Curtis RE, et al. Chronic lymphocytic leukaemia and small lymphocytic lymphoma: overview of the descriptive epidemiology. Br J Haematol 2007;139(5):809–19.
2. Hallek M, Cheson BD, Catovsky D, et al. Guidelines for the diagnosis and treatment of chronic lymphocytic leukemia: a report from the International Workshop on Chronic Lymphocytic Leukemia updating the National Cancer Institute-Working Group 1996 guidelines. Blood 2008;111(12):5446–56.
3. Binet JL, Auquier A, Dighiero G, et al. A new prognostic classification of chronic lymphocytic leukemia derived from a multivariate survival analysis. Cancer 1981; 48(1):198–206.
4. Rai KR, Han T. Prognostic factors and clinical staging in chronic lymphocytic leukemia. Hematol Oncol Clin North Am 1990;4(2):447–56.
5. Oscier DG, Matutes E, Copplestone A, et al. Atypical lymphocyte morphology: an adverse prognostic factor for disease progression in stage A CLL independent of trisomy 12. Br J Haematol 1997;98(4):934–9.
6. Frater JL, McCarron KF, Hammel JP, et al. Typical and atypical chronic lymphocytic leukemia differ clinically and immunophenotypically. Am J Clin Pathol 2001; 116(5):655–64.
7. Bennett JM, Catovsky D, Daniel MT, et al. Proposals for the classification of chronic (mature) B and T lymphoid leukaemias. French-American-British (FAB) Cooperative Group. J Clin Pathol 1989;42(6):567–84.
8. Mueller-Hermelink HK, Montserrat E, Catovsky D, et al. Chronic lymphocytic leukemia/small lymphocytic lymphoma. In: Swerdlow SH, Campo E, Harris NL, et al, editors. WHO classification of tumours of the haematopoietic and lymphoid tissues. Lyon, France: IARC; 2008. p. 180–2.
9. Vallespi T, Montserrat E, Sanz MA. Chronic lymphocytic leukaemia: prognostic value of lymphocyte morphological subtypes. A multivariate survival analysis in 146 patients. Br J Haematol 1991;77(4):478–85.
10. Lens D, Dyer MJ, Garcia-Marco JM, et al. p53 abnormalities in CLL are associated with excess of prolymphocytes and poor prognosis. Br J Haematol 1997; 99(4):848–57.
11. Matutes E, Oscier D, Garcia-Marco J, et al. Trisomy 12 defines a group of CLL with atypical morphology: correlation between cytogenetic, clinical and laboratory features in 544 patients. Br J Haematol 1996;92(2):382–8.
12. Montserrat E, Villamor N, Reverter JC, et al. Bone marrow assessment in B-cell chronic lymphocytic leukaemia: aspirate or biopsy? A comparative study in 258 patients. Br J Haematol 1996;93(1):111–6.
13. Raphael M, Chastang C, Binet JL. Is bone marrow biopsy a prognostic parameter in B-CLL? Nouv Rev Fr Hematol 1988;30(5–6):377–8.
14. Rozman C, Montserrat E, Rodriguez-Fernandez JM, et al. Bone marrow histologic pattern–the best single prognostic parameter in chronic lymphocytic leukemia: a multivariate survival analysis of 329 cases. Blood 1984;64(3): 642–8.
15. Kjeldsberg CR, Marty J. Prolymphocytic transformation of chronic lymphocytic leukemia. Cancer 1981;48(11):2447–57.
16. Bessudo A, Kipps TJ. Origin of high-grade lymphomas in Richter syndrome. Leuk Lymphoma 1995;18(5–6):367–72.
17. Foucar K, Rydell RE. Richter's syndrome in chronic lymphocytic leukemia. Cancer 1980;46(1):118–34.

18. Nakamura N, Abe M. Richter syndrome in B-cell chronic lymphocytic leukemia. Pathol Int 2003;53(4):195–203.
19. Foon KA, Gale RP. Clinical transformation of chronic lymphocytic leukemia. Nouv Rev Fr Hematol 1988;30(5–6):385–8.
20. Fayad L, Robertson LE, O'Brien S, et al. Hodgkin's disease variant of Richter's syndrome: experience at a single institution. Leuk Lymphoma 1996;23(3–4): 333–7.
21. Kanzler H, Kuppers R, Helmes S, et al. Hodgkin and Reed-Sternberg-like cells in B-cell chronic lymphocytic leukemia represent the outgrowth of single germinal-center B-cell-derived clones: potential precursors of Hodgkin and Reed-Sternberg cells in Hodgkin's disease. Blood 2000;95(3):1023–31.
22. Rubin D, Hudnall SD, Aisenberg A, et al. Richter's transformation of chronic lymphocytic leukemia with Hodgkin's-like cells is associated with Epstein-Barr virus infection. Mod Pathol 1994;7(1):91–8.
23. Ohno T, Smir BN, Weisenburger DD, et al. Origin of the Hodgkin/Reed-Sternberg cells in chronic lymphocytic leukemia with "Hodgkin's transformation". Blood 1998;91(5):1757–61.
24. McCarron KF, Hammel JP, Hsi ED. Usefulness of CD79b expression in the diagnosis of B-cell chronic lymphoproliferative disorders. Am J Clin Pathol 2000; 113(6):805–13.
25. Matutes E, Owusu-Ankomah K, Morilla R, et al. The immunological profile of B-cell disorders and proposal of a scoring system for the diagnosis of CLL. Leukemia 1994;8(10):1640–5.
26. Damle RN, Wasil T, Fais F, et al. Ig V gene mutation status and CD38 expression as novel prognostic indicators in chronic lymphocytic leukemia. [In Process Citation]. Blood 1999;94(6):1840–7.
27. Hamblin TJ, Orchard JA, Ibbotson RE, et al. CD38 expression and immunoglobulin variable region mutations are independent prognostic variables in chronic lymphocytic leukemia, but CD38 expression may vary during the course of the disease. Blood 2002;99(3):1023–9.
28. Del Poeta G, Maurillo L, Venditti A, et al. Clinical significance of CD38 expression in chronic lymphocytic leukemia. Blood 2001;98(9):2633–9.
29. Hsi ED, Kopecky KJ, Appelbaum FR, et al. Prognostic Significance of CD38 and CD20 expression as assessed by quantitative flow cytometry in chronic lymphocytic leukemia (CLL). Br J Haematol 2003;120:1017–25.
30. Admirand JH, Rassidakis GZ, Abruzzo LV, et al. Immunohistochemical detection of ZAP-70 in 341 cases of non-Hodgkin and Hodgkin lymphoma. Mod Pathol 2004;17:954–61.
31. Orchard JA, Ibbotson RE, Davis Z, et al. ZAP-70 expression and prognosis in chronic lymphocytic leukaemia. Lancet 2004;363(9403):105–11.
32. Rassenti LZ, Huynh L, Toy TL, et al. ZAP-70 compared with immunoglobulin heavy-chain gene mutation status as a predictor of disease progression in chronic lymphocytic leukemia. N Engl J Med 2004;351(9):893–901.
33. Rassenti LZ, Jain S, Keating MJ, et al. Relative value of ZAP-70, CD38, and immunoglobulin mutation status in predicting aggressive disease in chronic lymphocytic leukemia. Blood 2008;112(5):1923–30.
34. Marti G, Orfao A, Goolsby C. ZAP-70 in CLL: towards standardization of a biomarker for patient management: history of clinical cytometry special issue. Cytometry B Clin Cytom 2006;70(4):197–200.
35. Hamblin TJ. Prognostic markers in chronic lymphocytic leukaemia. Best Pract Res Clin Haematol 2007;20(3):455–68.

36. Dohner H, Stilgenbauer S, Benner A, et al. Genomic alterations and survival in chronic lymphocytic leukemia. N Engl J Med 2000;343:1910–6.
37. Hamblin TJ, Davis Z, Gardiner A, et al. Unmutated Ig V(H) genes are associated with a more aggressive form of chronic lymphocytic leukemia [see comments]. Blood 1999;94(6):1848–54.
38. Tobin G, Soderberg O, Thunberg U, et al. V(H)3–21 gene usage in chronic lymphocytic leukemia–characterization of a new subgroup with distinct molecular features and poor survival. Leuk Lymphoma 2004;45(2):221–8.
39. Tobin G, Thunberg U, Johnson A, et al. Somatically mutated Ig V(H)3–21 genes characterize a new subset of chronic lymphocytic leukemia. Blood 2002;99(6): 2262–4.
40. Rosenwald A, Alizadeh AA, Widhopf G, et al. Relation of gene expression phenotype to immunoglobulin mutation genotype in B cell chronic lymphocytic leukemia. J Exp Med 2001;194(11):1639–47.
41. Wiestner A, Rosenwald A, Barry TS, et al. ZAP-70 expression identifies a chronic lymphocytic leukemia subtype with unmutated immunoglobulin genes, inferior clinical outcome, and distinct gene expression profile. Blood 2003;101:4944–51.
42. Matutes E, Morilla R, Owusu-Ankomah K, et al. The immunophenotype of splenic lymphoma with villous lymphocytes and its relevance to the differential diagnosis with other B-cell disorders. Blood 1994;83(6):1558–62.
43. Lush CJ, Vora AJ, Campbell AC, et al. Polyclonal CD5 + B-lymphocytosis resembling chronic lymphocytic leukaemia. Br J Haematol 1991;79(1):119–20.
44. Delage R, Roy J, Jacques L, et al. All patients with persistent polyclonal B cell lymphocytosis present Bcl-2/Ig gene rearrangements. Leuk Lymphoma 1998; 31(5–6):567–74.
45. Galton DA, Goldman JM, Wiltshaw E, et al. Prolymphocytic leukemia. Br J Haematol 1974;27:7–23.
46. Schlette E, Bueso-Ramos C, Giles F, et al. Mature B-cell leukemias with more than 55% prolymphocytes. A heterogeneous group that includes an unusual variant of mantle cell lymphoma. Am J Clin Pathol 2001;115(4):571–81.
47. Hsi ED, Frater JL. Advances in the diagnosis and classification of chronic lymphoproliferative disorders. Cancer Treat Res 2004;121:145–65.
48. Wong KF, So CC, Chan JK. Nucleolated variant of mantle cell lymphoma with leukemic manifestations mimicking prolymphocytic leukemia. Am J Clin Pathol 2002;117(2):246–51.
49. Melo JV, Catovsky D, Galton DA. The relationship between chronic lymphocytic leukaemia and prolymphocytic leukaemia. I. Clinical and laboratory features of 300 patients and characterization of an intermediate group. Br J Haematol 1986;63(2):377–87.
50. Campo E, Catovsky D, Montserrat E, et al. Prolymphocytic leukemia. In: Swerdlow SH, Campo E, Harris NL, et al, editors. WHO classification of tumours of the haematopoietic and lymphoid tissues. Lyon, France: IARC; 2008. p. 183–4.
51. Lens D, Matutes E, Catovsky D, et al. Frequent deletions at 11q23 and 13q14 in B cell prolymphocytic leukemia (B-PLL). Leukemia 2000;14(3):427–30.
52. Lens D, De Schouwer PJ, Hamoudi RA, et al. p53 abnormalities in B-cell prolymphocytic leukemia. Blood 1997;89(6):2015–23.
53. Hercher C, Robain M, Davi F, et al. A multicentric study of 41 cases of B-prolymphocytic leukemia: two evolutive forms. Leuk Lymphoma 2001;42(5):981–7.
54. McCune SL, Gockerman JP, Moore JO, et al. Alemtuzumab in relapsed or refractory chronic lymphocytic leukemia and prolymphocytic leukemia. Leuk Lymphoma 2002;43(5):1007–11.

55. Saven A, Lee T, Schlutz M, et al. Major activity of cladribine in patients with de novo B-cell prolymphocytic leukemia. J Clin Oncol 1997;15(1):37–43.
56. Shvidel L, Shtalrid M, Bassous L, et al. B-cell prolymphocytic leukemia: a survey of 35 patients emphasizing heterogeneity, prognostic factors and evidence for a group with an indolent course. Leuk Lymphoma 1999;33(1–2):169–79.
57. Marti G, Abbasi F, Raveche E, et al. Overview of monoclonal B-cell lymphocytosis. Br J Haematol 2007;139(5):701–8.
58. Rawstron AC, Bennett FL, O'Connor SJ, et al. Monoclonal B-cell lymphocytosis and chronic lymphocytic leukemia. N Engl J Med 2008;359(6):575–83.
59. Goodman GR, Bethel KJ, Saven A. Hairy cell leukemia: an update. Curr Opin Hematol 2003;10(4):258–66.
60. Goodman GR, Burian C, Koziol JA, et al. Extended follow-up of patients with hairy cell leukemia after treatment with cladribine. J Clin Oncol 2003;21(5):891–6.
61. Kraut EH. Clinical manifestations and infectious complications of hairy-cell leukaemia. Best Pract Res Clin Haematol 2003;16(1):33–40.
62. Bethel KJ, Sharpe RW. Pathology of hairy-cell leukaemia. Best Pract Res Clin Haematol 2003;16(1):15–31.
63. Macon WR, Kinney MC, Glick AD, et al. Marrow mast cell hyperplasia in hairy cell leukemia. Mod Pathol 1993;6(6):695–8.
64. Burke JS, Rappaport H. The diagnosis and differential diagnosis of hairy cell leukemia in bone marrow and spleen. Semin Oncol 1984;11(4):334–46.
65. DiGiuseppe JA, Borowitz MJ. Clinical utility of flow cytometry in the chronic lymphoid leukemias. Semin Oncol 1998;25(1):6–10.
66. Matutes E, Morilla R, Owusu-Ankomah K, et al. The immunophenotype of hairy cell leukemia (HCL). Proposal for a scoring system to distinguish HCL from B-cell disorders with hairy or villous lymphocytes. Leuk Lymphoma 1994;14(Suppl 1): 57–61.
67. Robbins BA, Ellison DJ, Spinosa JC, et al. Diagnostic application of two-color flow cytometry in 161 cases of hairy cell leukemia. Blood 1993;82(4):1277–87.
68. de Boer CJ, Kluin-Nelemans JC, Dreef E, et al. Involvement of the CCND1 gene in hairy cell leukemia. Ann Oncol 1996;7(3):251–6.
69. Specht K, Kremer M, Muller U, et al. Identification of cyclin D1 mRNA overexpression in B-cell neoplasias by real-time reverse transcription-PCR of microdissected paraffin sections. Clin Cancer Res 2002;8(9):2902–11.
70. Del GI, Matutes E, Morilla R, et al. The diagnostic value of CD123 in B-cell disorders with hairy or villous lymphocytes. Haematologica 2004;89(3):303–8.
71. Falini B, Tiacci E, Liso A, et al. Simple diagnostic assay for hairy cell leukaemia by immunocytochemical detection of annexin A1 (ANXA1). Lancet 2004; 363(9424):1869–70.
72. Jasionowski TM, Hartung L, Greenwood JH, et al. Analysis of CD10+ hairy cell leukemia. Am J Clin Pathol 2003;120(2):228–35.
73. Andersen CL, Gruszka-Westwood A, Ostergaard M, et al. A narrow deletion of 7q is common to HCL, and SMZL, but not CLL. Eur J Haematol 2004;72(6): 390–402.
74. Sole F, Woessner S, Florensa L, et al. Cytogenetic findings in five patients with hairy cell leukemia. Cancer Genet Cytogenet 1999;110(1):41–3.
75. Forconi F, Poretti G, Kwee I, et al. High density genome-wide DNA profiling reveals a remarkably stable profile in hairy cell leukaemia. Br J Haematol 2008;141(5):622–30.
76. Arons E, Sunshine J, Suntum T, et al. Somatic hypermutation and VH gene usage in hairy cell leukaemia. Br J Haematol 2006;133(5):504–12.

77. Tiacci E, Liso A, Piris M, et al. Evolving concepts in the pathogenesis of hairy-cell leukaemia. Nat Rev Cancer 2006;6(6):437–48.
78. Basso K, Liso A, Tiacci E, et al. Gene expression profiling of hairy cell leukemia reveals a phenotype related to memory B cells with altered expression of chemokine and adhesion receptors. J Exp Med 2004;199(1):59–68.
79. Grever MR, Doan CA, Kraut EH. Pentostatin in the treatment of hairy-cell leukemia. Best Pract Res Clin Haematol 2003;16(1):91–9.
80. Tallman MS, Hakimian D, Kopecky KJ, et al. Minimal residual disease in patients with hairy cell leukemia in complete remission treated with 2-chlorodeoxyadenosine or 2-deoxycoformycin and prediction of early relapse. Clin Cancer Res 1999;5(7):1665–70.
81. Cawley JC, Burns GF, Hayhoe FG. A chronic lymphoproliferative disorder with distinctive features: a distinct variant of hairy-cell leukaemia. Leuk Res 1980; 4(6):547–59.
82. Matutes E, Wotherspoon A, Brito-Babapulle V, et al. The natural history and clinico-pathological features of the variant form of hairy cell leukemia. Leukemia 2001;15(1):184–6.
83. Matutes E, Wotherspoon A, Catovsky D. The variant form of hairy-cell leukaemia. Best Pract Res Clin Haematol 2003;16(1):41–56.
84. Munoz L, Nomdedeu JF, Lopez O, et al. Interleukin-3 receptor alpha chain (CD123) is widely expressed in hematologic malignancies. Haematologica 2001;86(12):1261–9.
85. Traverse-Glehen A, Baseggio L, Bauchu EC, et al. Splenic red pulp lymphoma with numerous basophilic villous lymphocytes: a distinct clinicopathologic and molecular entity? Blood 2008;111(4):2253–60.
86. McKenna RW, Parkin J, Kersey JH, et al. Chronic lymphoproliferative disorder with unusual clinical, morphologic, ultrastructural and membrane surface marker characteristics. Am J Med 1977;62(4):588–96.
87. Loughran TP Jr, Kadin ME, Starkebaum G, et al. Leukemia of large granular lymphocytes: association with clonal chromosomal abnormalities and autoimmune neutropenia, thrombocytopenia, and hemolytic anemia. Ann Intern Med 1985;102(2):169–75.
88. Loughran TP Jr. Clonal diseases of large granular lymphocytes. Blood 1993; 82(1):1–14.
89. Lamy T, Loughran TP Jr. Clinical features of large granular lymphocyte leukemia. Semin Hematol 2003;40(3):185–95.
90. Karadimitris A, Li K, Notaro R, et al. Association of clonal T-cell large granular lymphocyte disease and paroxysmal nocturnal haemoglobinuria (PNH): further evidence for a pathogenetic link between T cells, aplastic anaemia and PNH. Br J Haematol 2001;115(4):1010–4.
91. Lamy T, Loughran TP Jr. Current concepts: large granular lymphocyte leukemia. Blood Rev 1999;13(4):230–40.
92. Evans HL, Burks E, Viswanatha D, et al. Utility of immunohistochemistry in bone marrow evaluation of T-lineage large granular lymphocyte leukemia. Hum Pathol 2000;31(10):1266–73.
93. Morice WG, Kurtin PJ, Tefferi A, et al. Distinct bone marrow findings in T-cell granular lymphocytic leukemia revealed by paraffin section immunoperoxidase stains for CD8, TIA-1, and granzyme B. Blood 2002;99(1):268–74.
94. Langerak AW, van Den BR, Wolvers-Tettero IL, et al. Molecular and flow cytometric analysis of the Vbeta repertoire for clonality assessment in mature TCRalpha-beta T-cell proliferations. Blood 2001;98(1):165–73.

95. Lima M, Almeida J, Santos AH, et al. Immunophenotypic analysis of the TCR-Vbeta repertoire in 98 persistent expansions of CD3(+)/TCR-alphabeta(+) large granular lymphocytes: utility in assessing clonality and insights into the pathogenesis of the disease. Am J Pathol 2001;159(5):1861–8.

96. Beck RC, Stahl S, O'Keefe CL, et al. Detection of mature T-cell leukemias by flow cytometry using anti-T-cell receptor V beta antibodies. Am J Clin Pathol 2003; 120(5):785–94.

97. Ingen-Housz-Oro S, Bussel A, Flageul B, et al. A prospective study on the evolution of the T-cell repertoire in patients with Sezary syndrome treated by extracorporeal photopheresis. Blood 2002;100(6):2168–74.

98. Lundell R, Hartung L, Hill S, et al. T-cell large granular lymphocyte leukemias have multiple phenotypic abnormalities involving pan-T-cell antigens and receptors for MHC molecules. Am J Clin Pathol 2005;124(6):937–46.

99. Bourgault-Rouxel AS, Loughran TP Jr, Zambello R, et al. Clinical spectrum of gammadelta+ T cell LGL leukemia: analysis of 20 cases. Leuk Res 2008; 32(1):45–8.

100. Posnett DN, Sinha R, Kabak S, et al. Clonal populations of T cells in normal elderly humans: the T cell equivalent to "benign monoclonal gammapathy". J Exp Med 1994;179(2):609–18.

101. Pandolfi F, Loughran TP Jr, Starkebaum G, et al. Clinical course and prognosis of the lymphoproliferative disease of granular lymphocytes. A multicenter study. Cancer 1990;65(2):341–8.

102. Dhodapkar MV, Li CY, Lust JA, et al. Clinical spectrum of clonal proliferations of T-large granular lymphocytes: a T-cell clonopathy of undetermined significance? Blood 1994;84(5):1620–7.

103. Morice WG, Leibson PJ, Tefferi A. Natural killer cells and the syndrome of chronic natural killer cell lymphocytosis. Leuk Lymphoma 2001;41(3–4): 277–84.

104. Rabbani GR, Phyliky RL, Tefferi A. A long-term study of patients with chronic natural killer cell lymphocytosis. Br J Haematol 1999;106(4):960–6.

105. Zambello R, Trentin L, Ciccone E, et al. Phenotypic diversity of natural killer (NK) populations in patients with NK-type lymphoproliferative disease of granular lymphocytes. Blood 1993;81(9):2381–5.

106. Ohno Y, Amakawa R, Fukuhara S, et al. Acute transformation of chronic large granular lymphocyte leukemia associated with additional chromosome abnormality. Cancer 1989;64(1):63–7.

107. Imamura N, Kusunoki Y, Kawa-Ha K, et al. Aggressive natural killer cell leukaemia/lymphoma: report of four cases and review of the literature. Possible existence of a new clinical entity originating from the third lineage of lymphoid cells. Br J Haematol 1990;75(1):49–59.

108. Matutes E, Brito-Babapulle V, Swansbury J, et al. Clinical and laboratory features of 78 cases of T-prolymphocytic leukemia. Blood 1991;78(12):3269–74.

109. Hoyer JD, Ross CW, Li CY, et al. True T-cell chronic lymphocytic leukemia: a morphologic and immunophenotypic study of 25 cases. Blood 1995;86(3): 1163–9.

110. Matutes E, Catovsky D. Similarities between T-cell chronic lymphocytic leukemia and the small-cell variant of T-prolymphocytic leukemia. Blood 1996;87(8): 3520–1.

111. Garand R, Goasguen J, Brizard A, et al. Indolent course as a relatively frequent presentation in T-prolymphocytic leukaemia. Groupe Francais d'Hematologie Cellulaire. Br J Haematol 1998;103(2):488–94.

112. Matutes E, Garcia TJ, O'Brien M, et al. The morphological spectrum of T-prolymphocytic leukemia. Br J Haematol 1986;64:111–24.
113. Mallett RB, Matutes E, Catovsky D, et al. Cutaneous infiltration in T-cell prolymphocytic leukaemia. Br J Dermatol 1995;132(2):263–6.
114. Valbuena JR, Herling M, Admirand JH, et al. T-cell prolymphocytic leukemia involving extramedullary sites. Am J Clin Pathol 2005;123(3):456–64.
115. Herling M, Khoury JD, Washington LT, et al. A systematic approach to diagnosis of mature T-cell leukemias reveals heterogeneity among WHO categories. Blood 2004;104(2):328–35.
116. Maljaei SH, Brito-Babapulle V, Hiorns LR, et al. Abnormalities of chromosomes 8, 11, 14, and X in T-prolymphocytic leukemia studied by fluorescence in situ hybridization. Cancer Genet Cytogenet 1998;103(2):110–6.
117. Virgilio L, Lazzeri C, Bichi R, et al. Deregulated expression of TCL1 causes T cell leukemia in mice. Proc Natl Acad Sci U S A 1998;95(7):3885–9.
118. Gritti C, Dastot H, Soulier J, et al. Transgenic mice for MTCP1 develop T-cell prolymphocytic leukemia. Blood 1998;92(2):368–73.
119. Johnson AJ, Lucas DM, Muthusamy N, et al. Characterization of the TCL-1 transgenic mouse as a preclinical drug development tool for human chronic lymphocytic leukemia. Blood 2006;108(4):1334–8.
120. Laine J, Kunstle G, Obata T, et al. The protooncogene TCL1 is an Akt kinase coactivator. Mol Cell 2000;6(2):395–407.
121. Pekarsky Y, Zanesi N, Aqeilan R, et al. Tcl1 as a model for lymphomagenesis. Hematol Oncol Clin North Am 2004;18(4):863–79, ix.
122. Pekarsky Y, Koval A, Hallas C, et al. Tcl1 enhances Akt kinase activity and mediates its nuclear translocation. Proc Natl Acad Sci U S A 2000;97(7):3028–33.
123. Soma L, Cornfield DB, Prager D, et al. Unusually indolent T-cell prolymphocytic leukemia associated with a complex karyotype: is this T-cell chronic lymphocytic leukemia? Am J Hematol 2002;71(3):224–6.
124. Yokohama A, Karasawa M, Takada S, et al. Prolonged survival in two cases of T-prolymphocytic leukemias with complex hypodiploid chromosomal abnormalities. J Med 2000;31(3–4):183–94.
125. Herling M, Patel KA, Teitell MA, et al. High TCL1 expression and intact T-cell receptor signaling define a hyperproliferative subset of T-cell prolymphocytic leukemia. Blood 2008;111(1):328–37.
126. Cao TM, Coutre SE. T-cell prolymphocytic leukemia: update and focus on alemtuzumab (Campath-1H). Hematology 2003;8(1):1–6.
127. Dearden CE, Matutes E, Cazin B, et al. High remission rate in T-cell prolymphocytic leukemia with CAMPATH-1H. Blood 2001;98(6):1721–6.
128. Fraser-Andrews EA, Russell-Jones R, Woolford AJ, et al. Diagnostic and prognostic importance of T-cell receptor gene analysis in patients with Sezary syndrome. Cancer 2001;92(7):1745–52.
129. Duncan SC, Winkelmann RK. Circulating Sezary cells in hospitalized dermatology patients. Br J Dermatol 1978;99(2):171–8.
130. Bogen SA, Pelley D, Charif M, et al. Immunophenotypic identification of Sezary cells in peripheral blood. Am J Clin Pathol 1996;106(6):739–48.
131. Harmon CB, Witzig TE, Katzmann JA, et al. Detection of circulating T cells with CD4+CD7- immunophenotype in patients with benign and malignant lymphoproliferative dermatoses. J Am Acad Dermatol 1996;35(3 Pt 1):404–10.
132. Vonderheid EC, Bigler RD, Kotecha A, et al. Variable CD7 expression on T cells in the leukemic phase of cutaneous T cell lymphoma (Sezary syndrome). J Invest Dermatol 2001;117(3):654–62.

133. Jones D, Dang NH, Duvic M, et al. Absence of CD26 expression is a useful marker for diagnosis of T-cell lymphoma in peripheral blood. Am J Clin Pathol 2001;115(6):885–92.
134. Bernengo MG, Novelli M, Quaglino P, et al. The relevance of the CD4+ CD26- subset in the identification of circulating Sezary cells. Br J Dermatol 2001; 144(1):125–35.
135. Bahler DW, Hartung L, Hill S, et al. CD158k/KIR3DL2 is a useful marker for identifying neoplastic T-cells in Sezary syndrome by flow cytometry. Cytometry B Clin Cytom 2008;74(3):156–62.
136. Schwab C, Willers J, Niederer E, et al. The use of anti-T-cell receptor-Vbeta antibodies for the estimation of treatment success and phenotypic characterization of clonal T-cell populations in cutaneous T-cell lymphomas. Br J Haematol 2002; 118(4):1019–26.
137. Klemke CD, Brade J, Weckesser S, et al. The diagnosis of Sezary syndrome on peripheral blood by flow cytometry requires the use of multiple markers. Br J Dermatol 2008;159(4):871–80.
138. Vermeer MH, van Doorn R, Dijkman R, et al. Novel and highly recurrent chromosomal alterations in Sezary syndrome. Cancer Res 2008;68(8):2689–98.
139. Willemze R, Jaffe ES, Burg G, et al. WHO-EORTC classification for cutaneous lymphomas. Blood 2005;105(10):3768–85.
140. Matutes E. Adult T-cell leukaemia/lymphoma. J Clin Pathol 2007;60(12):1373–7.
141. Karube K, Ohshima K, Tsuchiya T, et al. Expression of FoxP3, a key molecule in CD4CD25 regulatory T cells, in adult T-cell leukaemia/lymphoma cells. Br J Haematol 2004;126(1):81–4.
142. Shimauchi T, Kabashima K, Tokura Y. Adult T-cell leukemia/lymphoma cells from blood and skin tumors express cytotoxic T lymphocyte-associated antigen-4 and Foxp3 but lack suppressor activity toward autologous CD8+ T cells. Cancer Sci 2008;99(1):98–106.
143. Kamihira S, Sugahara K, Tsuruda K, et al. Proviral status of HTLV-1 integrated into the host genomic DNA of adult T-cell leukemia cells. Clin Lab Haematol 2005;27(4):235–41.

Bone Marrow Involvement by Hodgkin and Non-Hodgkin Lymphomas

Qian-Yun Zhang, MD, PhD[a],*, Kathryn Foucar, MD[b]

KEYWORDS

- Bone marrow lymphoma • Hodgkin
- Non-Hodgkin lymphomas • Immunophenotype
- Molecular genetic assessment of non-Hodgkin lymphomas

INDICATIONS FOR BONE MARROW EXAMINATION

Bone marrow examination (BME) can provide significant diagnostic and prognostic information in patients with either Hodgkin lymphomas (HL) or non-Hodgkin lymphomas (NHL). However, there are no set rules regarding if and when BME is required in patients with confirmed or suspected lymphoma or in patients with inaccessible extramedullary disease. In recent years, radiologic modalities, especially positron emission tomography (PET) scans and magnetic resonance imaging (MRI), have assumed a greater role in staging and ongoing monitoring of lymphoma patients.[1,2] However, BME remains a cornerstone in the evaluation and monitoring of many lymphoma patients; indications for BME in patients with lymphoma are diverse (**Box 1**). In a patient with unexplained cytopenias/symptoms, the bone marrow may even be the initial site of detection of disease, although confirmation of a primary bone marrow diagnosis of the either HL or NHL by examination of an extramedullary site is always recommended, whenever feasible.

BONE MARROW EXAMINATION: SPECIMENS AND SPECIALIZED TECHNIQUES

Because each specimen type provides complementary information, optimal BM evaluation should include complete blood count (CBC) data, blood smear, BM aspirate smears and touch (imprint) preparations, clot sections, and core biopsy sections (**Fig. 1**).[3–5] Ideally, a single diagnostician should review and interpret all specimen

[a] Department of Pathology, Health Sciences Center, School of Medicine, University of New Mexico, MSC08 4640, 1 University of New Mexico, Albuquerque, NM 87131-0001, USA
[b] Department of Pathology, Health Sciences Center, University of New Mexico, TriCore Reference Laboratory, 1001 Woodward Place NE, Albuquerque, NM 87102, USA
* Corresponding author.
E-mail address: qzhang@salud.unm.edu (Q-Y. Zhang).

Hematol Oncol Clin N Am 23 (2009) 873–902
doi:10.1016/j.hoc.2009.04.014
0889-8588/09/$ – see front matter © 2009 Elsevier Inc. All rights reserved.
hemonc.theclinics.com

Box 1
Indications for BME in lymphoma patients

Initial assessment for cytopenias of unclear cause

Inaccessible extramedullary sites of disease

Atypical, yet nondiagnostic, lymphoid infiltrate in extramedullary site

Initial staging of NHL and HL with diagnosis established in an extramedullary site

Follow-up assessment of response to therapy in patients with Stage IV disease

Assessment for possible lymphoma relapse

Clinical questions regarding hematopoietic reserve

Required at various time points for protocol studies

Abbreviation: BME, bone marrow examination.

---

types to promote a comprehensive integrated diagnosis as well as the most cost-effective use of expensive specialized tests (**Table 1**).

Flow cytometric immunophenotyping can complement morphologic interpretation in cases in which abnormal cells are detected either in blood or on BM aspirate smears (**Fig. 2**). Targeted fluorescence in situ hybridization (FISH) for selected genetic findings is potentially useful in cases in which abnormal cells are present in liquid specimens or on air-dried, unfixed slide smear preparations (blood, touch preparation, or BM aspirate smears). Some FISH tests can be performed on paraffin-imbedded specimens. All specialized studies should target logical differential diagnostic considerations and use of these techniques should be predicated on evidence that the abnormal cell population is adequately represented in the potential study sample. Reflexive esoteric testing on morphology negative specimens is generally noninformative. Because small clonal lymphoid populations of uncertain significance are common in the BM of elderly patients, the detection of a clone in these cases might lead to an erroneous interpretation of stage IV NHL.[6] In contrast, some investigators have described cases positive by flow cytometry, but negative by morphology, especially in patients with follicular lymphoma.[7] Similarly, false-positive or false-negative results from molecular/genetic studies may provoke misdiagnosis, especially if these specialized studies are *not* integrated with morphology and immunohistochemical results.

Step sections of generous bilateral (or double unilateral) core biopsy specimens are especially valuable in the identification of focal BM lesions. Once an abnormal infiltrate has been identified, immunohistochemical/in situ hybridization studies may provide additional information about the lineage and stage of maturation of this abnormal infiltrate (see **Fig. 1**).[5,8]

Bone marrow core biopsy specimens are also crucial for establishing the pattern and extent of BM infiltration by lymphoma (**Fig. 3** and **Table 2**). The pattern of infiltration is designated as focal, nonparatrabecular, focal, paratrabecular, intrasinusoidal, diffuse interstitial or diffuse, and solid (see **Fig. 1**, **Table 2**). This pattern is often a clue to a specific lymphoma subtype as noted in **Table 2** and subsequent tables in this review.[5,8,9] The detection of BM involvement virtually always advances lymphoma patients to Stage IV disease. The exception to this general rule occurs in cases in which there is a discordance between large cell lymphoma in the extranodal site versus small clonal B cells in the BM. This type of discordance may occur in lymphomas of follicular center cell derivation (see later discussion).[9]

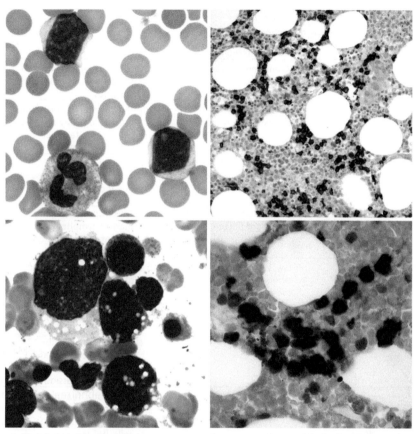

Fig. 1. Peripheral blood and bone marrow from a patient with leukemic mantle cell lymphoma illustrating the morphologic overlap with chronic lymphocytic leukemia in the peripheral blood (*upper left*), the morphologic features of mantle cell lymphoma on a bone marrow aspirate smear from this same patient (*lower left*), the patchy interstitial infiltrates of mantle cell lymphoma highlighted by immunoperoxidase (IPOX) for CD20 on the bone marrow core biopsy (*upper right*), and nuclear cyclin D1 positivity on the BM core biopsy from this same patient (*lower right*).

BONE MARROW INVOLVEMENT IN HODGKIN LYMPHOMA

Most young patients with classic HL have localized, node-based disease. In patients with localized disease by clinical/radiographic examination and no evidence of B symptoms (fever, night sweats, weight loss), the likelihood of BM involvement is low (**Table 3**). Consequently, routine BME may not be warranted in these low-stage patients.[11–13] In contrast, older patients with HL often present with B symptoms, unexplained cytopenias, and inaccessible sites of extramedullary disease (ie, retroperitoneum). In these patients, the yield of a positive BME is substantially higher. Indeed, the BM may be the initial site of detection of disease. Similarly, immunodeficient patients are at a greater risk for the development of HL with BM involvement. Likewise the type of HL is predictive of the incidence of BM involvement in that nodular lymphocyte predominant HL (NLPHL) only rarely involves BM, whereas BM involvement by classic HL is substantially more common, especially in symptomatic or immunodeficient patients (see **Table 3**).[11,13,14]

Table 1
Bone marrow examination in lymphoma

Specimen	Evaluation/Technique	Comments/Caveats
Blood	CBC and morphology review	Circulating lymphoma cells identified in selected NHL subtypes
Blood	Flow cytometry, FISH, cytogenetics, molecular	Only indicated if circulating morphologically atypical cells noted; targeted special studies
BM aspirate (touch preparation)	Differential count, morphology, detection of abnormal cells. A touch preparation may include inaspirable cells from fibrotic lesions	Assess for distinctive lymphoma cells; assess HP lineages. May be challenging to distinguish lymphoma cells from normal bone marrow lymphocytes in patients with small cell neoplasms
BM aspirate	Flow cytometry, cytogenetics, FISH, molecular	Selected use in cases with abnormal cells noted on aspirate smears. Special studies must target specific differential diagnostic considerations. Not recommended for routine use in all cases regardless of morphologic assessment
BM clot section	Morphology/IHC, limited FISH	Morphologic features for extent of infiltration and assessment of residual HP cells; IHC to assess abnormal infiltrates
BM core biopsy sections, 1–2 cm, bilateral	Morphology/IHC	Pattern and extent of infiltration of lymphoma. Associated bone, vessel and stromal changes; assess individual HP lineages. IHC to assess abnormal infiltrates

Abbreviations: FISH, fluorescence in situ hybridization; NHL, non-Hodgkin lymphoma; HP, hematopoietic; IHC, immunohistochemistry.

The successful identification of HL in BM requires the integration of morphologic and immunohistochemical (IHC)/in situ hybridization (ISH) features (**Figs. 4–6**). Large mononuclear or binucleate cells with prominent eosinophilic nucleoli within the appropriate cellular milieu are essential for diagnosis (**Table 4**). These cells are either classic Reed Sternberg (RS) cells or mononuclear RS variant cells (see **Fig. 5**). By IHC, RS cells in classic HL are CD30-positive, CD15 positive, CD45-negative, and variably CD20 positive.[14] T cell antigens are not usually expressed. By Epstein Barr virus-encoded RNA (EBER) ISH, Epstein-Barr virus (EBV) is detected within the nuclei of these

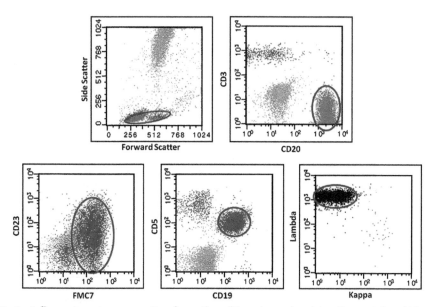

Fig. 2. A flow cytometry composite of mantle cell lymphoma involving the peripheral blood mimicking chronic lymphocytic leukemia morphologically showing positivity for FMC7 and CD23 in conjunction with CD5 coexpression, bright CD20, and lambda light chain restriction. Despite the morphologic overlap with chronic lymphocytic leukemia, this immunophenotypic profile is more characteristic of mantle cell lymphoma.

cells in some, but not all cases (see **Fig. 6**). As noted in **Table 5**, there are many caveats in BME for HL, and one notable problem is the degradation of IHC/ISH due to decalcification or fixation techniques.[19,20] Consequently, false-negative results for expression of CD30 and notably EBER are not uncommon in BM core biopsy sections. Because normal internal positive cells are not typically present, negative results for

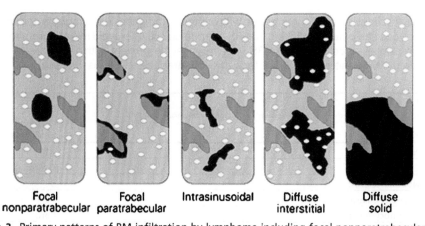

Focal nonparatrabecular Focal paratrabecular Intrasinusoidal Diffuse interstitial Diffuse solid

Fig. 3. Primary patterns of BM infiltration by lymphoma including focal nonparatrabecular, focal paratrabecular, sinusoidal, diffuse interstitial (with some preservation of hematopoiesis among lymphoma infiltrates), and diffuse solid infiltrates of lymphoma filling the entire area between bony trabeculae and completely effacing hematopoietic cells. (*From* Foucar K. Non-Hodgkin lymphoma and Hodgkin lymphoma (disease) in bone marrow. In: Bone marrow pathology. 2nd edition. Chicago (IL): ASCP Press; 2001. p. 438–83; with permission.)

Table 2
Patterns of BM involvement in HL and NHL

Pattern Type	Features	Lymphoma Types
Focal, nonparatrabecular	Discrete aggregates of lymphoma cells in random intertrabecular space	Common pattern exhibited by small lymphoid NHL cell types and HL
Focal, paratrabecular	Discrete aggregates of lymphoma cells molded against bony trabeculae	Common pattern exhibited by follicular NHL and occasional mantle cell or other types of NHL
Intravascular, intrasinusoidal	Serpiginous, linear abnormal lymphoid infiltrates within identifiable sinuses, or less often, vessel lumina	Common pattern in splenic marginal zone lymphoma, and rare intrasinusoidal large cell lymphomas. Often noted in conjunction with other patterns in many NHL subtypes
Diffuse, interstitial	Patchy, variably subtle, poorly delineated regions of abnormal lymphoid cell infiltrates, which are dispersed among hematopoietic and fat cells	Can be seen in many types of NHL but more prevalent in aggressive/blastic lesions
Diffuse, solid	Complete effacement of HP and fat cells between bony trabeculae	May be seen in many types of HL and NHL in which there is extensive BM effacement

Abbreviations: HL, Hodgkin lymphoma; NHL, non-Hodgkin lymphoma.
Data from Refs.[5,8–10]

these two stains must be interpreted with caution. In addition, immunoblasts and other cell types can potentially mimic true RS morphologically. To avoid misinterpretation of these lookalike cells; RS cells/RS variants must be present within discrete foci of altered BM architecture. These focal, nonparatrabecular lesions of classic HL are

Table 3
Incidence of bone marrow involvement in Hodgkin lymphoma (HL)

Type	Incidence (%)
NLPHL	<1
Classic HL	Overall 4–10
Nodular sclerosis	3
Mixed cellularity	10
Lymphocyte rich	Rare
Lymphocyte depleted	>50
Immunodeficiency-associated (often lymphocyte depleted)	>60

Abbreviations: HL, Hodgkin lymphoma; NLPHL, nodular lymphocyte predominant Hodgkin lymphoma.
Data from Refs.[11–17]

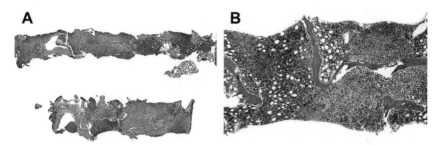

Fig. 4. Low (*A*) and high (*B*) magnification of core biopsy specimens showing discrete effacing infiltrates of Hodgkin lymphoma. Note extensive areas of diffuse, solid effacement (hematoxylin-eosin).

often associated with fibrosis and, therefore, inaspirable (see **Fig. 4**). Reed Sternberg cells generally account for only a minority of the total cells within these discrete focal or diffuse solid lesions, except in cases of lymphocyte depletion in which RS cells and variants are abundant.[21] The cellular milieu of HL includes admixed lymphocytes, histiocytes, plasma cells, and eosinophils with only a small component of RS cells/ RS variants (see **Fig. 5**).

Caution should be used in making a primary diagnosis of HL in a BM specimen; lymph node biopsy should always be recommended, if clinically feasible. In addition, bone marrow involvement by HL may be masked by a concurrent prominent histiocyte infiltrate; again lymph node biopsy should be pursued (see **Fig. 6**). In rare, usually immunocompromised patients, the bone marrow will be the only site of disease.[22]

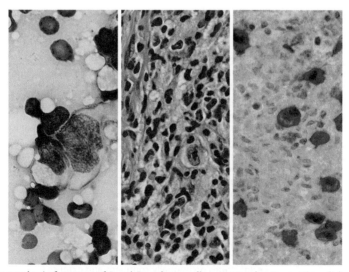

Fig. 5. The cytologic features of Reed Sternberg cells on a touch preparation slide (*left*), the admixture of Reed Sternberg cells with lymphocytes and histiocytes on the bone marrow core biopsy section (*center*), and the coexpression of membrane and cytoplastic CD30 and weak nuclear PAX5 typical of Reed Sternberg cells by IPOX staining for CD30/PAX5 on the BM core biopsy section (*right*).

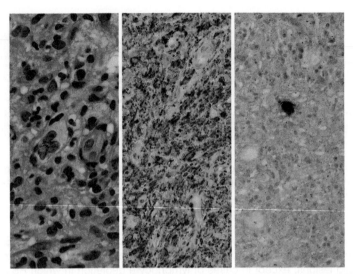

Fig. 6. The morphologic and immunohistochemical features of histiocyte rich classic Hodgkin lymphoma in a bone marrow core biopsy section. Note rare Reed Sternberg cells admixed with numerous histiocytes (hematoxylin-eosin) (*left*), the abundant histiocytes are readily apparent by CD68 immunohistochemical staining (*center*), the rare Reed Sternberg cells are positive for EBV by in situ hybridization staining (*right*).

BONE MARROW INVOLVEMENT IN B CELL NON-HODGKIN LYMPHOMA

The incidence of B cell non-Hodgkin lymphoma (B-NHL) involving bone marrow varies by the subtype (**Table 6**). In general, indolent small cell B-NHL involves BM much more frequently than aggressive B-NHL (see **Table 6**). Small lymphocytic lymphoma

Table 4 Bone marrow findings in Hodgkin lymphoma	
Specimen	**Comments**
Aspirate	• Marrow may be inaspirable in cases with extensive involvement due to associated fibrosis • RS cells only rarely noted on aspirate smears
Touch preparation	• RS cells and the associated HL milieu (plasma cells, lymphocytes, histiocytes, eosinophils) are more likely to be present on touch preparations than aspirate smears
Core biopsy	• Involvement of BM in classic HL is usually characterized by discrete lesions detectable on low magnification • Lesions are focal, nonparatrabecular • Lesions polymorphous and RS cells/variants may be infrequent • RS variant cells, large with prominent nucleoli; may be mono-nuclear or bi-/multinucleated • IHC of RS cells: CD30-positive, CD15-positive, PAX5-dim, CD20-variable, CD45-negative, EBER-positive in a subset of cases • Reticulin/collagen fibrosis associated with lesions • Infiltrates occasionally confluent and extensive • BM involvement in nodular lymphocyte predominate HL is rare; consists of large B cells with abundant small T cells

Abbreviations: IHC, immunohistochemical; RS cells, Reed Sternberg cells.
   Data from Refs.[5,8,11,15–18]

Table 5	
Caveats in the identification of Hodgkin lymphoma in bone marrow	
Finding	**Comments**
Striking predominance of histiocytes without identifiable RS cells	Histiocytes may mask BM infiltrates of HL, especially in immunodeficient patients; recommend lymph node biopsy
Striking predominance of plasma cell masking RS cells	More problematic on small core biopsy specimens
Atypical large cells with some morphologic features of RS cells	Abnormal cells must be in appropriate milieu (ie, discrete lesion with plasma cells, eosinophils, and so forth); peripheral T-NHL/other NHL may closely mimic HL in BM
Inconclusive IHC/ISH assessment	Antigenicity may be lost with decalcification; fixation techniques (false-negatives common)

Abbreviations: IHC, immunohistochemical; ISH, in situ hybridization.
Data from Joshi A, Aqel NM. Hodgkin's disease of bone marrow masquerading as a heavy plasma cell infiltration and fibrosis. Br J Haematol 2003;122(3):343.

involves bone marrow (BM) in more than 80% of cases[5,9] and follicular lymphoma (FL) involves BM in about 40% to 70% of cases depending on the study.[23,24,30] Splenic marginal zone lymphoma (SMZL) almost always involves BM.[5,9,31] In contrast, aggressive lymphomas such as T cell/histiocyte rich large B cell lymphoma involves marrow in 15% to 60% of cases,[25,26] whereas diffuse large B cell lymphoma (DLBCL) involves marrow in only 10% to 30% of cases.[27,28]

The pattern of involvement of bone marrow also varies by B-NHL subtype (see **Table 6**). In general, small lymphocytic lymphoma (SLL) and lymphoplasmacytic lymphoma (LPL) show predominantly interstitial and diffuse patterns of infiltration, FL exhibits predominantly paratrabecular infiltrates, mantle cell lymphoma (MCL) exhibits paratrabecular and nonparatrabecular lymphoid nodules, marginal zone lymphoma (MZL) shows predominantly nonparatrabecular lymphoid nodules, whereas SMZL may exhibit intrasinusoidal infiltrates, nonparatrabecular lymphoid nodules or both.

B-Lymphoblastic Leukemia/Lymphoma

Precursor B-lymphoblastic leukemia/lymphoma (B-LBL) is an immature B cell neoplasm and is primarily a disease of children. When this neoplasm involves primarily blood and bone marrow, which is in most cases, it is designated as B-acute lymphoblastic leukemia (B-ALL). When the primary disease is extramedullary based and there are less than 25% lymphoblasts in the marrow, it is arbitrarily designated as B-lymphoblastic lymphoma (B-LBL).[32] As expected, precursor B-ALL involves marrow in all cases with predominantly interstitial, diffuse infiltrate. B-LBL also involves marrow in most, but not all cases. When involved, the bone marrow aspirate shows a population of lymphoblasts (<25% of total cells) with morphology identical to ALL cells. The cytologic features are described in **Table 6**. The bone marrow core biopsy reveals a patchy interstitial infiltration pattern, similar to B-ALL but with a much lower extent of effacement. Immunophenotypic and genetic features of B-LBL are identical to B-ALL (see **Table 6**).[32] The caveat in assessing bone marrow involvement in B-LBL is the potential to mistake hematogones for lymphoma cells. Hematogones share some morphologic and immunophenotypic features with leukemic blasts and can

Table 6
Features of bone marrow involvement in B cell non-Hodgkin lymphomas

Lymphoma Subtype	Incidence of BM Involvement (%)	1st Pattern of BM Core Biopsy (2nd Patterns)	Cytologic Features	Immunophenotypic Features	Genotype
B-LBL	40–60	Patchy, interstitial (diffuse, focal nodules)	Small- to medium-sized blasts, high nuclear/cytoplasmic ratio, fine chromatin, small nucleoli, subset with cytoplasmic vacuoles	Immature B cell, CD19, CD79a, CD20, CD22, CD10, CD34, TdT, HLA-DR, no surface Ig	Clonal *IGH* and *TCR* gene rearrangement may be detected; ALL type translocations in a minority
SLL	85	Nodular, nonparatrabecular predominant (focal patchy interstitial)	Small, round nuclei, condensed chromatin with bandlike clearing, inconspicuous nucleoli, occasional large paraimmunoblasts or prolymphocytes	Weak sIg, CD19, CD79a, weak CD20, weak CD22, CD5, CD23, BCL2	Clonal *IGH* gene rearrangement, mutated or unmutated *IgVH*, trisomy 12, del(13q), del(17p)
MCL	50–80	Focal nonparatrabecular, (focal paratrabecular)	Small to intermediate, irregular nuclei, inconspicuous nucleoli, usually with cytologic heterogeneity	sIg, CD19, CD79a, CD20, CD22, CD5, FMC7, cyclin D1, BCL2	Clonal *IGH* gene rearrangement, t(11;14)(q13;q32)/*CYCLIN D1-IGH*
FL	40–70	Focal paratrabecular	Small cleaved admixed with large cleaved and large noncleaved	sIg,[a] CD19, CD79a, CD20, CD10, BCL2, CD22, FMC7	Clonal *IGH* gene rearrangement, t(14;18)(q32;q21)/*BCL2-IGH*

LPL	100	Focal nonparatrabecular, interstitial, diffuse	Spectrum of small lymphocytes, plasmacytoid lymphocytes, and plasma cells with occasional intracytoplasmic or intranuclear pseudoinclusions, increased mast cells	Monoclonal lymphoma cells with cIg, CD19, CD79a, variable sIg, CD22, FMC7, variable CD23, CD25, CD103 and CD11c. Monoclonal plasma cells with cIg	Clonal *IGH* gene rearrangement, t(9;14)(p13;q32)/ *PAX5-IGH* in half of the cases, monosomy 8, del(6q)
SMZL	70–100	Usually mixed pattern, focal nonparatrabecular, interstitial, intrasinusoidal/ intravascular (focal paratrabecular, diffuse)	Small to intermediate cells with moderate to abundant pale gray-blue cytoplasm, occasionally form cytoplasmic projections or "villi," condensed chromatin, inconspicuous nucleoli	sIg, sometimes cIg, CD19, CD79a, CD20, CD22, FMC7, BCL2	Clonal *IGH* gene rearrangement, deletion 7q in 30%–50% cases, some cases may harbor trisomy 3, or trisomy 18
EMZL	3–20	Usually mixed pattern, focal nonparatrabecular, paratrabecular, interstitial	Moderate to abundant cytoplasm, noncleaved nuclei	sIg, CD19, CD79a, CD20, CD22, BCL2	Clonal *IGH* gene rearrangement, t(11;18) (q21;q21)/ *API2-MALT1*, some cases have trisomy 3
NMZL	30–40	Single pattern predominant, focal nonparatrabecular, paratrabecular, interstitial	Moderate to abundant cytoplasm, noncleaved nuclei	sIg, CD19, CD79a, CD20, CD22, BCL2	Clonal *IGH* gene rearrangement, some cases have trisomy 3

(continued on next page)

Table 6
(continued)

Lymphoma Subtype	Incidence of BM Involvement (%)	1st Pattern of BM Core Biopsy (2nd Patterns)	Cytologic Features	Immunophenotypic Features	Genotype
DLBCL	10–30	Focal nonparatrabecular, focal paratrabecular, diffuse	Large cells, moderatecytoplasm, small to prominent nucleoli, discordant morphology with concurrent extramedullary tissue may exist	sIg, CD19, CD79a, CD20, CD22, BCL2, vCD10, vCD5, vCD43	Clonal *IGH* gene rearrangement, cytogenetic abnormality depends on subtype, t(14;18)(q32;q21)/ *BCL2-IGH* in 20%–30% cases, *BCL6* rearrangement in 30% cases, may show complex karyotypes
TCRBCL	15–60	Paratrabecular, diffuse	Heterogeneity infiltrate, scattered large atypical cells in a mixed small lymphocytic/histiocytic background	sIg, CD19, CD79a, CD20, BCL6, negative for CD15, CD30 and EBV	Clonal *IGH* gene rearrangement
BL	15–35	Diffuse interstitial, diffuse solid	Intermediate, deep basophilic cytoplasm with distinct vacuoles, round nuclei, variable number of inconspicuous nucleoli	sIg, CD19, CD79a, CD20, CD22, CD10, CD43	Clonal *IGH* gene rearrangement, t(8;14)(q24;q32)/ *MYC-IGH*, less likely t(2;8)(p12;q24)/ *KAPPA-MYC* or t(8;22)(q24;q11)/ *MYC- LAMBDA*

Abbreviations: BL, Burkitt lymphoma; B-LBL, B-lymphoblastic lymphoma; cIg, cytoplasmic immunoglobulin; DLBCL, diffuse large B cell lymphoma; EBV, Epstein Barr virus; EMZL, extranodal marginal zone lymphoma of mucosa-associated lymphoid tissue (MALT lymphoma); FL, follicular lymphoma; IgVH, immunoglobulin heavy chain variable region; LPL, lymphoplasmacytic lymphoma; MCL, mantle cell lymphoma; NMZL, nodal marginal zone lymphoma; SLL, small lymphocytic lymphoma; SMZL, splenic B cell marginal zone lymphoma; sIg, surface immunoglobulin; vCD, variably present.

[a] Some cases of FL can be surface Ig negative.

Data from Refs.[5,9,23–29]

mimic ALL.[33–35] Hematogones are usually more abundant in BM from children, particularly when there has been marrow damage or insult.[33] Flow cytometric and molecular studies can help to distinguish hematogones from B-LBL cells. Lymphoma cells usually demonstrate a distinct tight population of immature cells and lack the characteristic maturation spectrum that hematogones exhibit by flow cytometry. Lymphoma cells may also express aberrant myeloid markers.[34,35]

Small Lymphocytic Lymphoma

Chronic lymphocytic leukemia (CLL) and small lymphocytic lymphoma (SLL) are synonymous diseases with different manifestations. By definition, CLL is a disease of peripheral blood and bone marrow, whereas SLL is a node-based disease with a high frequency of secondary BM involvement (see **Table 6**). In an international lymphoma study group classification, SLL comprises 6.7% of all NHL.[36] The cell morphology and bone marrow infiltration pattern are described in **Table 6**. Flow cytometry reveals a monoclonal B cell population with CD23 expression, aberrant CD5 coexpression, weak surface immunoglobulin light chain, and weak CD20 expression.[37]

Mantle Cell Lymphoma

Mantle cell lymphoma (MCL) accounts for 4% to 10% of NHL, affects men frequently, and typically shows an aggressive clinical course with short survival times. The features of BM involvement, cytologic morphology, and immunophenotype are described in **Table 6**. Paratrabecular and nonparatrabecular focal lesions may be seen (see **Figs. 1** and **2**). Occasionally, MCL patients may present with significant blood and BM involvement, mimicking leukemia (see **Fig. 1**). The characteristic flow cytometric findings for MCL are shown in **Fig. 2**. Rarely, BM involvement can be subtle and easily overlooked. If flow cytometric analysis is not available, generous use of cyclin D1 in conjunction with CD20 immunostaining can be helpful (see **Fig. 1**). The clinically aggressive blastic variant MCL is rare and is comprised of predominantly intermediate to large cells mimicking acute leukemia.[38] A definitive diagnosis of MCL is established by demonstration of overexpression of cyclin D1 by immunohistochemical study or documentation of translocation of t(11;14)(q13;q32)/BCL1/IgH fusion by cytogenetics or FISH (See **Fig. 1**).[39]

Follicular Lymphoma

Follicular lymphoma (FL) is the most common small lymphocytic B cell NHL and comprises approximately 35% of all NHL in the United States. Follicular lymphoma is an indolent but incurable tumor affecting adults with a median age of onset of 59 years and a median overall survival of 7 to 10 years.[30] The incidence of BM involvement, cytologic features, bone marrow infiltration patterns, and immunophenotype of FL are described in **Table 6**. FL is typically distinctive on low power review of the bone marrow core biopsy due to the paratrabecular localization of infiltrates. Although nuclei are typically clefted, this is often more evident on blood smears or core biopsy sections rather than aspirate smears (**Fig. 7**). Bone marrow examination for FL staging can be challenging in several respects (**Table 7**). First, expression of BCL2, although classic for FL, can be seen in many other neoplastic and non-neoplastic lymphocytes. Nonetheless, the concurrent coexpression of BCL2 and germinal center associated markers BCL6 or CD10 is compatible with FL. Second, there can be discordance between the size of lymphoma cells seen in lymph node compared with those in BM. Cytogenetic and FISH studies for t(14;18)(q32;q21)/*BCL2-IGH* fusion are helpful in diagnosing FL.[40] The successful diagnosis of FL in BM requires specific comments

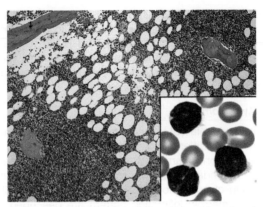

Fig. 7. Follicular lymphoma cells circulating in peripheral blood (inset) and exhibiting focal paratrabecular infiltrates on bone marrow core biopsy section (Wrights and hematoxylin-eosin).

about the size of the lymphoma cells within the bone marrow; a comparison with concurrent lymph node specimens is optimal (see **Table 7**).

Lymphoplasmacytic Lymphoma

Lymphoplasmacytic lymphoma (LPL) is an indolent B cell lymphoproliferative disorder with variable plasmacytoid differentiation.[41] A related disease, Waldenstrom

Table 7
Caveats of bone marrow staging in follicular lymphoma

Specimen	Comment
Bone marrow aspirate	Paratrabecular lymphoid infiltrate closely appose to the bony trabeculae and are frequently accompanied by fibrosis. The bone marrow aspirate is often poorly representative. Consequently, flow cytometric immunophenotype and morphologic assessment of BM aspirate may be falsely negative
Bone marrow core biopsy	Lymphoma cells coexpress germinal center associated antigen CD10. If the surface immunoglobulin is weak or indeterminate in the lymphoma cells, it is difficult to distinguish the lymphoma cells from the normal counterpart germinal center cells. FISH may be needed to distinguish between benign and malignant infiltrates
Lymph node	There may be morphologic discordance between bone marrow and lymph node. The bone marrow involvement may reveal a small cell process whereas the concurrent lymphoid tissue biopsy could show, eg, a higher grade follicular lymphoma or a diffuse large B cell lymphoma (DLBCL). This is called "discordant" or "down-graded" lymphoma (details in Table 8). Rarely, the marrow and lymph node disparity is the opposite, with a predominance of large cells in the BM and smaller cells in the node

Data from Arber DA, George TI. Bone marrow biopsy involvement by non-Hodgkin's lymphoma: frequency of lymphoma types, patterns, blood involvement, and discordance with other sites in 450 specimens. Am J Surg Pathol 2005;29(12):1549–57.

macroglobulinemia (WM), is regarded as a distinct clinicopathologic entity, and diagnosis should be confined to those patients with LPL who have demonstrable serum IgM monoclonal protein.[42] LPL comprises approximately 5% of NHLs and is associated with hepatitis C virus infection in 26% of cases with or without cryoglobulinemia.[8,41] LPL affects middle-aged to older adults with a male predominance and the median overall survival is 4 to 5 years. Classic LPL/WM typically involves the bone marrow and spleen. The cytologic features, bone marrow infiltration patterns, and immunophenotype are described in **Table 6**. In blood and bone marrow, a spectrum of small lymphocytes, plasmacytoid lymphocytes and plasma cells is typical (**Fig. 8**). Translocation t(9;14)(p13;q32) is rarely detected in LPL cases; 6q21 deletion is observed in approximately 50% of LPL cases and is associated with adverse prognosis.[41]

Marginal Zone Lymphoma

Marginal zone lymphoma (MZL) includes splenic marginal zone lymphoma (SMZL), extranodal marginal zone lymphoma (EMZL) of mucosa-associated lymphoid tissue (MALT) and nodal marginal zone lymphoma (NMZL). SMZL is an indolent B cell lymphoproliferative disorder and comprises approximately 2% of cases of B-NHL.[43] The cell morphology, bone marrow infiltration pattern, and immunophenotype are described in **Table 6**. A predilection for sinusoidal infiltration is highly characteristic of SMZL in BM (**Fig. 9**). There is no specific genetic abnormality for SMZL (see **Table 6**). A subset of SMZL has been shown to be associated with hepatitis C infection.[44]

EMZL of MALT (MALT lymphoma) and NMZL are also indolent B-NHLs. EMZL is common and comprises about 8% of NHLs. NMZL is rare and accounts for less than 1% of all lymphomas.[43] The bone marrow findings for ENMZ and NMZ are listed in **Table 6**. The bone marrow involvement in marginal zone lymphoma can be inconspicuous. Flow cytometric studies with or without immunohistochemical staining can be valuable in those cases.

Diffuse Large B Cell Lymphoma

Diffuse large B cell lymphoma (DLBCL) is an aggressive intermediate to high grade B cell lymphoma. DLBCL comprises a clinically, morphologically, and genetically heterogeneous group of large B cell lymphomas. DLBCL constitutes 30% to 40% of

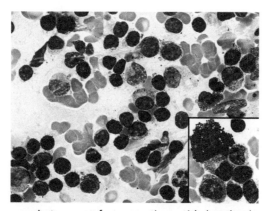

Fig. 8. Bone marrow aspirate smear from a patient with lymphoplasmacytic lymphoma shows the spectrum of small lymphocytes, plasmacytoid lymphocytes, and plasma cells. Increased mast cells are frequently present in lymphoplasmacytic lymphoma (Wrights).

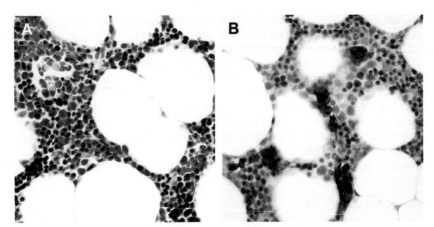

Fig. 9. (*A*) Bone marrow core biopsy of a patient with splenic marginal zone lymphoma showing normocellular marrow without overt lymphoid infiltrates. (*B*) The same case stained with antibody CD20 reveals the intrasinusoidal pattern of involvement (hematoxylin-eosin, CD20).

NHLs in western countries and an even higher proportion in developing countries. The median age of diagnosis is in the seventh decade.[45] Recent gene expression profile studies have identified 2 major subtypes of DLBCL, a germinal center B cell subtype and an activated B cell subtype, which may use different oncogenic pathways.[46] Patients with germinal center B cell–like DLBCL have significantly better overall survival than those with activated B cell–like DLBCL. The incidence of BM involvement, morphology, BM infiltration pattern, and immunophenotype are listed in **Table 6**. The BM infiltration pattern and cytologic features are illustrated in **Fig. 10**. Although large lymphoma cells are evident in the BM in most cases, discordant marrow involvement in DLBCL is observed in up to 25% of cases.[9,27,47] The morphology and clinical significance of discordant morphology are described in **Table 8**. Cytogenetic and molecular studies reveal t(14;18)/BCL2-IgH in approximately 10% to 30% of germinal center B cell–like DLBCL.[48] The outcome of DLBCL is highly variable, reflecting the

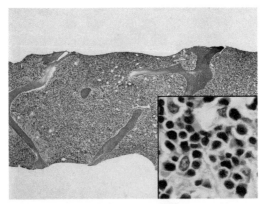

Fig. 10. Bone marrow core biopsy of a patient with diffuse large B cell lymphoma showing extensive replacement. The lymphoma cells are moderate to large and show moderate pleomorphism and increased mitoses (inset) (hematoxylin-eosin).

Table 8		
Discordant bone marrow morphology in diffuse large B cell lymphoma		
Bone Marrow Morphology	**Lymph Node Morphology**	**Comment**
Small or mixed small and large cells	Predominantly large cells	"Discordant" BM infiltrates in DLBCL represent a heterogeneous group of disorders, encompassing cases with a clonally related, clinically occult small cell component, as well as cases with two clonally distinct, unrelated B cell neoplasms presenting synchronously at different locations. Therefore the presence of discordant disease, irrespective of the clonal relatedness, should not be equated with disseminated (stage IV) large cell lymphoma
Predominantly large cells	Predominantly large cells	"Concordant" bone marrow involvement (the true stage IV disease) is relatively infrequent and it carries poor prognosis

Data from Refs.[9,27,47]

heterogeneity of this tumor.[42] Biomarkers and gene expression profiling have been used in assessment of prognosis.[49,50]

T Cell Rich B Cell Lymphoma

T cell rich B cell lymphoma (TCRBCL) is a subtype of DCBCL with characteristic morphologic and immunophenotypic features.[51] The frequency of BM involvement by TCRBCL in different studies is variable.[25,26] Research has shown that the TCRBCL lymphoma cells are derived from germinal center cells.[25,52] The cell morphology and bone marrow infiltration patterns are described in **Table 6**. Flow cytometry has limited use in TCRBCL and is almost always negative due to the low number of lymphoma cells (<10%) within the marrow infiltrates. The diagnosis of TCRBCL can be challenging and the presence of predominantly small lymphocytes and histiocytes can be mistaken as a benign lymphoid or histiocytic infiltrate. Diagnosis is based on immunohistochemical stains (see **Table 6, Fig. 11**). Another major differential diagnostic consideration is HL, because TRCBCL and HL characteristically show abundant benign cells with only rare neoplastic cells. However, TCRBCL shows strong uniform CD20 expression and is typically negative for the HL-associated markers CD15, CD30, and EBV stain.

Burkitt Lymphoma

Burkitt lymphoma (BL) is an aggressive B cell lymphoma with unique clinical, morphologic, immunophenotypic, and cytogenetic features (ie, translocation t(8;14) or its variants).[53] BL has endemic, sporadic, and AIDS-associated forms.[53] The rate of bone marrow involvement, cell morphology, immunophenotype, and infiltration patterns are described in **Table 6** and **Fig. 12**. On tissue sections, BL exhibits diffuse growth of medium-sized cells with brisk mitoses and apoptosis. A starry sky pattern is usually apparent due to numerous macrophages ingesting tumor cells or cell debris. Cytogenetic or FISH studies confirm the diagnosis by finding translocation t(8;14)(q24;q32)/ *MYC-IGH* or its variant translocations t(2;8)(q12;q24)/*KAPPA-MYC* or t(8;22) (q24;q11)/*MYC-LAMBDA*.[29,54]

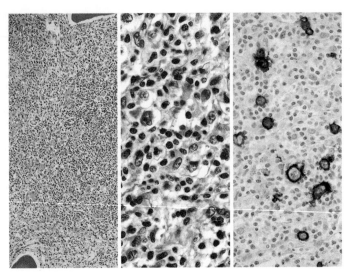

Fig. 11. (A) Bone marrow core biopsy from a patient with T cell rich B cell lymphoma showing diffuse marrow replacement by lymphoma. (B) The large atypical lymphoma cells are sparse and admixed with background small lymphocytes and histiocytes. (C) The same case stained with antibody CD20 reveals scattered lymphoma cells (hematoxylin-eosin, CD20).

BONE MARROW INVOLVEMENT IN T CELL AND NATURAL KILLER CELL LYMPHOMAS

Although many types of mature T and natural killer (NK) cell neoplasms are included in the recent WHO classification,[55] only those disorders that manifest primarily as lymphomas are included in this review. Furthermore, the discussion focuses on those mature T cell and NK cell neoplasms with either a propensity for BM involvement or a propensity for systemic cytokine-mediated hematologic manifestations (**Table 9**).[56] As a group, mature T cell and NK cell lymphomas account for only 7% of all NHLs with a broad range in the incidence of BM involvement.[5,9] The immature T cell

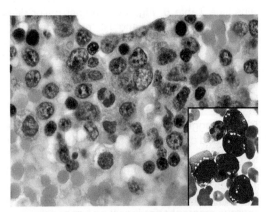

Fig. 12. Bone marrow clot section from a patient with Burkitt lymphoma showing a prominent lymphoma cell infiltrate. The lymphoma cells are large and nuclei show a vesicular chromatin pattern with multiple small nucleoli. The lymphoma cells have scant deep blue cytoplasm with sharp cytoplasmic vacuoles (inset) (hematoxylin-eosin, Wrights).

neoplasms consist of only precursor T lymphoblastic lymphomas (T-LBL) and leukemias (T-ALL).

T Lymphoblastic Lymphoma

T lymphoblastic lymphomas (T-LBL) are genetically and biologically similar to T acute lymphoblastic leukemia (T-ALL) differing primarily in disease distribution. Those cases with prominent BM effacement are designated as leukemias; BM involvement should be less than 25% lymphoblasts on differential cell counting for a lymphoma designation.[32,65] With modern treatment protocols this arbitrary distinction is largely irrelevant and the designation of T lymphoblastic lymphoma/leukemia is used. The cytologic, histologic, immunophenotypic, and genetic features of T-LBL and T-ALL are similar (see **Table 9**).[32,65] Morphologic and immunophenotypic evidence of immaturity characterize T-LBL. In the BM, the lymphoblastic infiltrate, if present, is much less conspicuous than T-ALL by definition. Interstitial patches of blasts may be highlighted by immunohistochemical assessment for CD99, TdT, CD3, or CD1a. Documentation of weak CD45 and CD34 expression may require flow cytometric immunophenotyping. None of these antigens alone is specific for T-LBL but rather a panel of antibodies must be used to distinguish T-LBL from NK leukemias and other blastic neoplasms. Genetic abnormalities in T-LBL generally involve the various T cell receptor genes.[32,65]

Mycosis Fungoides/Sézary Syndrome

Although mycosis fungoides (MF) and Sézary syndrome (SS) are likely separate entities, from the perspective of cytologic features in blood and infiltrates within BM they are similar.[66–68] The incidence of BM involvement is highly variable across the clinical spectrum of MF, whereas blood involvement is a defining feature in patients with erythoderma-associated SS (see **Table 9**).[65,66] Circulating Sézary cells are distinctive in that these cells have dark nuclei secondary to subtle cerebriform nuclear folding, best appreciated by focusing up and down (**Fig. 13**). The overall size is highly variable and large, so-called monstrosity cells, have been described. Bone marrow infiltrates are often subtle and may be highlighted by immunohistochemical assessment (see **Fig. 13**). Sézary cells are mature, classically CD4 positive helper T cells that often lack CD7 expression. Various criteria to detect and quantitate SS in blood have been proposed.[69,70] Genetic features are not distinctive or disease-defining.[67] A recent report describes significant array comparative genomic hybridization (CGH) and gene expression profiling differences between MF and SS.[68]

Anaplastic Large Cell Lymphoma

Bone marrow infiltrates of anaplastic large cell lymphoma (ALCL) are often inconspicuous and can be overlooked if the large pleomorphic, individually dispersed cells are mistaken for megakaryocytes (see **Table 9**). Although the term ALCL is used for anaplastic kinase (ALK)-positive and ALK-negative disorders, only ALK-positive ALCL represents a distinctive entity with a profile of unique features. The defining feature of ALK-positive ALCL is t(2;5)(p23;q35), which results in the chimeric fusion of the ALK gene and the nucleophosmin (NPM) gene. Variant translocations have also been described.[57] The distinctive aberrant nuclear positivity for ALK by immunohistochemical staining is the result of this translocation. Other typical immunohistochemical features include strong membrane CD30 positivity with variable expression of CD45, T cell antigens, epithelial membrane antigen (EMA), and T cell intracellular antigen-1 (TIA-1). Differences in flow cytometric immunophenotyping have been described between ALK-positive and ALK-negative cases, in terms of the proportion of cases expressing various T cell antigens.[71] ALK-positive ALCL

Table 9
Bone marrow manifestations in T and NK cell neoplasms

Lymphoma Subtype	Incidence of BM Involvement (%)	Patterns of Involvement	Cytologic Findings	Associated Hematologic Manifestation	Prototypic IP
T lymphoblastic lymphoma	Variable (30–50)	Diffuse or patchy, interstitial	Blastic features with scant cytoplasm	Not typical	Weak CD45, cytoplasmic CD3, TdT, CD1a; variable CD34, and T lineage antigens
Mycosis fungoides/ Sézary syndrome	Highest in de novo Sézary syndrome	Patchy, interstitial (may be subtle highlighted by IHC)	Mature cells with subtle nuclear convolutions, condensed chromatin, variable size and amount of cytoplasm	Blood or bone marrow eosinophilia common	Mature helper T cell; loss of CD7
Anaplastic large cell lymphoma	Variable, highest in patients with small cell variant (15–25)	Often isolated individual cells admixed with normal HP cells (may be occult by morphology)	Variable cell size; prototypic cells are large with multilobated nuclei, prominent nucleoli and moderate amounts of cytoplasm	May see hemophagocytic syndrome; leukemic picture in some children	CD30-positive T cell (variable T cell antigen expression) ALK-positive in cases with t(2;5) (p23; q35)

Hepatosplenic T cell lymphoma	>95	Intravascular/intrasinusoidal (subtle; may be occult)	Small- to medium-sized cells with some nuclear irregularity and scant cytoplasm	May see hemophagocytic syndrome, abnormal megakaryocytes or abnormal myelomonocytic proliferations	Mature γδ T cell (CD3+ 4−, 8−, TIA-1+ CD56+)
Angioimmunoblastic T cell lymphoma	>50	Focal nonparatrabecular	Neoplastic cells large with variably prominent nucleoli and moderate amounts of cytoplasm Polymorphous with many plasma cells/immunoblasts	May see hemolytic anemia picture; may see extensive infiltrates of EBV-positive B cells. Extensive plasma cell infiltrate may mask lymphoma	Mature T cell; CD4> CD8, CD10+, variable EBER+
Aggressive NK cell leukemia	>95	Subtle to extensive interstitial	Blood and BM involvement characteristic, but may be occult. Spectrum of cytologic features includes blastic cells mimicking acute leukemia	May see florid hemophagocytic syndrome	True NK cell (CD56+ TIA1+, cytoplasmic CD3+) EBER+

Abbreviations: HP, hematopoietic; IHC, immunohistochemical; IP, immunophenotype.
Data from Refs.[5,8,56–64]

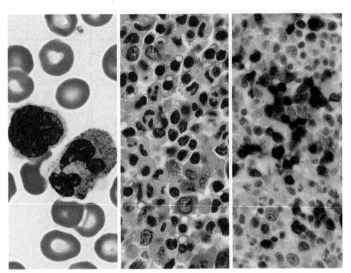

Fig. 13. The features of Sezary cells in peripheral blood (*left*), bone marrow core biopsy section (*center*), and immunohistochemical staining for CD3 (*right*). Infiltrates are subtle on routine H&E staining (*center*) (Wrights, hematoxylin-eosin, CD3).

predominates in children and adolescents; BM involvement is common in this group and blood involvement is also common, especially when sensitive molecular techniques are used.[58] In some pediatric cases, the ALCL cells are small; there is a greater propensity for a leukemic blood picture in these children (**Figs. 14** and **15**).[59] A recent report describes ALK-positive histiocytes in the BM of infants; this rare disorder must be distinguished from ALCL.[72]

Hepatosplenic T Cell Lymphoma

Virtually all patients with hepatosplenic T cell lymphoma (HSTC) will exhibit BM involvement, but the detection of HSTC in BM is even more challenging than ALCL

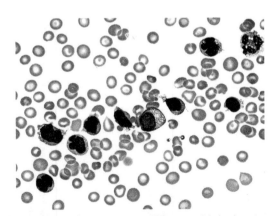

Fig. 14. Peripheral blood smears from a 17-year-old man with leukemic anaplastic large cell lymphoma who presented with a white blood cell count of 40×10^9/L (Wrights). (*Courtesy of* Chris Chong, MD, Minneapolis, MN.)

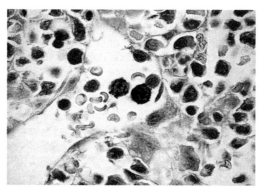

Fig. 15. Nuclear ALK-positive intrasinusoidal cells in a child with ALCL with a leukemic presentation (ALK 1).

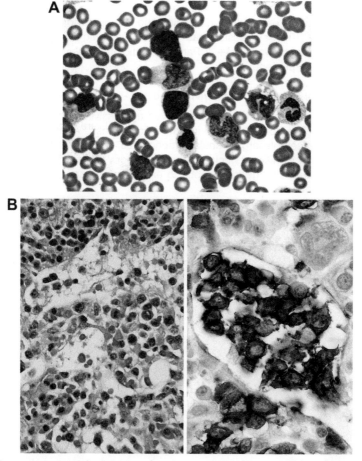

Fig. 16. Bone marrow aspirate smear showing cytologic features of hepatosplenic T cell lymphoma (*A*). Composite of core biopsy H&E and UCHL1 staining to highlight the intrasinusoidal infiltrates of hepatosplenic T cell lymphoma, which can be subtle by hematoxylin-eosin alone (*B*) (Wrights, hematoxylin-eosin, UCHL1).

(see **Table 9** and **Fig. 16**). The patchy, intrasinusoidal/intravascular infiltrates of small-to medium-sized lymphoid cells can be completely inconspicuous by hematoxylin and eosin (H&E) staining; generally a high index of suspicion and immunohistochemical assessment of CD3 are required for detection (see **Fig. 16**).[60] Hepatosplenic T cell lymphoma (HTCL) is unique among the mature T cell neoplasms in that this aggressive, typically disseminated, tumor is derived from a gamma/delta T cell. Consequently these tumor cells are CD3+, whereas CD4 and CD8 are characteristically negative. CD56 and TIA-1 expression are common. Most cases of gamma/delta HSTC lymphoma exhibit isochromosome 7(q10); rare cases are derived from alpha/beta T cells.[61] Paraneoplastic changes include BM hematopoietic hypercellularity with abnormal megakaryocytes.[60] In rare cases a prominent myelomonocytic infiltrate in blood and BM can mask HTCL.

Angioimmunoblastic T Cell Lymphoma

Bone marrow involvement is common in angioimmunoblastic T cell lymphoma (AILT), although the large neoplastic T cells are typically admixed with numerous non-neoplastic plasma cells, histiocytes, and lymphocytes. Consequently, recognition of these neoplastic infiltrates may be challenging and immunohistochemical staining is often required. CD10 coexpression has been documented for neoplastic CD3+ T cells, which are usually also CD4+.[56] Paraneoplastic phenomena such as hemolytic anemia may also be present.

Aggressive Natural Killer Cell Leukemia/Lymphoma

Although rare in western countries, EBV-derived aggressive NK cell neoplasms are more prevalent in Asian countries and in Native Americans.[62] Although the leukemic cells may closely resemble large granular lymphocytes, aggressive NK cell leukemias (ANKL) often exhibit significant nuclear immaturity more akin to blasts (**Fig. 17**).[62,73] Bone marrow infiltrates range from subtle to extensive and are best highlighted by

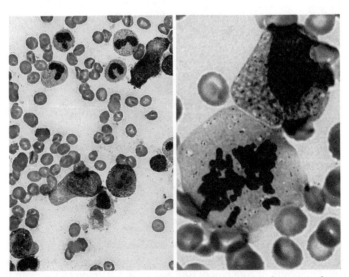

Fig. 17. Medium and high magnifications illustrate the cytologic features of aggressive NK cell leukemia/lymphoma on bone marrow aspirate smears (Wrights).

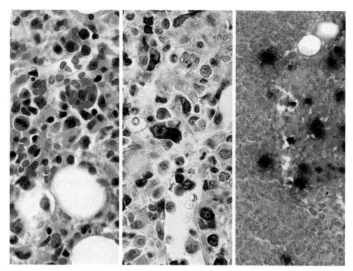

Fig. 18. The morphologic and immunohistochemical features of aggressive NK cell leukemia/lymphoma on bone marrow core biopsy sections. Infiltrates may be subtle on hematoxylin-eosin stain (*left*) but are highlighted by immunohistochemical staining for CD3 (*center*) and notably EBV (*right*) (hematoxylin-eosin, CD3, and EBER).

immunohistochemical/in situ hybridization staining for CD3, TIA-1, CD56, granzyme, and EBER (**Fig. 18**).[62,73] ANKL is also linked to florid hemophagocytic syndrome in BM, which can mask more occult leukemia cell infiltrates. This phenomenon can also be seen in other T/NK cell neoplasms (**Fig. 19**).

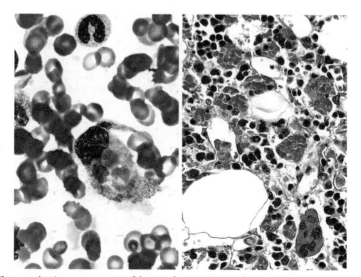

Fig. 19. The cytologic appearance of hemophagocytic syndrome on bone marrow aspirate (*left*) and bone marrow core biopsy sections (*right*) (Wrights, hematoxylin-eosin).

SUMMARY

The successful diagnosis of BM lymphoma is essential for staging, prognosis, and therapy. The diagnostician must be aware of the characteristic blood and BM features of lymphomatous infiltrates of B-NHL, T-NHL, NK cell neoplasms, and HL. An integrated approach correlating clinical findings, CBC and blood smear findings, BM aspirate, and core biopsy features, in addition to the immunophenotypic and genotypic features of these diverse neoplasms is essential. The diagnostician must have a high index of suspicion for those lymphomas that are characteristically occult in blood or bone marrow. Similarly, it is essential for the diagnostician to appreciate that paraneoplastic phenomena, notably hemophagocytic syndromes, can mask occult lymphomatous infiltrates. Finally, lymph node biopsy should be considered for cases in which bone marrow is the initial site of detection of disease.

ACKNOWLEDGMENTS

The authors thank Julianna Evans and Michael Grady for excellent support in preparing this manuscript.

REFERENCES

1. Cheson BD. Staging and evaluation of the patient with lymphoma. Hematol Oncol Clin North Am 2008;22(5):825–37, vii–viii.
2. Kwee TC, Kwee RM, Verdonck LF, et al. Magnetic resonance imaging for the detection of bone marrow involvement in malignant lymphoma. Br J Haematol 2008;141(1):60–8.
3. Hasserjian RP. Reactive versus neoplastic bone marrow: problems and pitfalls. Arch Pathol Lab Med 2008;132(4):587–94.
4. Viswanatha D. Procurement and interpretation of the bone marrow specimen. In: King D, Gardner W, Sobin L, et al, editors. Non-neoplastic disorders of bone marrow (AFIP fascicle). Washington, DC: American Registry of Pathology; 2008. p. 41–55.
5. Viswanatha D, Foucar K. Hodgkin and non-Hodgkin lymphoma involving bone marrow. Semin Diagn Pathol 2003;20(3):196–210.
6. Rawstron AC, Bennett FL, O'Connor SJ, et al. Monoclonal B-cell lymphocytosis and chronic lymphocytic leukemia. N Engl J Med 2008;359(6):575–83.
7. Perea G, Altes A, Bellido M, et al. Clinical utility of bone marrow flow cytometry in B-cell non-Hodgkin lymphomas (B-NHL). Histopathology 2004;45(3):268–74.
8. Foucar K. Non-Hodgkin lymphoma and Hodgkin lymphoma (disease) in bone marrow. In: Bone marrow pathology. 2nd edition. Chicago (IL): ASCP Press; 2001. p. 438–83.
9. Arber DA, George TI. Bone marrow biopsy involvement by non-Hodgkin's lymphoma: frequency of lymphoma types, patterns, blood involvement, and discordance with other sites in 450 specimens. Am J Surg Pathol 2005;29(12):1549–57.
10. Costes V, Duchayne E, Talb J, et al. Intrasinusoidal bone marrow infiltration: a common growth pattern for different lymphoma subtypes. Br J Haematol 2002;119(4):916–22.
11. Howell SJ, Grey M, Chang J, et al. The value of bone marrow examination in the staging of Hodgkin's lymphoma: a review of 955 cases seen in a regional cancer centre. Br J Haematol 2002;119(2):408–11.
12. Simpson CD, Gao J, Fernandez CV, et al. Routine bone marrow examination in the initial evaluation of paediatric Hodgkin lymphoma: the Canadian perspective. Br J Haematol 2008;141(6):820–6.

13. Vassilakopoulos TP, Angelopoulou MK, Constantinou N, et al. Development and validation of a clinical prediction rule for bone marrow involvement in patients with Hodgkin lymphoma. Blood 2005;105(5):1875–80.
14. Stein H, Delsol G, Pileri SA, et al. Classical Hodgkin lymphoma. In: Swerdlow S, Campo E, Harris N, editors. WHO classification of tumours: pathology & genetics: tumours of haematopoietic and lymphoid tissues. Lyon, France: IARC Press; 2008. p. 326–9.
15. Khoury JD, Jones D, Yared MA, et al. Bone marrow involvement in patients with nodular lymphocyte predominant Hodgkin lymphoma. Am J Surg Pathol 2004; 28(4):489–95.
16. Poppema S, Delsol G, Pileri SA, et al. Nodular lymphocyte predominant Hodgkin lymphoma. In: Jaffe E, Harris N, Stein H, et al, editors. WHO classification of tumours: tumours of haematopoietic and lymphoid tissues. Lyon, France: IARC Press; 2008. p. 323–5.
17. Weiss LM, von Wasielewski R, Delsol G, et al. In: Jaffe E, Harris N, Stein H, et al, editors. WHO classification of tumours: tumours of haematopoietic and lymphoid tissues. Lyon, France: IARC Press; 2008. p. 331.
18. Joshi A, Aqel NM. Hodgkin's disease of bone marrow masquerading as a heavy plasma cell infiltration and fibrosis. Br J Haematol 2003;122(3):343.
19. Taylor CR, Levenson RM. Quantification of immunohistochemistry – issues concerning methods, utility and semiquantitative assessment II. Histopathology 2006;49(4):411–24.
20. Walker RA. Quantification of immunohistochemistry–issues concerning methods, utility and semiquantitative assessment I. Histopathology 2006;49(4):406–10.
21. Bernharroch D, Stein H, Peh S-C. Lymphocyte-depleted classical Hodgkin lymphoma. In: Swerdlow S, Campo E, Harris N, et al, editors. WHO classification of tumours: pathology & genetics: tumours of haematopoietic and lymphoid tissues. Lyon, France: IARC Press; 2008. p. 334.
22. Ponzoni M, Fumagalli L, Rossi G, et al. Isolated bone marrow manifestation of HIV-associated Hodgkin lymphoma. Mod Pathol 2002;15(12):1273–8.
23. Canioni D, Brice P, Lepage E, et al. Bone marrow histological patterns can predict survival of patients with grade 1 or 2 follicular lymphoma: a study from the Groupe d'Etude des Lymphomes Folliculaires. Br J Haematol 2004;126(3):364–71.
24. Schmidt B, Kremer M, Gotze K, et al. Bone marrow involvement in follicular lymphoma: comparison of histology and flow cytometry as staging procedures. Leuk Lymphoma 2006;47(9):1857–62.
25. Abramson JS. T-cell/histiocyte-rich B-cell lymphoma: biology, diagnosis, and management. Oncologist 2006;11(4):384–92.
26. Rodriguez J, Pugh WC, Cabanillas F. T-cell-rich B-cell lymphoma. Blood 1993; 82(5):1586–9.
27. Chung R, Lai R, Wei P, et al. Concordant but not discordant bone marrow involvement in diffuse large B-cell lymphoma predicts a poor clinical outcome independent of the International Prognostic Index. Blood 2007;110(4):1278–82.
28. Talaulikar D, Dahlstrom JE, Shadbolt B, et al. Role of immunohistochemistry in staging diffuse large B-cell lymphoma (DLBCL). J Histochem Cytochem 2008; 56(10):893–900.
29. Braziel R, Arber D, Slovak M, et al. The Burkitt-like lymphomas: a Southwest Oncology Group study delineating phenotypic, genotypic, and clinical features. Blood 2001;97(12):3713–20.
30. Harris NL, Swerdlow SH, Jaffe ES, et al. Follicular lymphoma. In: Swerdlow S, Campo E, Harris N, editors. WHO classification of tumours: pathology &

genetics: tumours of haematopoietic and lymphoid tissues. 4th edition. Lyon, France: IARC Press; 2008. p. 220–6.

31. Isaacson P, Piris M, Berger F, et al. Splenic marginal zone lymphoma. In: Swerdlow S, Campo E, Harris N, editors. WHO classification of tumours: pathology & genetics: tumours of haematopoietic and lymphoid tissues. Lyon, France: IARC Press; 2008. p. 185–7.

32. Borowitz M, Chan J. Precursor lymphoid neoplasms. In: Swerdlow S, Campo E, Harris N, et al, editors. WHO classification of tumours: pathology & genetics: tumours of haematopoietic and lymphoid tissues. Lyon, France: IARC Press; 2008. p. 167–78.

33. Foucar K. Reactive lymphoid proliferations in blood and bone marrow. In: Foucar K, editor. Bone marrow pathology. 2nd edition. Chicago: ASCP Press; 2001. p. 344–63.

34. McKenna RW, Washington LT, Aquino DB, et al. Immunophenotypic analysis of hematogones (B-lymphocyte precursors) in 662 consecutive bone marrow specimens by 4-color flow cytometry. Blood 2001;98(8):2498–507.

35. Rimsza L, Larson R, Winter S, et al. Benign hematogone-rich lymphoid proliferations can be distinguished from B-lineage acute lymphoblastic leukemia by integration of morphology, immunophenotype, adhesion molecule expression, and architectural features. Am J Clin Pathol 2000;11466–75.

36. Anon. A clinical evaluation of the International Lymphoma Study Group classification of non-Hodgkin's lymphoma. The Non-Hodgkin's Lymphoma Classification Project. Blood 1997;89(11):3909–18.

37. Müller-Hermelink HK, Montserrat E, Catovsky D, et al. Chronic lymphocytic leukemia/small lymphocytic lymphoma. In: Swerdlow S, Campo E, Harris N, et al, editors. WHO classification of tumours: pathology & genetics: tumours of haematopoietic and lymphoid tissues. Lyon, France: IARC Press; 2008. p. 180–2.

38. Bernard M, Gressin R, Lefrere F, et al. Blastic variant of mantle cell lymphoma: a rare but highly aggressive subtype. Leukemia 2001;15(11):1785–91.

39. Swerdlow S, Campo E, Seto M, et al. Mantle cell lymphoma. In: Swerdlow S, Campo E, Harris N, editors. WHO classification of tumours: pathology & genetics: tumours of haematopoietic and lymphoid tissues. Lyon, France: IARC Press; 2008. p. 229–32.

40. Gu K, Chan WC, Hawley RC. Practical detection of t(14;18)(IgH/BCL2) in follicular lymphoma. Arch Pathol Lab Med 2008;132(8):1355–61.

41. Vitolo U, Ferreri AJ, Montoto S. Lymphoplasmacytic lymphoma – Waldenstrom's macroglobulinemia. Crit Rev Oncol Hematol 2008;67(2):172–85.

42. Dimopoulos MA, Merlini G, Leblond V, et al. How we treat Waldenstrom's macroglobulinemia. Haematologica 2005;90(1):117–25.

43. Zucca E, Bertoni F, Stathis A, et al. Marginal zone lymphomas. Hematol Oncol Clin North Am 2008;22(5):883–901, viii.

44. Takeshita M, Sakai H, Okamura S, et al. Splenic large B-cell lymphoma in patients with hepatitis C virus infection. Hum Pathol 2005;36(8):878–85.

45. Hunt KE, Reichard KK. Diffuse large B-cell lymphoma. Arch Pathol Lab Med 2008;132(1):118–24.

46. Lenz G, Wright GW, Emre NC, et al. Molecular subtypes of diffuse large B-cell lymphoma arise by distinct genetic pathways. Proc Natl Acad Sci U S A 2008; 105(36):13520–5.

47. Kremer M, Spitzer M, Mandl-Weber S, et al. Discordant bone marrow involvement in diffuse large B-cell lymphoma: comparative molecular analysis reveals a heterogenous group of disorders. Lab Invest 2003;83(1):107–14.

48. Gascoyne RD. Pathologic prognostic factors in diffuse aggressive non-Hodgkin's lymphoma. Hematol Oncol Clin North Am 1997;11(5):847–62.
49. Lossos IS, Morgensztern D. Prognostic biomarkers in diffuse large B-cell lymphoma. J Clin Oncol 2006;24(6):995–1007.
50. Shipp MA, Ross KN, Tamayo P, et al. Diffuse large B-cell lymphoma outcome prediction by gene-expression profiling and supervised machine learning. Nat Med 2002;8(1):68–74.
51. De Wolf-Peeters C, Delabie J, Campo E, et al. T cell/histiocyte-rich large B-cell lymphoma. In: Swerdlow S, Campo E, Harris N, et al, editors. WHO classification of tumours: pathology & genetics: tumours of haematopoietic and lymphoid tissues. Lyon, France: IARC Press; 2008. p. 238–9.
52. Lim M, Beaty M, Sorbara L, et al. T-cell/histiocyte-rich large B-cell lymphoma: a heterogeneous entity with derivation from germinal center B cells. Am J Surg Pathol 2002;26(11):1458–66.
53. Leonchini L, Raphael M, Stein H, et al. Burkitt lymphoma. In: Swerdlow S, Campo E, Harris N, et al, editors. WHO classification of tumours: pathology & genetics: tumours of haematopoietic and lymphoid tissue. Lyon, France: IARC Press; 2008. p. 262–3.
54. Kelly GL, Rickinson AB. Burkitt lymphoma: revisiting the pathogenesis of a virus-associated malignancy. Hematology Am Soc Hematol Educ Program 2007;2007: 277–84.
55. Swerdlow S, Campo E, Harris N, et al. WHO classification of tumours: pathology & genetics: tumours of haematopoietic and lymphoid tissues. Lyon, France: IARC Press; 2008.
56. Dogan A, Morice WG. Bone marrow histopathology in peripheral T-cell lymphomas. Br J Haematol 2004;127(2):140–54.
57. Delsol G, Falini B, Muller-Hermelink H, et al. Anaplastic large cell lymphoma (ALCL), ALK-positive. In: Swerdlow S, Campo E, Harris N, editors. WHO classification of tumours: pathology & genetics: tumours of haematopoietic and lymphoid tissues. Lyon, France: IARC Press; 2008. p. 312–6.
58. Mussolin L, Pillon M, d'Amore ES, et al. Prevalence and clinical implications of bone marrow involvement in pediatric anaplastic large cell lymphoma. Leukemia 2005;19(9):1643–7.
59. Onciu M, Behm FG, Raimondi SC, et al. ALK-positive anaplastic large cell lymphoma with leukemic peripheral blood involvement is a clinicopathologic entity with an unfavorable prognosis. Report of three cases and review of the literature. Am J Clin Pathol 2003;120(4):617–25.
60. Vega F, Medeiros LJ, Bueso-Ramos C, et al. Hepatosplenic gamma/delta T-cell lymphoma in bone marrow. A sinusoidal neoplasm with blastic cytologic features. Am J Clin Pathol 2001;116(3):410–9.
61. Gaulard P, Jaffe E, Krenacs L, et al. Hepatosplenic T-cell lymphoma. In: Swerdlow S, Campo E, Harris N, editors. WHO classification of tumours: pathology & genetics: tumours of haematopoietic and lymphoid tissues. Lyon, France: IARC Press; 2008. p. 292–3.
62. Chan J, Jaffe E, Ralfkiaer E, et al. Aggressive NK-cell leukaemia. In: Jaffe E, Harris N, Stein H, editors. WHO classification of tumours: tumours of haematopoietic and lymphoid tissues. Lyon, France: IARC Press; 2008. p. 276–7.
63. Allory Y, Challine D, Haioun C, et al. Bone marrow involvement in lymphomas with hemophagocytic syndrome at presentation: a clinicopathologic study of 11 patients in a Western institution. Am J Surg Pathol 2001;25(7):865–74.

64. Grogg KL, Morice WG, Macon WR. Spectrum of bone marrow findings in patients with angioimmunoblastic T-cell lymphoma. Br J Haematol 2007;137(5):416–22.
65. Good DJ, Gascoyne RD. Classification of non-Hodgkin's lymphoma. Hematol Oncol Clin North Am 2008;22(5):781–805, vii.
66. Ralfkiaer E, Cerroni L, Sander CA, et al. Mycosis fungoides. In: Swerdlow S, Campo E, Harris N, et al, editors. WHO classification of tumours: pathology & genetics: tumours of haematopoietic and lymphoid tissue. Lyon, France: IARC Press; 2008. p. 296–8.
67. Ralfkiaer E, Willemze R, Whittaker SJ. Sézary syndrome. In: Swerdlow S, Campo E, Harris N, et al, editors. WHO classification of tumours: pathology & genetics: tumours of haematopoietic and lymphoid tissues. Lyon, France: IARC Press; 2008. p. 299.
68. van Doorn R, van Kester MS, Dijkman R, et al. Oncogenomic analysis of mycosis fungoides reveals major differences with Sezary syndrome. Blood 2009;113(1):127–36.
69. Morice WG, Katzmann JA, Pittelkow MR, et al. A comparison of morphologic features, flow cytometry, TCR-Vbeta analysis, and TCR-PCR in qualitative and quantitative assessment of peripheral blood involvement by Sezary syndrome. Am J Clin Pathol 2006;125(3):364–74.
70. Vonderheid EC. On the diagnosis of erythrodermic cutaneous T-cell lymphoma. J Cutan Pathol 2006;33(Suppl):127–42.
71. Muzzafar T, Wei EX, Lin P, et al. Flow cytometric immunophenotyping of anaplastic large cell lymphoma. Arch Pathol Lab Med 2009;133(1):49–56.
72. Chan JK, Lamant L, Algar E, et al. ALK+ histiocytes: a novel type of systemic histiocytic proliferative disorder of early infancy. Blood 2008;112(7):2965–8.
73. Foucar K, Osuji N, Matutes E, et al. T-cell large granular lymphocytic leukemia, indolent NK lymphocytosis and aggressive NK cell leukemia. In Armitage J, Coiffer B, Dalla-Favera R, et al, editors. Non-Hodgkin lymphoma, 2nd edition. Baltimore (MD): Lippincott Williams & Wilkins; 2009, in press.

Molecular Diagnosis of Hematopoietic and Lymphoid Neoplasms

Dragan Jevremovic, MD, PhD, David S. Viswanatha, MD*

KEYWORDS

- Gene rearrangements • Clonality • Chromosome translocation
- Polymerase chain reaction • Fluorescence in situ hybridization
- Minimal residual disease

In recent decades, advances in our understanding of tumor genetics, as well as the ability to manipulate nucleic acids in increasingly sophisticated ways, have translated into an ever-growing number of clinical tests in molecular hematopathology. The result of these investigative efforts is an ongoing expansion of disease classifications; acute myeloid leukemia (AML), for example, is increasingly viewed as a syndrome encompassing numerous related entities with distinct pathobiologic and clinical features. The impact of molecular diagnostics continues to evolve in at least four important areas: (1) the continuing discovery of new disease associations with specific genetic changes; (2) the assessment of multiple tumor genetic abnormalities to refine prognosis and relapse risk for patients using current standard therapies; (3) the routine use of highly sensitive and reproducible molecular techniques for detecting minimal residual disease (MRD) burden after therapy; (4) a shift toward a more "holistic" approach to elucidating the molecular pathogenesis of hematolymphoid neoplasms based on a multiparametric understanding of interacting abnormal genetic and epigenetic alterations. This article does not constitute a comprehensive overview of molecular genetics of the hematopoietic cancers but rather is a précis of the most common and frequently assessed abnormalities encountered in the clinical molecular diagnostics laboratory. The first section presents an overview of major molecular testing methods and principles, followed by discussions concerning the application of molecular analyses to specific myeloid and lymphoid neoplasms.

Division of Hematopathology, Department of Laboratory Medicine and Pathology, Mayo Clinic, 200 First Street SW, Rochester, MN 55905, USA
* Corresponding author.
E-mail address: viswanatha.david@mayo.edu (D.S. Viswanatha).

Hematol Oncol Clin N Am 23 (2009) 903–933
doi:10.1016/j.hoc.2009.04.011
0889-8588/09/$ – see front matter © 2009 Elsevier Inc. All rights reserved.

TECHNIQUES IN MOLECULAR HEMATOPATHOLOGY
Antigen Receptor Gene Rearrangements

Immunoglobulin (Ig) and T-cell receptors (TCRs) are encoded by clusters of gene segments, which undergo somatic recombination events during B- and T-cell development in bone marrow and thymus, respectively. This recombination process results in a tremendous diversity in the variety and specificities of the antigen receptors.[1] Antigen receptor gene structure is defined by variable (V), diverse (D), joining (J), and constant (C) regions. D gene regions are associated with the Ig heavy chain genes and beta TCR genes. Each of the regions in the antigen receptor genes contains multiple exon segments with polymorphic DNA sequences. These segments are joined into a potentially functional V(D)JC coding sequence by the process of gene rearrangement and excision of the intervening DNA regions (**Fig. 1**). In addition to the combinatorial process of segmental recombination, further sequence diversity is obtained by (1) imperfection in junction site splices and (2) action of the enzyme terminal deoxynucleotidyl transferase (TdT), which adds random nucleotides to the joining ends. As a result, each antigenically naïve B or T lymphocyte has a uniquely different antigen receptor expressed on its surface. When a lymphocyte encounters an antigen for which it has a high enough affinity (eg, a native antigen for Ig or processed peptide for TCR), it starts an activation program that includes rapid division and expansion of a "clonal" population with single epitope specificity. Additional sequence modifications can be added to the peptide-encoding sequences of B cells by the process of somatic hypermutation, occurring during the germinal center (GC) reaction in lymphoid tissues. Reactive lymphoid conditions are polyclonal, given that numerous different clonotypic populations are formed by lymphocytes recognizing different foreign or self-antigens (eg, in autoimmune disorders). These polyclonal proliferations are self-limiting and reversible, because proliferating cells are programmed to die when the target antigen is eliminated or contained. On the other hand, neoplastic lymphoid expansions are by definition monoclonal; that is, a single lymphocyte acquiring deleterious mutations can proliferate without control. As a result, essentially all, or a very large proportion, of the total lymphocyte pool is represented by a single clonal population. It is important to understand that apparent monoclonality in a lymphoid population does not always imply a neoplastic process, as certain reactive or nonmalignant conditions can result in restricted lymphoid repertoires. The latter scenario is particularly encountered in some older people who, due to aging of the immune system, have a contraction of the available range of receptor diversity. Nevertheless, the concept of polyclonality versus monoclonality is routinely applied in the diagnostic assessment of lymphoid disorders.

Two techniques are used in the molecular hematopathology laboratory to detect clonality status in lymphocyte populations: Southern blot hybridization (SBH) analysis and polymerase chain reaction (PCR) technique. SBH technique involves restriction endonuclease enzyme digestions of a DNA sample from the lymphocyte population of interest, followed by electrophoretic fragment separation and immobilization on a membrane. The affixed DNA fragments are then hybridized under stringent conditions with a labeled DNA probe complementary to the specific target region of interest.[2,3] For a structurally unaltered (non-rearranged) locus of DNA, probe hybridization analysis will reveal a certain pattern of fragment sizes or bands, termed a "germline" configuration, based on the distribution of particular restriction enzyme sites flanking or within the region in question (see **Fig. 1**B). If the specific DNA locus has undergone somatic rearrangement, as in the case of the B- and T-cell antigen receptor loci, a different banding pattern will be produced (as a result of changes in the locations of usual restriction enzyme sites), and these changes can be readily recognized as distinct from the expected germline result.

Rearrangements of the immunoglobulin and TCR genes can be identified by PCR methods as well. In contrast to SBH, which detects relatively large structural genomic alterations, PCR is designed to amplify short regions of the DNA encompassing the immediate area of V-(D)-J gene segment fusion in the rearranged antigen receptor genes. Under standard PCR conditions, a germline antigen receptor gene configuration is not successfully amplified due to the very large intervening areas of DNA between primer sites. However, when coding V-(D)-J segments are juxtaposed in a rearranged gene, amplification of the region between the now closely related primers is readily accomplished by PCR (see **Fig. 1**C). Although tremendous recombination diversity exists in rearranged lymphocyte antigen receptor genes, PCR assessment of clonality is feasible because of the presence of "consensus" sequence motifs flanking the core rearrangement loci, to which the amplification primers can be directed. The most widely used loci for PCR determination of B- and T-lymphoid clonality are the immunoglobulin heavy chain (*IGH*) and kappa light chain (*IGK*) genes and TCR gamma (*TRG*) gene, respectively.[4–7]

SBH and PCR can be considered complementary methods in the evaluation of blood or tissue samples for the presence of a clonal lymphoid population. However, the application of each technique is subject to several limitations determined by technical complexity, efficiency, specimen requirements, and clinical and analytic sensitivity. SBH requires a relatively large quantity of high molecular weight DNA, typically 5 micrograms for each enzymatic digestion, per probe. The method is laborious and technically challenging. Furthermore, provision of SBH results typically requires a delay in finalizing hematopathology case evaluation. PCR in contrast is rapid, analytically very sensitive, requires minimal DNA, can be performed using paraffin-embedded sample material, and is technically straightforward. The benefits of PCR analysis are somewhat offset by the finding that not all clonotypic gene rearrangements can be detected by consensus primer strategies. GC-associated B-cell lymphomas typically contain *IGH* genes with extensive somatic hypermutation, which often inhibits the ability of primers to effectively bind to their target sites. In contrast, PCR amplification of physiologically restricted antigen receptor gene rearrangement populations (eg, with age-related changes in T-cell production) may produce skewed rearrangement patterns mimicking a monoclonal result known as "pseudoclonality," a phenomenon not infrequently encountered when amplifying rearrangements of the T-cell gamma (*TRG*) locus. Although SBH can overcome limitations of the PCR technique, the latter approach for clonality assessment has been significantly improved by the advent of more comprehensive primer sets targeting multiple antigen receptor loci[6–10] and improvements in PCR product resolution (eg, heteroduplex and fluorescent capillary electrophoresis analyses). Lymphoid clonality analysis by PCR can also detect the so-called "cross-lineage" gene rearrangements,[6] wherein TCR gene rearrangements can be seen in B-cell malignancies and vice versa. This is most commonly observed in B-lineage acute leukemias, in which up to 50% of cases can have TCR gene rearrangements. Consequently, it is important to appreciate that a monoclonal antigen receptor gene rearrangement cannot be used on its own for the purpose of defining cell lineage in a neoplastic lymphoid proliferation.

Chromosome Translocations, Deletions, and Numerical Abnormalities

Translocations involve recombination of large segments of DNA, which can (1) result in the formation of a new (composite) gene, or (2) lead to protein overexpression by juxtaposing positive regulatory elements from one gene to coding sequences of another.

Large translocations are easily detectable by conventional cytogenetics. However, this technique requires fresh tissue for cell culture and production of metaphase chromosomes. The two most common molecular-based methods for detecting translocations are PCR and fluorescent in situ hybridization (FISH). Principles of PCR in detecting translocations using genomic DNA are similar to those described for antigen receptor gene rearrangements. Selection of oligonucleotide primers flanking the abnormal gene fusion locus enables specific amplification of the altered DNA region. Knowledge of specific DNA break points is necessary to design adequate primers for successful amplification. The main limitations of DNA-based PCR for detecting translocations include the lack of highly conserved genomic break points in the rearranging genes and the presence of very long intervening areas of DNA between possible primer sites, precluding efficient PCR. DNA PCR assays are most often used for translocations resulting in gene overexpression abnormalities, as seen in some lymphoid

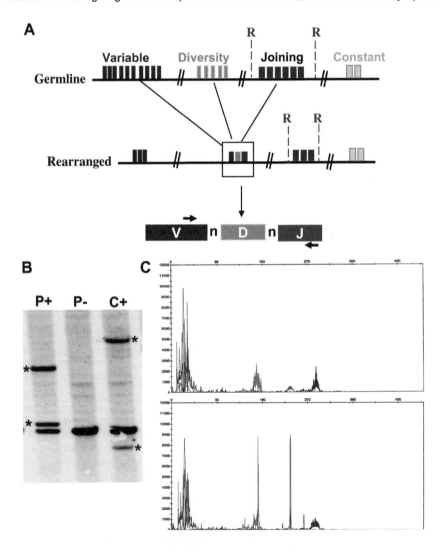

tumors. Alternatively, translocations that result in the formation of chimeric mRNA species can be sensitively and specifically identified using RNA as the starting material and reverse transcription followed by PCR (reverse transcriptase polymerase chain reaction [RT-PCR]). The latter situation is encountered in myeloid and B-lymphoblastic leukemias.

FISH enables the targeted detection of large DNA recombinations, other structural alterations, and numerical chromosome changes, without the need for knowledge of specific sequence-level details.[11] FISH involves the base pairing of large (ie, kilobase to megabase), fluorescently labeled nucleic acid probes complementary to DNA sequences in tissue or cell nuclear preparations, followed by direct visualization of probe-specific signals using fluorescence microscopy. For detection of translocations, deletions, or inversions, FISH methods using locus-specific probes are employed. Translocation detection is typically accomplished by either dual-color/dual-fusion probe (D-FISH) or break-apart probe (BAP) techniques, the latter being of value in situations where a single genetic locus can potentially be translocated to a large number of partner genes. Enumeration probes are employed to identify changes in chromosome number. FISH analysis is a very powerful way to identify numerical and structural rearrangements in hematolymphoid tumors at diagnosis, and one can use fresh, frozen, or fixed tissue sources. The major drawbacks to FISH include a limited analytic sensitivity (1%–5%) and the inability to resolve submegabase changes in DNA. When deciding the proper choice of FISH versus PCR in detection of major chromosomal aberrations, one has to appreciate the pros and cons of each method. FISH is a rapid and technically straightforward methodology, and many probes are now readily available for most clinically important aberrations. On the other hand, FISH is a relatively expensive technology, requiring the use of an individual probe per target region (unlike conventional cytogenetics, which can concurrently assess whole genome changes). PCR techniques have an advantage

◄━━━━━━━━━━━━━━━━━━━━━━━━━━━━━━━━━━━━━━

Fig. 1. Rearrangement of antigen receptor genes: (A) schematically demonstrates the basic process of somatic rearrangement of the antigen receptor genes in developing lymphocytes. Selection and rearrangement of diversity (D) and joining (J) gene segments first occur over a large region of intervening DNA, followed by the recruitment of a variable region (V) exon to complete a VDJ coding cassette. (At some loci, including the T-cell receptor gamma (TRG) and immunoglobulin light chain genes (IGK and IGL), D regions are absent, and initial rearrangements involve only V- and J segments). Substantial diversity is generated at the nucleotide level because of the recombination potential of the many V, (D), and J segments. In addition, the activity of the enzyme TdT, which inserts a random number of "nontemplated" (N) nucleotides at the rearranged junctions, adds to this diversity. The V(D)J rearranged segment is then joined with the constant region (C) to complete the gene-coding unit. If genetic rearrangements fail to produce a functional antigen receptor protein at one allele, the mechanism proceeds at the second allelic locus. Label R represents restriction enzyme sites informative for SBH analysis. Horizontal arrows indicate strategy for placement of consensus primers for PCR-based clonality analysis. (B) depicts T-cell beta (TRB) SBH analysis using a chemiluminescently labeled probe. Lane P+ shows a patient lymphoma sample with a positive (monoclonal) result, indicating a biallelic rearrangement (asterisks demonstrate nongermline rearranged bands). Lane P- shows a nonclonal result with a nonrearranged (germline) band. Lane C+ is a positive cell line control (asterisks demonstrate nongermline rearranged bands). (C) displays typical results of a PCR analysis using oligonucleotide consensus primers specific for the T-cell receptor gamma (TRG) locus. The upper diagram shows a negative result with normal (polyclonal) distribution of PCR products. The lower diagram shows amplification of a monoclonal population (distinct peaks, biallelic pattern) as well as a minimal polyclonal T-cell background.

in analytic sensitivity, turnaround time (in some cases), and simplicity of technique. However, PCR is impractical or not feasible for chromosome translocations and inversions in which the breakpoint sites are spread over large genomic areas, as is often the case for aberrations associated with many malignant lymphomas. The sensitivity of PCR is valuable for patient follow-up during and posttherapy, particularly when employing quantitative PCR techniques (see later section on MRD monitoring).

Single Nucleotide (Point) Mutations and Small Sequence Variations

Point mutations and other small sequence variations (ie, short insertions or deletions) occurring in oncogenes and tumor suppressor genes are well-known pathogenic events in a number of hematologic disorders. Many new diagnostic and prognostic associations continue to emerge from the identification of acquired single nucleotide or oligonucleotide sequence changes. There are many techniques capable of detecting these events. Direct sequencing of PCR-amplified products (either Sanger-type cycle sequencing or pyrosequencing) can specifically identify point mutation changes of diagnostic significance. Sanger sequencing methods are limited by a relatively low analytic sensitivity (20%) and by the presence of tumor heterogeneity. Analytic sensitivity for point mutation detection can be substantially improved using a variety of PCR-based methods, including allele-specific PCR (AS-PCR), allele-specific primer extension, and amplification refractory mutation systems (ARMS). As with diagnostic PCR assays, the starting material can be DNA or RNA. Post-PCR analytic capabilities have also greatly expanded in this regard, with the use of highly accurate PCR amplicon sizing using capillary electrophoresis and high-resolution melting of PCR products. The former analytic platform is useful for detecting small recurrent sequence variations, whereas melting analysis can substitute for direct sequencing in some situations. Other techniques, such as ligation-based assays, isothermal amplification, denaturing high-performance liquid chromatography, or flow cytometric bead array platforms, have each found a place in the molecular diagnostic laboratory, but the specifics are beyond the scope of this article.

Quantitative Minimal Residual Disease Monitoring

Although the qualitative PCR technique can achieve remarkable sensitivity and specificity, it is not reliable for quantification of rare or low-level molecular events. Real-time quantitative (RQ-PCR) analytic platforms have become commonplace in most molecular laboratories, offering a combination of high reproducibility, wide dynamic range for specified targets, and semiautomated functionality. Two major chemistries are employed in the process of quantitative PCR. In the hydrolysis probe approach, a dual-labeled and quenched fluorescence probe is situated within a short amplicon target flanked by specific PCR primers. During repeated PCR cycles, the 5' exonuclease activity of thermostable (Taq) DNA polymerase hydrolyzes the probe during primer extension, generating an increasing fluorescent signal that is quantitatively related to the amount of starting DNA or RNA target of interest. This technology, pioneered by Applied Biosystems Incorporated (ABI, Foster City, CA), is also known as "Taq-Man" RQ-PCR. In another variation advanced commercially by Roche Diagnostics ("LightCycler," Roche, Indianapolis IN), the principle of fluorescence resonance energy transfer (FRET) is exploited during the annealing phase of PCR, using two fluorescent oligonucleotides to generate a particular wavelength emission when they are in close proximity, which happens only if both probes hybridize to the target region of the DNA being amplified. Using either RQ-PCR platform, frequent fluorescence measurements are captured over time, and the appearance of a signal in the early exponential segment of the PCR curve (the crossing threshold) becomes a highly reproducible measurement related to the initial target quantity.[12] RQ-PCR is rapidly performed in a closed, automated system and has the advantage of multiwell plate analysis, permitting the simultaneous evaluation of numerous patient samples and all appropriate controls. The analytic sensitivity of RQ-PCR ranges from 10^{-3} to 10^{-4} for clone-specific antigen receptor gene rearrangements[13] to 10^{-6} for transloca-tion-related chimeric mRNA targets, such as breakpoint cluster region (BCR)-ABL1 transcripts. Once adequately controlled and validated for linearity and dynamic range, RQ-PCR experiments show remarkable intrarun precision and very good between-run correlations for a given nucleic acid target. RQ-PCR techniques have been developed primarily for monitoring MRD in several hematologic malignancies, including child-hood B-cell lymphoblastic leukemia, acute promyelocytic leukemia (APL), and chronic myelogenous leukemia. In each scenario, the measurement of MRD provides informa-tion critical to prognosis and ongoing patient management. In addition to consider-ations of technical standardization, other factors influencing the impact of MRD analysis include the timing of measurement (eg, end of induction chemotherapy versus end of treatment) and the frequency of interval assessment. For some tumors, even a single MRD result will provide important clinical information that may alter ther-apeutic intent, whereas ongoing monitoring of low-level disease burden is more typical of neoplasms with a chronic course. The recognition that chromosomal trans-location events can be detected at very low levels in healthy subjects might raise concern regarding the interpretation of low abundance MRD levels in patients;[14] however, current RQ-PCR methods, although sensitive, are not optimized for extremely low-level detection but are rather designed to detect specified targets in a clinically relevant range. RQ-PCR methods are also valuable to quantify mutated alleles in heterogeneous tumor populations and to validate transcript level results derived from mRNA gene expression profiling.

MOLECULAR DIAGNOSIS IN MYELOID MALIGNANCIES
Myeloproliferative Neoplasms

Chronic myeloid leukemia

Chronic myeloid leukemia (CML) is defined by the well known t(9;22)(q34;q11) or Philadelphia chromosome (Ph), producing the BCR-ABL1 gene fusion.[15–17] The BCR-ABL1 chimeric gene is also central to the pathogenesis of 20% to 25% of adult B-lineage acute lymphoblastic leukemia (ALL) and approximately 2% to 3% of precursor B-cell ALL of childhood, in either case associated with very poor prog-nosis.[18] Although the functional role of the normal BCR gene product is not completely understood, the abnormal genetic fusion protein disrupts the localization and highly regulated activity of the ABL1 tyrosine kinase, producing complex effects on cellular signal transduction pathways, proliferation, apoptosis control, and cell adhesion. Two major forms of the BCR-ABL1 exist mainly based on the predominant break-point-fusion sites occurring within the BCR gene (**Fig. 2**).[19,20] The major breakpoint cluster region (M-BCR) is involved in essentially all cases of CML, resulting in the production of either an e14(b3)-a2 or e13(b2)-a2 fusion transcript, with a correspond-ing chimeric protein, p210. The minor breakpoint cluster region (m-BCR), located further upstream in the BCR gene, is associated with most Ph+ ALL and the formation of an e1-a2–type fusion mRNA, giving rise to a p190 oncogenic protein. However, BCR gene break sites and disease associations are not exactly correlated, given that approximately one-third of adult Ph+ ALL (and a lesser number of pediatric cases) are associated with breakpoints in the "CML-associated" M-BCR. Similarly, very rare occurrences of CML with e1-a2 (p190) fusions have been identified. A number

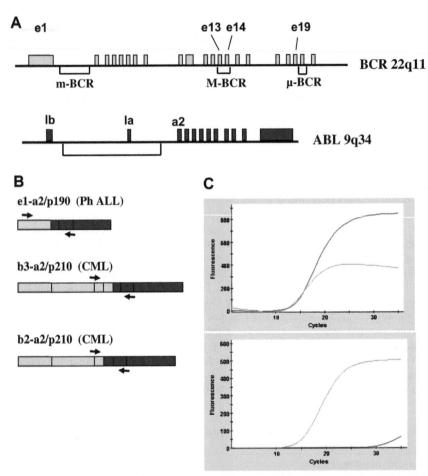

Fig. 2. t(9;22)/*BCR-ABL* abnormality in chronic myeloid leukemia and Ph+ acute lympho-blastic leukemia. (*A*) demonstrates an exon map of the translocated *BCR* and *ABL1* genes. Three major breakpoint regions are recognized in the *BCR* gene: the minor breakpoint cluster region (m-BCR), the major breakpoint cluster region (M-BCR), and the μ-BCR. The M-BCR is involved in nearly all cases of chronic myeloid leukemia (CML) and approximately one-third of de novo adult Ph+ acute lymphoblastic leukemias (Ph+ ALL). A small percentage of pediatric Ph+ ALL may have BCR breakpoints at this site as well. The m-BCR is typically associated with the vast majority of pediatric Ph+ ALL and most adult Ph+ ALL. Breakpoints at the μ-BCR have been associated with the entity "chronic neutro-philic leukemia," a rare variant of CML. For the *ABL1* gene, breakpoints are distributed throughout a large region 5′ of exon 2 (a2), encompassing the first exon region. (*B*) shows the principal BCR-ABL1 chimeric transcripts arising from these various translocation fusion gene breakpoints. The exon-exon fusions are indicated for these transcripts, and the corre-sponding chimeric protein product sizes are shown in kilodaltons (eg, e1-a2/p190). The arrows indicate relative positions of PCR primers to detect these various forms in reverse transcription (RT)-PCR assays. (*C*) illustrates a real-time quantitative PCR (RQ-PCR) result for detection of transcripts. The upper panel shows a high level of BCR-ABL1 transcripts (*blue tracing*) and this result is typically observed at the diagnosis. The lower panel shows a minimal residual disease (MRD) detection of a relatively small amount of BCR-ABL1 tran-scripts (*blue tracing*). The green tracings in each panel represent amplification of control ABL1 transcripts, used to normalize the BCR-ABL1 levels for reproducible quantitative MRD measurements.

of very infrequent alternative BCR-ABL1 transcripts have also been described in CML, including e6-a2, e19-a2, e13-a3, and e14-a3 types.

The naturally poor prognosis of CML changed dramatically with the introduction of imatinib (Gleevec[R], Novartis Inc.), a competitive small-molecule tyrosine kinase inhibitor (TKI) targeting the adenosine triphosphate (ATP) binding pocket of BCR-ABL1.[21,22] As such, the management of CML has become transformed truly in the manner of a "chronic" disease, requiring the continuous involvement of treating clinicians and ongoing molecular hematopathology investigations, particularly RQ-PCR. The algorithms for monitoring response to TKI therapy in CML continue to evolve and become better refined. At diagnosis, current recommendations for patients include performing conventional bone marrow karyotype studies or FISH testing to confirm the presence of the BCR-ABL1 abnormality. Conventional cytogenetics can reveal additional chromosomal abnormalities, including del(9q)i(17q), and +8, which are associated with treatment resistance and higher risk of progression to accelerated and blast phase. An initial BCR-ABL1 transcript level (normalized to a control gene transcript, such as ABL1 itself) is often obtained at this time, also to verify the transcript type for monitoring disease. In general, therapeutic milestones with TKI therapy in CML include attainment of partial and complete cytogenetic responses (CCRs) by 6 and 12 months, respectively, as assessed by cytogenetics and/or FISH. Complete cytogenetic eradication of t(9;22) is a requisite goal for longer-term disease-free survival. At this juncture, patients achieving greater than 2 log reduction in quantitative BCR-ABL1 levels measured by RQ-PCR typically achieve durable treatment responses;[23] FISH does not have a role in quantitative BCR-ABL1 detection following a CCR. Molecular analysis by RQ-PCR is itself a powerful indicator of outcome.[24–27] Patients achieving greater than 3 log reduction of BCR-ABL1 from baseline or, more appropriately, 0.1% BCR-ABL1/ABL1 (normalized) levels or lower on the proposed international standard scale (ie, a major molecular response [MMR]) have long-term disease-free survival and an extremely low relapse risk.[25] A major effort at present concerns the establishment of international standards for RQ-PCR analysis of BCR-ABL1 transcript levels,[28] and, generally, follow-up studies by the same molecular hematopathology laboratory are recommended.

Suboptimal TKI therapy is reflected by the inability to attain a CCR, loss of a CCR, or loss of a MMR. These situations imply TKI resistance, which can be mediated through a variety of tumor-related mechanisms. Approximately 50% of TKI resistance is thought to arise from acquired mutations in the ABL1 kinase domain (KD) region of the chimeric BCR-ABL1 gene. These KD mutations target critical areas involving ATP binding, activation, catalytic function, or direct drug contact. Although a large number of mutations are now described in patients on imatinib therapy, fewer than 20 account for 80% to 90% of clinically significant drug resistance. RQ-PCR has proven valuable in predicting patients with resistance to imatinib therapy; individuals with serially increasing BCR-ABL1 levels (>0.5–1 log) have been shown to have a strong association with the presence of mutations in the translocated ABL1 gene conferring resistance to the drug, whereas those with stable low levels of transcript have an exceedingly low incidence of imatinib resistance due to such mutations.[29–32] The effect of some mutations can be overcome with escalated imatinib dosage, whereas others are highly refractory. The advent of new generation TKI drugs (eg, dasatinib, nilotinib) can circumvent imatinib resistance in many of these cases, representing an alternative therapeutic choice for some individuals. Most significantly, CML patients with the T315I KD mutation are unresponsive to all currently employed TKI agents. The spectrum of molecular diagnostic management for patients treated with TKIs has therefore expanded to include *BCR-ABL1* KD mutation analysis when suboptimal responses are encountered, as indicated above. KD mutations are most often detected by RT-PCR and direct sequencing of the ABL1 region in the BCR-ABL1 transcript. Knowledge about specific mutations can therefore be helpful in prognosis as well as in tailoring therapy with the new-generation TKIs.

Non-chronic myeloid leukemia myeloproliferative neoplasms

The chronic myeloproliferative neoplasms (MPN) include polycythemia vera (PV), essential thrombocythemia (ET), and primary myelofibrosis (PMF). It has recently been shown that mutations in the Janus kinase 2 (*JAK2*) gene are highly prevalent in these diseases,[33–36] further strengthening the unique subclassification of these entities. The family of JAK tyrosine kinases are normally engaged by cytokine receptor dimerization events in the presence of growth ligands such as erythropoietin and thrombopoietin. JAK signaling results in phosphorylation of signal transducer and activator of transcription (STAT) proteins, leading to nuclear STAT translocation and potent effects on target gene regulation. The vast majority of *JAK2* mutations in MPN occur as a codon V617F substitution within exon 14, affecting the autoregulatory pseudokinase domain. This mutation produces a constitutively active tyrosine kinase capable of initiating downstream cell signaling independent of erythropoietin (and possibly other cytokine) induced receptor dimerization. In several reported series, the V617F mutation is observed in up to 95% of cases of PV, approximately one-third to one-half of ET and 75% of PMF patients. In the proper clinical setting (ie, erythrocytosis in the face of very low to absent serum erythropoietin), the additional presence of the *JAK2* V617F is virtually diagnostic of PV. A subset of patients with PV demonstrate biallelic *JAK2* V617F mutations, which have been shown to arise as a result of acquired uniparental disomy of chromosome 9p24 following the initial mutational event; homozygosity for *JAK2* V617F has been associated with poorer disease course in MPN patients. A small number of PV patients lack the *JAK2* V617F, but instead they have been shown to harbor small insertion or deletion events or point mutations in exon 12 of the gene.[37,38] More comprehensive screening of the entire pseudokinase region has revealed that additional *JAK2* mutations are rarely present in some MPN.[39] The V617F *JAK2* mutation can be detected by a number of standard molecular laboratory techniques, including PCR with direct sequencing, AS-PCR assays (including ARMS and RQ-PCR), restriction enzyme digestion of PCR-amplified products, and fluorescent melting curve analysis of PCR products. Sequencing, restriction digestion, and standard melting curve analyses are less analytically sensitive than other approaches. Quantitative methodologies are attractive given their ability to assess mutated allele burden. The uncommon exon 12 *JAK2* mutations are detected by PCR and sequencing, high-resolution melting analysis, or by precise size discrimination methods (eg, capillary electrophoresis of fluorescent PCR products).[38,40] In very rare cases of PMF and ET without detectable JAK2 alterations, mutations in the thrombopoietin receptor (*MPL*) have been described, at approximately 5% and 1% frequency, respectively.[41,42] The most common of these involves the W515 residue of *MPL* and also results in constitutional activation of the *JAK2* pathway. Unlike *JAK2* molecular testing, screening for mutations involving *MPL* have not been incorporated into routine patient evaluation for suspected MPN.

Several outstanding issues remain concerning the molecular analysis of non-CML MPNs. Foremost are the cases of ET and PMF that are not associated with *JAK2* mutations. As further aspects of the molecular pathogenesis of these tumors emerge, it is anticipated that additional diagnostic molecular markers will be identified in this regard. Second, for *JAK2* V617F-positive MPNs, quantifying mutation allele burden in addition to its presence may become an important prognostic factor.[43,44] Finally, the indications for quantitative *JAK2* mutation monitoring in the era of targeted TKI therapy need to be better defined and clarified.

Systemic mastocytosis and disorders of primary eosinophilia

Systemic mast cell disease (SM) is a relatively uncommon MPN characterized by a proliferation and accumulation of atypical neoplastic mast cells, with the clinical picture most often caused by cytokine dysregulation. This disorder is frequently accompanied by eosinophilia, raising the differential diagnosis of a myeloid neoplasm with eosinophilia, or a primary eosinophilic disorder. A specific D816V mutation in the receptor for stem cell factor, *cKIT*, is identified in most cases of systemic mastocytosis.[45,46] Several rarer mutations situated elsewhere in the *cKIT* gene have also been described in SM. The D816V mutation leads to constitutive activation of the receptor tyrosine kinase activity. Detection of D816V mutation is an integral aspect in the diagnosis of SM and is best accomplished by AS-PCR methods, to ensure adequate analytic sensitivity. Notably, a negative D816V mutation result does not preclude the diagnosis of SM, if other diagnostic criteria are clearly present. Importantly, this specific mutation renders transformed mast cells insensitive to imatinib therapy,[47] but other kinase inhibitors may be effective.[48] Hematologic neoplasms with eosinophilia and abnormalities of platelet-derived growth factor receptors (PDGFR) A and -B, or fibroblast growth factor receptor (FGFR)-1, constitute a new World Health Organization (WHO) diagnostic category that encompasses entities previously recognized as hypereosinophilic syndrome and chronic eosinophilic leukemia. Abnormalities and excessive proliferation of eosinophilic precursors result from the increased tyrosine kinase activity of deregulated PDGFR and FGFR1 in these cases. These diseases are grouped together, despite a range of morphologic and clinical features, due to the common occurrence of gene fusions involving receptor tyrosine kinases and the frequent component of abnormal eosinophilia. The most common *PDGFRA* abnormality is an interstitial deletion (or translocation) of the *CHIC2* gene region of chromosome 4(q12), resulting in juxtaposition of *FIP1L1* and *PDGFRA* genes.[49,50] This fusion can be detected by FISH for the loss of *CHIC2* signal or RT-PCR for the chimeric FIP1L1-PDGFRA transcript. PDGFRA overexpression is central to the pathogenesis of a primary hypereosinophilia, which in rare cases can progress to AML or T-cell lymphoblastic lymphoma/leukemia (T-ALL). Notably, a subset of PDGFRA-driven eosinophilias is also associated with a proliferation of mast cells in the bone marrow, although the D816V abnormality is not seen in this setting. The *PDGFRB* on chromosome 5q31-q32 recombines with the *ETV6 (TEL)* gene on chromosome 12p13 in rare cases of chronic myelomonocytic leukemia and eosinophilia with the t(5;12) abnormality.[51] While cytogenetic studies can readily identify t(5;12), not all tumors show translocation to the *PDGFRB* locus. Conversely, FISH analysis for *PDGFRB* gene rearrangements is occasionally negative in the presence of molecular gene alterations. For these reasons a PCR-based approach is the most comprehensive means to demonstrate the presence of the *ETV6-PDGFRB* fusion gene. Translocations of the *FGFR1* gene on chromosome 8p11 occur in several rare neoplasms, including T-ALL and AML, each characteristically associated with increased and/or abnormal eosinophils. Cytogenetic studies and FISH for *FGFR1* rearrangements are diagnostically helpful in these lesions.

Although SM patients with the *cKIT* D816V are unresponsive to imatinib, cases of *FIP1L1-PDGFRA*–positive hypereosinophilia are in contrast exquisitely sensitive to this drug, even at lower doses than those used for CML therapy. Patients with *PDGFRB-* and *FGFR1*-related hematologic diseases do not respond to imatinib. Molecular diagnostic and karyotypic evaluation of suspected SM and disorders of abnormal eosinophilia is therefore especially sought in the era of imatinib (and other TKI agent) therapy, particularly given the overlapping clinical and pathologic presentations that can be encountered.

Acute Myeloid Leukemias

AMLs have become increasingly defined by a variety of tumor genetic abnormalities with both diagnostic and prognostic significance, impacting the current WHO classification accordingly. In the broadest terms, genetic abnormalities in AML encompass recurring translocations or variants, normal karyotype AML, and complex karyotype tumors. The latter subset of AML is characterized by aggressive course and poor prognosis. Recurrent genetic abnormalities in AML have been the most extensively studied thus far, especially translocation events producing leukemogenic fusion genes. Normal karyotype AML accounts for nearly 50% of de novo AML occurrences, and this area has seen many recent advances revealing several small-scale genetic mutations that appear to be cooperative in determining biologic and clinical behavior. AML is clearly a remarkably heterogeneous set of diseases, the molecular characterization of which requires a combination of classical cytogenetics, molecular cytogenetics (ie, FISH), molecular diagnostics, and sensitive post-therapy molecular monitoring approaches. The following section briefly details the major AML entities and salient features as applicable to molecular diagnosis.

Acute promyelocytic leukemia

APL accounts for 5% to 10% of de novo AML and is a paradigm for the use of relatively nontoxic cell differentiation therapy based on its unique molecular pathogenesis. APL is defined by t(15;17)(q22;q21), resulting in the formation of a novel fusion gene *PML-RARA* on the derivative chromosome 15q.[52] Promyelocytic leukemia (*PML*) is a tumor suppressor involved in multiprotein nuclear body complexes regulating gene transcription and cellular apoptosis,[53] whereas the *RARA* gene encodes the alpha receptor for the nuclear transcription factor retinoic acid. The chimeric PML-RARA protein shows pleiotropic effects by disrupting normal PML function as well as retinoic acid transcriptional regulation. The major manifestation of the chimeric PML-RARa protein is the production of a maturation block at the promyelocyte stage of myeloid differentiation, with the accumulation of neoplastic blasts and promyelocytes. However, the clinical significance of the PML-RARa abnormality lies in the responsiveness of malignant APL cells to pharmacologic doses of all *trans* retinoic acid (atRA),[54] which, in combination with chemotherapy, leads to an excellent outcome in nearly 80% of patients. Mechanistically, atRA promotes derepression of transcriptional sites in genes that are critical for normal myeloid cell development by allowing dissociation of nuclear repressor factors, including histone deacetylase. This action also restores normal wild-type PML activity at regulatory foci within the nucleus. The resounding success of atRA-based therapy for APL has reversed the prognostic outlook for this disease, establishing it as a curable type of AML. However, rarely occurring mimickers of APL can occur with alternative translocations involving the *RARA* gene, such as the t(11;17)/*PLZF-RARA* abnormality. These APL-like AML cases are typically either poorly sensitive or nonresponsive to atRA-based therapy, with a correspondingly unfavorable clinical outcome.[55,56] The *PML-RARA* abnormality can be readily detected by FISH using dual-probe hybridization or by RT-PCR analysis for the fusion mRNA. There are several advantages of PCR methods, including the ability to detect the 3 major fusion transcripts (which arise through PML breakpoint heterogeneity), the ability to detect rare submicroscopic complex translocations and, most importantly, to monitor for MRD following treatment.[57] Quantitative PCR (RQ-PCR) assessment of PML-RARA transcript level at the end of consolidation therapy is highly predictive of relapse in this disease;[58] there is practically no role for FISH testing in this setting of treated APL. Typically, a negative RQ-PCR result should be confirmed by subsequent molecular studies in the first year, to detect a possible interval PCR-positive conversion. RQ-PCR measurements should be performed on bone marrow cells, given the 1-2 log difference in detection sensitivity compared with peripheral blood after hematologic remission is established. Treatment for "molecular relapse" in APL is an important aspect in this disease, in light of additional active agents against APL cells, like arsenic trioxide.

Acute myeloid leukemia involving core-binding factor abnormalities

This subgroup of AML has in common the dysregulation of components of the heterodimeric core-binding factor (CBF), a key transcriptional enhancer of genes involved in myeloid and lymphoid differentiation.[59] The 2 major abnormalities in this category are t(8;21)(q22;q22) and inv16(p13q22) [or related t(16;16)(p13;q22)], together accounting for approximately 15% to 20% of de novo AML cases. In t(8;21), the *AML1* gene (also designated *RUNX1* or *CBFA2*), encoding an isoform of the alpha subunit of CBF, is joined to a putative transcription factor *ETO* (or *MTG8*), to form the *AML1-ETO* (*RUNX1-MTG8*) gene fusion.[60] In the case of the inv16 or t(16;16), the gene producing the beta subunit of CBF (ie, *CBFB*) is juxtaposed to a smooth-muscle myosin heavy chain gene *MYH11* to form the hybrid *CBFB-MYH11*.[61] The intact CBF heterodimer is physiologically active at the promoter sites of many genes critically involved in myeloid and lymphoid cell development by recruiting other cofactors and enabling a normal gene expression program.[62] Disruption of the CBF pathway is thus thought to underlie the central pathogenesis of these distinctive leukemias. The prominence of CBF pathway alterations in leukemogenesis is additionally emphasized by the finding of *AML1* gene translocations or mutations in several other types of leukemia and myelodysplasia. AMLs with CBF abnormalities generally have a favorable chemotherapeutic response, and molecular analysis for the specific translocation-associated chimeric gene transcripts is not routinely sought beyond standard cytogenetics or FISH methods; the role of RQ-PCR for MRD assessment has been explored,[63] but it is also not commonly applied in hematopathology practice. Concurrent mutations in the c*KIT* gene (affecting exons 8 and 17) have been shown to positively correlate with the risk of progression and adverse outcome in CBF AML patients,[64] and other studies are beginning to dissect the roles of additional cooperating genetic mutations in determining clinical outcomes for this group.[65]

Acute myeloid leukemia with normal karyotype: FLT3, NPM1, and other recently described gene mutations

FLT3 gene mutations occur in 20% to 30% of "cytogenetically normal" AML. FLT3 is a receptor tyrosine kinase involved in the maintenance and propagation of early hematopoietic progenitor cells. Two types of *FLT3* gene mutations have been described: internal tandem duplications (ITD) occurring within the juxtamembrane domain and KD point mutations involving codons 835 or 836.[66–68] Both abnormalities cause constitutive activation of FLT3 tyrosine kinase activity, leading to deregulated cell proliferation. *FLT3*-ITD is a recognized adverse prognostic factor in AML, particularly the ratio of wild type to ITD alleles (ie, "gene dosage"); the effect of *FLT3* kinase point mutations remains less clear. DNA-based PCR amplification of exons 14 and 15 of

FLT3 with accurate amplicon sizing (eg, by fluorescent capillary electrophoresis technique) can identify the ITD abnormality, as these alterations are variably larger in fragment size than expected for this region in the wild-type gene. Semiquantitative PCR approaches have been described for estimating allelic wild type to ITD ratio. Different molecular approaches can be used to detect the *FLT3* point mutations, including DNA PCR followed by amplicon digestion with an informative restriction endonuclease, direct sequencing, or other sequence-specific methods. FLT3 kinase inhibitors continue to be studied as possible specific therapeutic agents for these AML patients, given the poor outcome conferred by *FLT3* mutations.

Mutations in the gene encoding nucleophosmin (*NPM1*) have been detected in as many as one-third or more of de novo AML patients with normal karyotype, establishing this abnormality as one of the most frequent recurrent genetic lesions in AML. Nucleophosmin is a nucleolar protein responsible for many important cellular functions, including nucleo-cytoplasmic transport of ribosomal proteins and the regulation of the tumor suppressor p53 and cell cycle proteins.[69,70] Mutations in *NPM1* occur in exon 12, most frequently observed as a TCTG duplication at position 956. This small nucleotide insertion event leads to frame shift in the C-terminus of NPM1, which is responsible for nucleolar localization; the mutant dysfunctional protein therefore abnormally accumulates in the cytoplasm. Many other small nucleotide insertions have been described in *NPM1*, but four common tetranucleotide insertions account for nearly 95% of cases. Given this scenario, PCR with fluorescent primer and capillary electrophoresis can sensitively distinguish wild type from mutated *NPM1* alleles at diagnosis. Other detection methods include post-PCR melting curve analysis and direct sequencing of PCR amplicons. RQ-PCR methods have also been described for quantifying *NPM1* mutation-positive cells for MRD analysis following therapy. *NPM1* mutations are associated with relatively good prognosis and treatment responsiveness in AML; however, the generally positive association of *NPM1* mutation with outcome is essentially nullified if a concurrent *FLT3* gene mutation is also present. Thus, molecular analysis of *NPM1* must always be performed in conjunction with *FLT3* mutation testing to establish its true prognostic value in normal karyotype AML.

Various other single gene mutations have been described in AML with normal cytogenetics, and these entities have recently been included in the 2008 WHO classification of AML. These new genetic aberrancies appear to have prognostic significance and include AML with mutations in *CEBPA* and *WT1* genes as well as overexpression/deregulation of *ERG*, *MN-1*, and *BAALC* genes. As the field of genetic characterization of normal karyotype AML expands, there is a growing need to be able to simultaneously analyze multiple genetic alterations and critically assess the biologic, therapeutic, and prognostic contributions of cooperating or interacting mutations. From a practical viewpoint, new analysis platforms need to be developed with true multiplex capacity and sufficient sensitivity to account for mutated gene dosage due to tumor heterogeneity. In conjunction with these laboratory considerations, sufficiently large and uniformly treated AML patient populations will be required for future study, with excellent bioinformatics and multivariate analyses, to more completely understand the complexity of this large group of AML.

MOLECULAR DIAGNOSIS IN LYMPHOID MALIGNANCIES
Mature B-Lymphoid Neoplasms

Follicular lymphoma: BCL2 gene rearrangements
Approximately 85% to 90% of follicular lymphoma (FL) are characterized by the presence of the t(14;18)(q32;q21) genetic abnormality. This translocation juxtaposes the

BCL2 gene to the *IGH* locus on the derivative chromosome 14. As a result, the BCL2 gene is strongly deregulated, leading in almost all cases to excess cellular production of this potent antiapoptotic protein.[71,72] Overexpression of BCL2 is thought to confer protection to the neoplastic B cell from ongoing genotoxic or oncogenic (proliferative) stress and is a factor in tumor chemoresistance. Of note, many other B-cell lymphomas overexpress BCL2 but through alternative pathogenic mechanisms unrelated to t(14;18). Clustering of breakpoints within the third exon of *BCL2* and the *IGH*-JH exon region permits detection of the *BCL2-IGH* gene fusion in nearly 70% of cases using genomic DNA-based PCR methods. However, the presence of additional distinct break sites 3' to the *BCL2* gene on chromosome 18q21 complicates typical PCR approaches, despite some described advances using multiple primer sets to enhance breakpoint coverage.[73–76] Thus, the dual-color fluorescence in situ hybridization technique (D-FISH) has become more frequently employed for the initial detection of *BCL2* gene rearrangements and specifically the *BCL2-IGH* abnormality.[77] D-FISH is applicable to fresh or frozen biopsies as well as interphase nuclei isolated from paraffin tissues. Although identification of the t(14;18)/*BCL2-IGH* abnormality is not typically required for the diagnosis of FL, its presence can be helpful to distinguish FL from atypical follicular hyperplasias or other B-cell lymphomas that can exhibit a follicular or nodular histologic pattern (eg, marginal zone lymphoma, mantle cell lymphoma [MCL]). *BCL2-IGH* rearrangements can also be employed as tumor-specific markers to sensitively monitor residual disease in individual FL patients treated with curative intent therapy, using quantitative PCR methods.[78] Conversely, a negative PCR or D-FISH study should not exclude the diagnosis of FL if other pathologic findings are supportive, given that a small proportion of FL lacks the t(14;18) and BCL2 gene rearrangements.

Mantle cell lymphomas: CCND1 gene rearrangements

MCL is essentially defined by the presence of the t(11;14)(q13;q32) abnormality, which results in the fusion of the *CCND1* gene with the *IGH* locus on 14(q32).[79] *CCND1* encodes the tightly regulated G1-phase–specific cell cycle protein cyclin D1. Cyclin D1 bound to cyclin-dependent kinase Cdk4 or Cdk6 forms an active holoenzyme complex that promotes the transition from G1 to S phase of the cell cycle in dividing cells, principally through phosphorylation of the retinoblastoma (RB) protein.[80] Deregulation of cyclin D1 expression as a consequence of juxtaposition with the *IGH* gene is thus considered a central factor underlying the proliferative phenotype of MCL. Chromosome 11q13 breakpoints are variably distributed within the so-called *BCL1* genomic region and are typically situated far from the actual *CCND1* gene. Nearly 50% of MCL cases show breakpoint clustering at the major translocation cluster (MTC) region, located approximately 120 kb centromeric to *CCND1*.[79] Additional break-fusion sites are found between the MTC and the *CCND1* gene, involving a large expanse of intervening DNA, without significant clustering. The *IGH* break sites are uniformly present within the JH region. Given the substantial heterogeneity of breakpoints in *BCL1*, D-FISH using broad coverage DNA probes is the method of choice for detecting more than 95% of *CCND1* rearrangements in MCL at diagnosis.[81,82] Genomic DNA-based PCR using *BCL1* and *IGH*-JH consensus primers flanking the MTC region can also be used to identify t(11;14), although this approach will detect slightly less than half of positive cases.[79,83] Immunohistochemistry using antibodies against cyclin D1 protein is alternatively a very specific means of identifying MCL, since normal B cells and nearly all B-cell malignancies (with the exception of some cases of hairy cell leukemia and myeloma) lack expression of this particular D-type cyclin. Cyclin D1 immunohistochemistry also identifies rare cases of MCL with a negative

CCND1-IGH FISH study. Although immunohistochemical detection of cyclin D1 protein expression has diminished the frequency of routine molecular and FISH analyses in MCL, molecular diagnostic assessment of the CCND1-IGH genetic abnormality continues to be of value, especially concerning fresh or frozen tissue biopsy sources (eg, peripheral blood). Gene expression profiling analysis of MCL has recently identified rare tumors that have the morphologic, immunophenotypic, and transcriptional features of MCL yet lack the t(11;14)/CCND1-IGH abnormality and cyclin D1 overexpression. These lymphomas are instead characterized by alterations in cyclin D2 or D3 expression.[84,85] The diagnosis of cyclin D1–negative MCL must nonetheless be approached with caution, given that many other B-cell lymphomas can show expression of cyclins D2 and D3, and further, because definitive diagnostic criteria for cyclin D1–negative MCL have not been defined at present beyond these experimental gene expression studies.

Extranodal marginal zone B-cell lymphomas: MALT1, BCL10, and FOXP1 gene rearrangements

The molecular pathogenesis of extranodal marginal zone B-cell lymphomas of mucosa-associated lymphoid tissue (MALT lymphomas) has become better understood, expanding the role for molecular diagnostics in this area of lymphoid tumor pathology. Recurrent gene rearrangements resulting from chromosomal translocations are associated with many MALT lymphomas and include the t(11;18)(q21;q21)/API2-MALT1, t(1;14)(p22;q32)/BCL10-IGH, and t(14;18)(q21;q32)/MALT1-IGH abnormalities.[86] These findings vary both in frequency and organ distribution among the typical MALT lymphoma sites, such as stomach, colon, lung, ocular adexa, and thyroid and salivary glands.[86–88] The t(11;18) creates a chimeric API2-MALT1 gene fusion and corresponding oncoprotein. API2 normally functions as an apoptosis inhibitor (API2, cIAP2) protein, whereas MALT1 is a paracaspase-like protein that is a critical component of normal NFκB pathway signaling.[89–91] MALT1 gene expression can also become deregulated by translocation to the IGH locus as a consequence of the t(14;18) abnormality. The rarely identified t(1;14) abnormality juxtaposes the BCL10 gene next to the IGH locus, resulting in overexpression of the BCL10 protein. BCL10 normally interacts with MALT1 in NFκB signaling and is important for normal lymphocyte development.[89,92] Each of these three translocation events results in constitutive activation of the NFκB signal transduction pathway, ultimately through degradation of the NFκB regulatory protein inhibitor of kappa B (IKB).[86] NFκB normally functions as a highly regulated pleiotropic transcription factor targeting genes involved in lymphocyte cell survival, activation, and proliferation; aberrant NFκB expression is thus now considered central to the pathophysiology of these lymphomas.[93] Further expanding the spectrum of genetic aberrations in MALT lymphomas is the discovery of t(3;14)(p13;q32), resulting in the FOXP1-IGH gene fusion and overexpression of the of the forkhead family transcription factor, FOXP1.[94] FOXP1 is normally involved in the regulation of Rag1 and Rag2 recombinase enzyme expression during B-cell development.[95]

The identification of recurrent translocations in MALT lymphomas can be accomplished most comprehensively using FISH techniques and appropriate locus-specific probes. The t(11;18)/API2-MALT1 can also be detected by RT-PCR amplification of the chimeric API2-MALT1 mRNA, although this approach is technically challenging because of the substantial breakpoint heterogeneity in both API2 and MALT1 genes. In many situations, the diagnosis of MALT lymphoma can be established without additional molecular diagnostic evaluation. Nonetheless, the presence of these abnormalities can be helpful to support the diagnosis of lymphoma in morphologically challenging small-tissue biopsies or to differentiate marginal zone lymphoma with follicular colonization from FL. Although the t(14;18) chromosome banding pattern is identical in both marginal zone lymphoma and FL, the *MALT1* gene is located slightly centromeric to the *BCL2* locus on 18q21, and the specific rearranged gene can be precisely delineated by FISH techniques. From a clinical standpoint, many cases of gastric MALT lymphoma associated with *Helicobacter pylori* infection can be successfully managed with intensive antibiotic therapy;[96] however, the presence of the t(11;18)/*API2-MALT1* is associated with a lack of tumor regression, and its detection can help identify patients requiring alternative treatment options. Finally, the central role of NFκB activation in the pathogenesis of many MALT lymphomas provides a rational premise for the development of novel therapeutic interventions using small-molecule–targeting drugs. Recently published investigations using gene expression profiling technology in pulmonary MALT lymphomas have provided additional novel observations concerning molecular pathogenesis, suggesting new diagnostic and therapeutic targets.[97]

Burkitt lymphomas and "high-grade" B-cell lymphomas: cMYC gene rearrangements
Burkitt lymphoma is a well-recognized high-grade B-cell lymphoma with characteristic morphologic and immunophenotypic features and the invariant presence of *cMYC* gene rearrangements in the absence of additional complex genetic anomalies. Most commonly, *cMYC* is juxtaposed with the *IGH* gene as a result of the t(8;14)(q24;q32) abnormality;[98,99] less frequently, translocations may involve the immunoglobulin light chain gene loci (*IGK* or *IGL*) on chromosomes 2p12 and 22q11, respectively. cMYC is a potent early response transcription factor, which initiates cell cycle entry and DNA replication responses following mitogenic signaling.[99,100] Breakpoints in the *cMYC* and immunoglobulin genes are highly variable and distributed over large genomic regions. Endemic-type BL (highly associated with Epstein-Barr virus infection) reveals *cMYC* break sites far upstream of the gene, with translocation to the JH region of *IGH*. Sporadic BL cases are instead characterized by *cMYC* breakpoints near or within the 5' part of the gene and involve the switch region (Sμ) of *IGH*. Although significant phenotypic or clinical differences do not seem to be associated with this variable molecular pathology, the heterogeneity in break-fusion events precludes the straightforward use of DNA PCR to detect *cMYC* gene translocations. FISH technique using a BAP probe strategy is highly sensitive and can be used to initially detect *cMYC* gene rearrangements. The presence of a translocation specifically involving the *IGH* gene can subsequently be discerned using a D-FISH approach.[101] Detection of a *cMYC* gene translocation is required to establish the diagnosis of BL in clinical cases with strong presumptive clinical and pathologic findings. Nevertheless, it is apparent that a subset of highly aggressive B-cell lymphomas may share partially overlapping morphologic and phenotypic features with classic BL and also harbor *cMYC* gene translocations. In the latter cases, additional FISH analyses for *BCL2* and *BCL6* gene rearrangements can be useful to distinguish true BL (ie, with *cMYC* translocation only) from "double hit," high-grade B-cell lymphoma (eg, with *cMYC* translocation plus a second genetic locus abnormality).[102–104]

Diffuse large B-cell lymphomas
The diagnosis of diffuse large B-cell lymphoma (DLBCL) seldom requires supplementary molecular genetic investigations. Indeed, much attention has instead focused on the discovery of pathobiologic features that will better distinguish patients with favorable versus poor outcome in a disease that appears morphologically and phenotypically quite homogeneous but is biologically rather diverse.

Among the well-known genetic abnormalities found in DLBCL, approximately 20% to 30% of DLBCL have the t(14;18) abnormality and accompanying *BCL2* gene rearrangements, with some of these cases representing transformations from an underlying FL. Structural rearrangements of the *BCL6* gene, located at chromosome 3q27, occur in a larger number of DLBCL (30%–40%) as well as a subset of FL (<20%). Translocations of *BCL6* can involve the immunoglobulin gene loci as well as several nonimmunoglobulin translocation gene partners,[105] in each case resulting in deregulation of *BCL6* expression. An even greater proportion of DLBCL and FL (either with or without *BCL6* translocations) demonstrate somatic mutations in the 5' noncoding regions of the gene, some of which abrogate the normal control of *BCL6* gene expression.[106] BCL6 is a zinc finger transcription factor essential for the formation of secondary B-cell follicles and T-cell–dependent antibody responses following antigenic stimulation; it is expressed exclusively in normal GC B cells and rapidly downregulated following B-cell exit from the GC environment.[107,108] Overexpression of BCL6 protein by aberrant genetic or epigenetic mechanisms is considered important in the pathogenesis of the GC-related B-cell lymphomas, by maintaining lymphocytes in a GC-like environment and creating a sustained proliferative setting in which additional genetic mutations can occur.[109–111] *BCL6* gene rearrangements arising from translocation events can be detected by the BAP FISH technique. A small subset (5%–10%) of large B-cell lymphoma is associated with *cMYC* gene translocations, and these individuals have a poor clinical outcome. As indicated, uncommon presentations of very aggressive high-grade B-cell lymphomas with blastoid nuclei (but not fulfilling precise morphologic or immunophenotypic criteria for Burkitt lymphoma) are characterized by *cMYC* translocations and may have accompanying rearrangements of *BCL2* or *BCL6*; an appropriate panel of FISH studies in these patients may therefore be of clinical prognostic value.[103,104] Rare occurrences of IgA-positive large B-cell lymphomas with plasmablastic or immunoblastic cytology have been associated with rearrangements involving the anaplastic lymphoma kinase (*ALK*) gene and the clathrin gene (*CLTC*), as a consequence of the t(2;17) cytogenetic abnormality.[112–114] The resultant CLTC-ALK fusion protein creates a distinctive immunostaining pattern of granular cell membrane positivity, corresponding to aberrant ALK localization within clathrin-coated pits. FISH analysis using an *ALK* gene BAP strategy can be helpful in classifying these lymphomas, although the characteristic histopathologic and immunophenotypic findings (including the pattern of ALK immunopositivity) are usually sufficient for the diagnosis.

Gene expression profiling analyses of DLBCL have generated interesting biologic and conceptual categories of these lymphomas that correspond to GC and "activated" B-cell (ABC) phenotypes.[115–117] In several studies, GC-type DLBCL have been associated with relatively favorable clinical outcome, in contrast to a poorer clinical course for ABC-type tumors. However, attempts to distill the expression profiling data to reproducible and clinically relevant prognostic assays in the hematopathology laboratory have been inconsistent and overall of questionable significance at the present time.[118] The reasons for this situation include methodological differences in immunohistochemical studies; variable choices of candidate markers; a general lack of corroborative, high-quality molecular diagnostic approaches (eg, quantitative PCR assays); insufficient large-scale clinical studies to confirm the GC versus ABC prognostic classification in the rituximab therapeutic era; and data from other gene expression DLBCL studies that provide alternative models of pathogenesis.[119] Although a standardized multiparameter strategy for identifying prognostically important subsets of DLBCL remains to be widely accepted, continuing investigations in this area show promise for delineating new markers of potential significance, as shown by the recent association of LMO2 gene and protein expression with favorable outcome.[120]

Chronic lymphocytic leukemia

Clinical outcome in chronic lymphocytic leukemia/small lymphocytic lymphoma (CLL/SLL) has become increasingly defined by several phenotypic and molecular abnormalities.[121–128] Cell markers of adverse prognosis include a high expression of surface CD38 and intracellular Zap70 protein kinase. The somatic mutational status of the clonal rearranged *IGH* gene also shows a strong correlation with disease course, in that unmutated *IGH* status (<2% deviation from germline sequence) describes a subset of patients with more aggressive clinical manifestations. *IGH* mutation evaluation is performed using standard PCR and sequencing techniques, but the process has been made particularly more feasible by the presence of comprehensive sequence analysis resources (ie, ImmunoGenetics; http://imgt.cines.fr). Four common and recurrent cytogenetic abnormalities are also associated with clinical course and response to treatment in CLL, including -13 or 13q-, +12, 11q-, and 17p-. Each deletion abnormality involves loss of 1 copy of a tumor suppressor gene: *RB* at 13q14; ataxia-telangiectasia-mutated at 11q22; and *TP53* at 17p13. In addition, 2 microRNA genes (miR-15 and miR-16) are associated with the minimally deleted region of 13q and may be important in CLL pathogenesis. Of these cytogenetic changes, isolated loss of 13q is observed in patients with a generally favorable prognosis, in contrast to 11q- and 17p-, which are seen in aggressive cases of CLL. Notably, these major genetic findings can often coexist in the same leukemia, complicating the assignment of prognostic value to some degree. However, loss of 17p, occurring in 5% to 10% of untreated CLL patients, confers a very poor prognosis regardless of additional genetic changes.[129–131] Most, but not all, CLL tumors with 17p- show point mutation inactivation of the remaining *TP53* allele. In rare patients, both 17p loci are cytogenetically present but show biallelic *TP53* gene mutations, in some cases due to mitotic recombination of 1 mutated allele (uniparental disomy). Although the major cytogenetic lesions are readily detected by FISH methods, molecular screening for *TP53* mutations also represents an important aspect of tumor genetic evaluation in CLL.[132] Evaluation of CLL patients thus involves the integration of many different prognostic factors and will typically include phenotyping, FISH, and molecular genetic analyses. At the present time, these ancillary studies are most informative for assessment of biologic behavior rather than to principally guide treatment options for CLL patients. One exception is the presence of *TP53* mutations, which portends significantly adverse clinical behavior and poor responsiveness to purine nucleoside analogs; these patients may be early candidates for alternative therapies.

Mature T-Lymphoid Neoplasms

Anaplastic large T-cell lymphoma

Anaplastic large cell lymphoma (ALCL) is a morphologically distinctive subtype of peripheral T-cell lymphoma, most of which are associated with overexpression of the *ALK* gene located on 2p23. ALK is normally not expressed in lymphoid cells but becomes constitutively activated as a consequence of aberrant rearrangements to one of several possible genetic loci. Most commonly, *ALK* is involved in a translocation with the nucleophosmin (*NPM1*) gene (5q35) forming a chimeric *NPM1-ALK* gene fusion, mRNA, and protein. Other translocations resulting in *ALK* deregulation include the t(1;2)(q25;p23)/*TPM3-ALK*, t(2;3)(p23;q35)/*TFG-ALK*, and inv(2)(p23q35)/*ATIC-ALK* abnormalities.[133,134] Importantly, the non-ALK component of a given chimeric oncoprotein determines its subcellular localization; thus NPM1, which functions in the processes of ribosomal synthesis and nucleolar-cytoplasmic transport, results in a distribution of NPM1-ALK within the nucleus and cytoplasm, whereas other ALK translocations (eg, with *TPM3*, tropomyosin-3) involve cytoplasmic protein components with a resultant diffuse cytoplasmic localization. These patterns can be demonstrated by anti-ALK immunohistochemistry.[135] ALCL with *ALK* rearrangements are associated with a relatively favorable prognosis compared with *ALK*-negative ALCL and peripheral T-cell lymphomas, unspecified. *ALK* rearrangements are most comprehensively detected by FISH using a BAP probe strategy; although this technique does not define the particular translocation in a given case of ALCL, there appears to be no additional prognostic significance in determining the non-*ALK* partner gene. The chimeric NPM1-ALK transcript can also be sensitively identified by RT-PCR methods, and this may have a role in minimal disease detection in bone marrow specimens.[136,137]

T-cell prolymphocytic leukemia

T-cell prolymphocytic leukemia (T-PLL) is an uncommon T-cell neoplasm with prominent peripheral blood, bone marrow, spleen, and lymph node involvement. Although often recognizable by peripheral smear cytology and immunophenotypic features, the diagnosis of T-PLL is now greatly enhanced by the detection of *TCL1* gene rearrangements. *TCL1* is an oncogene with incompletely understood functions, but it is implicated in cell survival and proliferation.[138,139] *TCL1* is not normally expressed in mature T cells and is not detected in peripheral T-cell neoplasms apart from T-PLL, thus providing a relatively specific marker for this tumor. Approximately 80% of T-PLL harbor either inv14(q11q32) or t(14;14)(q11;q32) rearrangements, placing the *TCL1* gene next to the TCR alpha (*TRA*) locus.[138,139] A minority of T-PLL show alternative abnormalities, including the t(X;14)(q28;q11) and t(X;7)(q28;q35); the latter translocations juxtapose the *TCL1*-related gene *MTCP1* to either the *TRA* or T-cell beta (*TRB*) loci respectively.[138,140] *TCL1* gene rearrangements are best identified by the FISH technique, as these abnormalities can be cytogenetically cryptic. Standard karyotyping analysis is of value to identify variant *MTCP1* translocations in other cases of T-PLL. Immunohistochemistry using anti-TCL1 antibodies can also be employed to help establish the diagnosis of T-PLL in tissue biopsies, although a small subset of T-PLL may lack both *TCL1* gene rearrangements and TCL1 protein expression.

Precursor Lymphoid Neoplasms

B-lymphoblastic leukemia/lymphoma

B-lymphoblastic leukemia/lymphoma (precursor B-cell acute lymphoblastic leukemia, B-ALL) is the most common childhood hematologic malignancy, but it occurs relatively rarely in adults. Childhood B-ALL has emerged as a paradigm for the use of multiple tumor genetic markers to provide prognostic, clinically important data to initially stratify patients for appropriately tailored treatment based on an estimated risk of disease relapse.[141] Several well-known cytogenetic and associated molecular genetic anomalies characterize nearly half of childhood B-ALL. These aberrancies can be broadly classified as numerical changes (ie, chromosomal hyperdiploidy and hypodiploidy) and structural translocation events. Approximately 25% of B-ALL patients have tumors with a hyperdiploid chromosome complement (>52 chromosomes), characteristically with trisomies of 4, 10, or 17; these individuals have excellent long-term survival. In contrast, a small number of patients (<5%) have lymphoblasts with modal chromosome numbers less than 45, and these hypodiploid tumors are associated with poor overall outcome.[142] These features of tumor aneuploidy can be demonstrated by standard karyotyping, FISH using multiple enumeration probes, or DNA content analysis by flow cytometry.

Recurrent chromosome translocations define a further 30% of childhood B-ALL, comprising the t(9;22)/*BCR-ABL1* (Ph+ B-ALL), t(1;19)/*E2A(TCF3)-PBX1*, t(12;21)/*ETV6(TEL)-RUNX1(CBFA2* or *AML1)*, and translocations involving the *MLL* gene at 11q23. The *BCR-ABL1* abnormality occurs in approximately 3% of childhood Ph+ B-ALL and is associated with distinctly aggressive tumor biology and poor outcome. In adults, this translocation is observed in 25% of B-ALL, with a similarly dismal prognostic relationship. In childhood Ph+ ALL, BCR gene breakpoints most often (>80%) involve the 5' m-bcr, producing an e1-a2 transcript and the so-called p190 BCR-ABL1 protein (see **Fig. 2**). A small proportion of pediatric cases (as well as nearly 40% of adult Ph+ B-ALL) show BCR breakage in the major breakpoint cluster (the region also associated with nearly all chronic myelogenous leukemias), producing an e13-a2– or e14-a2–type mRNA and corresponding p210 chimeric protein. Rare Ph+ ALL tumors may exhibit break sites that produce additional BCR-ABL1 variants (eg, e1-a3). Approximately 3% to 5% of childhood B-ALL demonstrate translocations of 11q23 involving the *MLL* gene. *MLL*-positive ALL is especially prevalent in infants (<1 year), and these leukemias are associated with poor outcome.[143] The *MLL* gene can be translocated to one of potentially dozens of partner genes; the most common abnormalities encountered are the t(4;11)/*MLL-AF4* and t(11;19)/*MLL-ENL*. Chimeric MLL fusion proteins display leukemogenic potential and are known to aberrantly stabilize HoxA9 and Meis1 transcription factors in stem/progenitor marrow cells, leading to abrogation of normal hematopoietic differentiation.[144] The frequent finding of *MLL* translocations in infant B-ALL indicates a short latency period before full manifestation of the leukemic disease. The t(12;21) is detected very infrequently (<0.1%) by classical cytogenetics but is found in 20% of childhood B-ALL using molecular techniques. The t(12;21) results in a fusion gene and transcript, *ETV6-RUNX1* (also known as *TEL-AML1*). The presence of the *ETV6-RUNX1* is associated with an excellent prognosis, although some patients can experience late leukemic recurrences.[145] The RUNX1 (AML1) protein is a key transcriptional regulator of hematopoietic differentiation, and its function is disrupted by fusion to ETV6. In many *ETV6-RUNX1*–positive B-ALL, the remaining *ETV6* allele is deleted, suggesting a tumor suppressor function for this gene as well. A small number of B-ALL cases (3%) show a characteristic "pre–B-cell" immunophenotype strongly associated with the presence of the *E2A* (or *TCF3)-PBX1* gene fusion. *E2A-PBX1*–positive leukemias have been associated with more aggressive disease, although improvements in treatment have now largely made this observation of historical significance.

These major chromosome translocation events can be accurately detected in B-ALL by standard FISH techniques on interphase (or metaphase) nuclei. Notably, all of the foregoing translocation events associated with B-ALL result in the production of a transcribed fusion gene with its corresponding chimeric mRNA and leukemogenic protein. The unique fusion mRNA transcripts can thus be sensitively and specifically detected by RT-PCR techniques. When designing RT-PCR assays, one must be aware of alternate breakpoint regions in the involved genes and alternative splicing events in the primary transcript, as exemplified by the *BCR-ABL1* abnormality. Accordingly, diagnostic RT-PCR assays should be sufficiently comprehensive to detect such variations, as prior knowledge of a particular transcript type helps guide appropriate MRD evaluations following therapy (see later section). In the case of *MLL* gene rearrangements, the most common t(4;11)/*MLL-AF4* can be readily detected by RT-PCR; however, given the marked proclivity for *MLL* translocations to occur with many other genes, FISH using a BAP strategy is a very useful alternative to reveal the presence of an *MLL* gene rearrangement at diagnosis.

Classification of childhood B-ALL according to these numerical or structural tumor genetic anomalies has helped to guide treatment type and duration for different groups of childhood B-ALL patients, when combined with standard measures of risk, such as age, gender, and presenting white blood cell count.[146] A significant proportion of children with ALL ($\sim$25%), regardless of pretherapy risk group assignment, still continue to fail therapy despite application of this sophisticated tumor genetic modeling approach. Earlier identification of these patients is clearly important. In this regard, highly sensitive quantitative PCR and flow cytometric methods have been developed to assess MRD in childhood leukemias, further refining the ability to determine treatment resistance and relapse risk. Automated quantitative PCR analyses can identify disease-specific targets in lymphoid leukemias, such as unique clonotypic B- or TCR gene rearrangements or chimeric transcripts arising from translocation-derived fusion genes.[12,147] Because molecular methods can suffer from some drawbacks such as labor-intensive preparatory procedures and a lack of uniform technical standardization, flow cytometric immunophenotyping techniques have also been developed for evaluating MRD in post-therapy samples with comparably high sensitivity and specificity.[148] Many studies in childhood B-ALL have now confirmed that early MRD measurements (typically in the period immediately following induction chemotherapy) have strong prognostic value and can help more accurately predict individual patient outcomes.[149–153] The addition of MRD studies to the clinical/tumor genetics prognostic framework has further extended the outcome prediction for childhood ALL and allows greater fine-tuning of therapeutic choices for additional subgroups of patients.

Recent studies of childhood B-ALL using genome-scale array hybridization methods have indicated that a majority of tumors show mutations in genes governing normal B-cell development. Of these changes, alterations of the *IKZF-1* gene, encoding the transcription factor Ikaros, define a subset of particularly high-risk patients, comparable to *BCR-ABL1*–positive B-ALL.[154,155] These investigations continue to expand our understanding of disease pathogenesis and also identify new targets for risk prediction and MRD analysis in childhood B-ALL. In contrast to childhood B-ALL, adult B-ALL is a disease that appears biologically distinct, with a relatively unfavorable prognosis overall. Apart from the very poor prognosis associated with the *BCR-ABL1* abnormality, tumor genetics have thus far been of limited value in the management of adult B-ALL patients. Newer genomic profiling studies therefore appear promising for pathobiologic discovery in this clinical group of B-ALL.

THE NEAR FUTURE: EMERGING TECHNOLOGIES FOR MOLECULAR DIAGNOSIS

Advances in technology and molecular genetics promise additional rapid progress in molecular diagnostic applications. Several methods for genome-scale evaluation are emerging with the potential to change our concepts of how routine molecular testing will be performed in hematopathology. Of these, array-based oligonucleotide comparative genomic hybridization and single nucleotide polymorphism arrays are exciting platforms, providing genomic analyses that bridge the gap in resolution between sequencing and FISH approaches.[156,157] Both technologies can identify intermediate-level changes in DNA structure termed copy number variations that are increasingly felt to be important in disease pathogenesis. Both methods also allow identification of copy neutral loss of heterozygosity, occurring as a result of pathologic uniparental disomy. These technologies are very sensitive in detection of small-to-medium–sized duplications, amplifications, and deletions, which are missed by conventional cytogenetics or FISH; so-called array karyotyping cannot, however, detect balanced translocations. Gene chip expression profiling (GEP) assessing the global transcriptome of tumors has found many research applications and is a potentially powerful tool in understanding molecular abnormalities and pathways in hematologic malignancies.[158] GEP methods are currently too cumbersome and lack reproducibility for routine diagnostic purposes; however, this may not preclude the development of limited mRNA expression analyses for specific tumor types or prognostic classification, possibly employing multiplexed RQ-PCR assays. Massive parallel genome sequencing platforms are now within reach of cost-effective applications. The ability to sequence large regions of DNA or whole genomes with highly redundant and accurate coverage is exemplified by the recent complete sequencing of a patient AML tumor genome,[159] establishing a precedent for potential future use in clinical practice. The landscape of biologic discovery is also changing with the demonstration of many new regulatory RNA species, including microRNAs. MicroRNAs are small non–protein-coding RNAs that are capable of decreasing protein expression by either translational interference or binding to target mRNA molecules and enhancing their degradation.[160,161] Profiling of microRNAs in some hematologic tumors has revealed some provocative associations with outcome in CLL/SLL[162] and other hematologic malignancies.[163]

Although these new technologies have a great potential to influence the practice of laboratory hematology and hematopathology, their scope is currently largely limited to research endeavors. Furthermore, the abundance of data generated by newer "–omics" approaches makes it necessary to employ increasingly sophisticated bioinformatics algorithms for data analysis. Additionally, validation of complex data generated by high-throughput techniques requires a large number of samples, without which it is impossible to establish statistically significant associations. Finally, the cost of these new technologies, although ever decreasing, remains prohibitive for wider clinical use. Despite these issues, the future for new frontiers of molecular diagnosis in hematopathology is certainly bright.

REFERENCES

1. Bassing CH, Swat W, Alt FW. The mechanism and regulation of chromosomal V(D)J recombination. Cell 2002;109(Suppl):S45–55.
2. Cossman J, et al. Molecular genetics and the diagnosis of lymphoma. Arch Pathol Lab Med 1988;112(2):117–27.
3. Medeiros LJ, Carr J. Overview of the role of molecular methods in the diagnosis of malignant lymphomas. Arch Pathol Lab Med 1999;123(12):1189–207.
4. Derksen PW, et al. Comparison of different polymerase chain reaction-based approaches for clonality assessment of immunoglobulin heavy-chain gene rearrangements in B-cell neoplasia. Mod Pathol 1999;12(8):794–805.
5. Liu H, et al. A practical strategy for the routine use of BIOMED-2 PCR assays for detection of B- and T-cell clonality in diagnostic haematopathology. Br J Haematol 2007;138(1):31–43.
6. van Dongen JJ, et al. Design and standardization of PCR primers and protocols for detection of clonal immunoglobulin and T-cell receptor gene recombinations in suspect lymphoproliferations: report of the BIOMED-2 Concerted Action BMH4-CT98-3936. Leukemia 2003;17(12):2257–317.
7. van Krieken JH, et al. Improved reliability of lymphoma diagnostics via PCR-based clonality testing: report of the BIOMED-2 Concerted Action BHM4-CT98-3936. Leukemia 2007;21(2):201–6.

8. Bruggemann M, et al. Powerful strategy for polymerase chain reaction-based clonality assessment in T-cell malignancies Report of the BIOMED-2 Concerted Action BHM4 CT98-3936. Leukemia 2007;21(2):215–21.
9. Evans PA, et al. Significantly improved PCR-based clonality testing in B-cell malignancies by use of multiple immunoglobulin gene targets. Report of the BIOMED-2 Concerted Action BHM4-CT98-3936. Leukemia 2007;21(2):207–14.
10. Langerak AW, et al. Polymerase chain reaction-based clonality testing in tissue samples with reactive lymphoproliferations: usefulness and pitfalls. A report of the BIOMED-2 Concerted Action BMH4-CT98-3936. Leukemia 2007;21(2):222–9.
11. Wolff DJ, et al. Guidance for fluorescence in situ hybridization testing in hematologic disorders. J Mol Diagn 2007;9(2):134–43.
12. van der Velden VH, et al. Detection of minimal residual disease in hematologic malignancies by real-time quantitative PCR: principles, approaches, and laboratory aspects. Leukemia 2003;17(6):1013–34.
13. van der Velden VH, et al. Analysis of minimal residual disease by Ig/TCR gene rearrangements: guidelines for interpretation of real-time quantitative PCR data. Leukemia 2007;21(4):604–11.
14. Bose S, et al. The presence of typical and atypical BCR-ABL fusion genes in leukocytes of normal individuals: biologic significance and implications for the assessment of minimal residual disease. Blood 1998;92(9):3362–7.
15. Heisterkamp N, et al. Structural organization of the bcr gene and its role in the Ph' translocation. Nature 1985;315(6022):758–61.
16. Nowell PC. The minute chromosome (PhI) in chronic granulocytic leukemia. Blut 1962;8:65–6.
17. Rowley JD. Letter: a new consistent chromosomal abnormality in chronic myelogenous leukaemia identified by quinacrine fluorescence and Giemsa staining. Nature 1973;243(5405):290–3.
18. Fletcher JA, et al. Translocation (9;22) is associated with extremely poor prognosis in intensively treated children with acute lymphoblastic leukemia. Blood 1991;77(3):435–9.
19. Deininger MW, Goldman JM, Melo JV. The molecular biology of chronic myeloid leukemia. Blood 2000;96(10):3343–56.
20. Melo JV. The diversity of BCR-ABL fusion proteins and their relationship to leukemia phenotype. Blood 1996;88(7):2375–84.
21. Druker BJ, et al. Five-year follow-up of patients receiving imatinib for chronic myeloid leukemia. N Engl J Med 2006;355(23):2408–17.
22. Kantarjian H, et al. Hematologic and cytogenetic responses to imatinib mesylate in chronic myelogenous leukemia. N Engl J Med 2002;346(9):645–52.
23. Press RD, et al. BCR-ABL mRNA levels at and after the time of a complete cytogenetic response (CCR) predict the duration of CCR in imatinib mesylate-treated patients with CML. Blood 2006;107(11):4250–6. doi: 10.1182/blood-2005-11-4406.
24. Branford S, Hughes TP, Rudzki Z. Monitoring chronic myeloid leukaemia therapy by real-time quantitative PCR in blood is a reliable alternative to bone marrow cytogenetics. Br J Haematol 1999;107(3):587–99.
25. Hughes TP, et al. Frequency of major molecular responses to imatinib or interferon alfa plus cytarabine in newly diagnosed chronic myeloid leukemia. N Engl J Med 2003;349(15):1423–32.
26. Ross DM, Hughes TP. Current and emerging tests for the laboratory monitoring of chronic myeloid leukaemia and related disorders. Pathology 2008;40(3):231–46.

27. Wang L, et al. Serial monitoring of BCR-ABL by peripheral blood real-time polymerase chain reaction predicts the marrow cytogenetic response to imatinib mesylate in chronic myeloid leukaemia. Br J Haematol 2002;118(3):771–7.
28. Branford S, et al. Rationale for the recommendations for harmonizing current methodology for detecting BCR-ABL transcripts in patients with chronic myeloid leukaemia. Leukemia 2006;20(11):1925–30.
29. Gorre ME, et al. Clinical resistance to STI-571 cancer therapy caused by BCR-ABL gene mutation or amplification. Science 2001;293(5531):876–80.
30. Hughes T, et al. Monitoring CML patients responding to treatment with tyrosine kinase inhibitors: review and recommendations for harmonizing current methodology for detecting BCR-ABL transcripts and kinase domain mutations and for expressing results. Blood 2006;108(1):28–37.
31. Jones D, et al. Laboratory practice guidelines for detecting and reporting BCR-ABL drug resistance mutations in chronic myelogenous leukemia and acute lymphoblastic leukemia: a report of the association for molecular pathology. J Mol Diagn 2009;11(1):4–11. doi: 10.2353/jmoldx.2009.080095.
32. O'Brien S, et al. Chronic myelogenous leukemia. J Natl Compr Canc Netw 2007; 5(5):474–96.
33. Baxter EJ, et al. Acquired mutation of the tyrosine kinase JAK2 in human myeloproliferative disorders. Lancet 2005;365(9464):1054–61.
34. James C, et al. A unique clonal JAK2 mutation leading to constitutive signalling causes polycythaemia vera. Nature 2005;434(7037):1144–8.
35. Kralovics R, et al. A gain-of-function mutation of JAK2 in myeloproliferative disorders. N Engl J Med 2005;352(17):1779–90.
36. Levine RL, et al. Activating mutation in the tyrosine kinase JAK2 in polycythemia vera, essential thrombocythemia, and myeloid metaplasia with myelofibrosis. Cancer Cell 2005;7(4):387–97.
37. Pietra D, et al. Somatic mutations of JAK2 exon 12 in patients with JAK2(V617F)-negative myeloproliferative disorders. Blood 2008;111(3):1686–9. doi: 10.1182/blood-2007-07-101576.
38. Scott LM, et al. JAK2 exon 12 mutations in polycythemia vera and idiopathic erythrocytosis. N Engl J Med 2007;356(5):459–68. doi: 10.1056/NEJMoa065202.
39. Ma W, et al. Mutation profile of JAK2 transcripts in patients with chronic myeloproliferative neoplasias. J Mol Diagn 2009;11(1):49–53.
40. Rapado I, et al. High resolution melting analysis for JAK2 Exon 14 and Exon 12 mutations: a diagnostic tool for myeloproliferative neoplasms. J Mol Diagn 2009;11(2):155–61. doi: 10.2353/jmoldx.2009.080110.
41. Pardanani AD, et al. MPL515 mutations in myeloproliferative and other myeloid disorders: a study of 1182 patients. Blood 2006;108(10):3472–6.
42. Pikman Y, et al. MPLW515L is a novel somatic activating mutation in myelofibrosis with myeloid metaplasia. PLoS Med 2006;3(7):e270.
43. Smith CA, Fan G. The saga of JAK2 mutations and translocations in hematologic disorders: pathogenesis, diagnostic and therapeutic prospects, and revised World Health Organization diagnostic criteria for myeloproliferative neoplasms. Hum Pathol 2008;39(6):795–810.
44. Vannucchi AM, et al. Prospective identification of high-risk polycythemia vera patients based on JAK2(V617F) allele burden. Leukemia 2007;21(9): 1952–9.
45. Longley BJ, et al. Somatic c-KIT activating mutation in urticaria pigmentosa and aggressive mastocytosis: establishment of clonality in a human mast cell neoplasm. Nat Genet 1996;12(3):312–4.

46. Nagata H, et al. Identification of a point mutation in the catalytic domain of the protooncogene c-kit in peripheral blood mononuclear cells of patients who have mastocytosis with an associated hematologic disorder. Proc Natl Acad Sci U S A 1995;92(23):10560–4.

47. Ma Y, et al. The c-KIT mutation causing human mastocytosis is resistant to STI571 and other KIT kinase inhibitors; kinases with enzymatic site mutations show different inhibitor sensitivity profiles than wild-type kinases and those with regulatory-type mutations. Blood 2002;99(5):1741–4.

48. Orfao A, et al. Recent advances in the understanding of mastocytosis: the role of KIT mutations. Br J Haematol 2007;138(1):12–30.

49. Cools J, et al. A tyrosine kinase created by fusion of the PDGFRA and FIP1L1 genes as a therapeutic target of imatinib in idiopathic hypereosinophilic syndrome. N Engl J Med 2003;348(13):1201–14.

50. Pardanani A, et al. CHIC2 deletion, a surrogate for FIP1L1-PDGFRA fusion, occurs in systemic mastocytosis associated with eosinophilia and predicts response to imatinib mesylate therapy. Blood 2003;102(9):3093–6.

51. Apperley JF, et al. Response to imatinib mesylate in patients with chronic myeloproliferative diseases with rearrangements of the platelet-derived growth factor receptor beta. N Engl J Med 2002;347(7):481–7.

52. Grignani F, et al. Acute promyelocytic leukemia: from genetics to treatment. Blood 1994;83(1):10–25.

53. Bernardi R, Papa A, Pandolfi PP. Regulation of apoptosis by PML and the PML-NBs. Oncogene 2008;27(48):6299–312.

54. Tallman MS, et al. All-trans-retinoic acid in acute promyelocytic leukemia. N Engl J Med 1997;337(15):1021–8.

55. Grimwade D, et al. Characterization of acute promyelocytic leukemia cases lacking the classic t(15;17): results of the European Working Party. Groupe Francais de Cytogenetique Hematologique, Groupe de Francais d'Hematologie Cellulaire, UK Cancer Cytogenetics Group and BIOMED 1 European Community-Concerted Action "Molecular Cytogenetic Diagnosis in Haematological Malignancies". Blood 2000;96(4):1297–308.

56. Melnick A, Licht JD. Deconstructing a disease: RARalpha, its fusion partners, and their roles in the pathogenesis of acute promyelocytic leukemia. Blood 1999;93(10):3167–215.

57. Grimwade D, Lo Coco F. Acute promyelocytic leukemia: a model for the role of molecular diagnosis and residual disease monitoring in directing treatment approach in acute myeloid leukemia. Leukemia 2002;16(10):1959–73.

58. Santamaria C, et al. Using quantification of the PML-RARalpha transcript to stratify the risk of relapse in patients with acute promyelocytic leukemia. Haematologica 2007;92(3):315–22.

59. Speck NA, et al. Core-binding factor: a central player in hematopoiesis and leukemia. Cancer Res 1999;59(7 Suppl):1789s–93s.

60. Downing JR. The AML1-ETO chimaeric transcription factor in acute myeloid leukaemia: biology and clinical significance. Br J Haematol 1999;106(2):296–308.

61. Liu PP, et al. Molecular pathogenesis of the chromosome 16 inversion in the M4Eo subtype of acute myeloid leukemia. Blood 1995;85(9):2289–302.

62. de Bruijn MF, Speck NA. Core-binding factors in hematopoiesis and immune function. Oncogene 2004;23(24):4238–48.

63. Krauter J, et al. Prognostic value of minimal residual disease quantification by real-time reverse transcriptase polymerase chain reaction in patients with core binding factor leukemias. J Clin Oncol 2003;21(23):4413–22.

64. Paschka P, et al. Adverse prognostic significance of KIT mutations in adult acute myeloid leukemia with inv(16) and t(8;21): a Cancer and Leukemia Group B Study. J Clin Oncol 2006;24(24):3904–11.
65. Mrozek K, et al. Advances in molecular genetics and treatment of core-binding factor acute myeloid leukemia. Curr Opin Oncol 2008;20(6):711–8.
66. Baldus CD, et al. BAALC expression and FLT3 internal tandem duplication mutations in acute myeloid leukemia patients with normal cytogenetics: prognostic implications. J Clin Oncol 2006;24(5):790–7.
67. Gilliland DG, Griffin JD. The roles of FLT3 in hematopoiesis and leukemia. Blood 2002;100(5):1532–42.
68. Yamamoto Y, et al. Activating mutation of D835 within the activation loop of FLT3 in human hematologic malignancies. Blood 2001;97(8):2434–9.
69. Borer RA, et al. Major nucleolar proteins shuttle between nucleus and cytoplasm. Cell 1989;56(3):379–90.
70. Colombo E, et al. Nucleophosmin regulates the stability and transcriptional activity of p53. Nat Cell Biol 2002;4(7):529–33.
71. Adams JM, Cory S. The Bcl-2 protein family: arbiters of cell survival. Science 1998;281(5381):1322–6.
72. Danial NN, Korsmeyer SJ. Cell death: critical control points. Cell 2004;116(2): 205–19.
73. Akasaka T, et al. Refinement of the BCL2/immunoglobulin heavy chain fusion gene in t(14;18)(q32;q21) by polymerase chain reaction amplification for long targets. Genes Chromosomes Cancer 1998;21(1):17–29.
74. Albinger-Hegyi A, et al. High frequency of t(14;18)-translocation breakpoints outside of major breakpoint and minor cluster regions in follicular lymphomas: improved polymerase chain reaction protocols for their detection. Am J Pathol 2002;160(3):823–32.
75. Buchonnet G, et al. Distribution of BCL2 breakpoints in follicular lymphoma and correlation with clinical features: specific subtypes or same disease? Leukemia 2002;16(9):1852–6.
76. Buchonnet G, et al. Characterisation of BCL2-JH rearrangements in follicular lymphoma: PCR detection of 3' BCL2 breakpoints and evidence of a new cluster. Leukemia 2000;14(9):1563–9.
77. Vega F, Medeiros LJ. Chromosomal translocations involved in non-Hodgkin lymphomas. Arch Pathol Lab Med 2003;127(9):1148–60.
78. Bowman A, et al. Quantitative PCR detection of t(14;18) bcl-2/JH fusion sequences in follicular lymphoma patients: comparison of peripheral blood and bone marrow aspirate samples. J Mol Diagn 2004;6(4):396–400.
79. Bertoni F, Zucca E, Cotter FE. Molecular basis of mantle cell lymphoma. Br J Haematol 2004;124(2):130–40.
80. Sherr CJ. The Pezcoller lecture: cancer cell cycles revisited. Cancer Res 2000; 60(14):3689–95.
81. Belaud-Rotureau MA, et al. A comparative analysis of FISH, RT-PCR, PCR, and immunohistochemistry for the diagnosis of mantle cell lymphomas. Mod Pathol 2002;15(5):517–25.
82. Remstein ED, et al. Diagnostic utility of fluorescence in situ hybridization in mantle-cell lymphoma. Br J Haematol 2000;110(4):856–62.
83. Chibbar R, et al. bcl-1 gene rearrangements in mantle cell lymphoma: a comprehensive analysis of 118 cases, including B-5-fixed tissue, by polymerase chain reaction and Southern transfer analysis. Mod Pathol 1998; 11(11):1089–97.

84. Fu K, et al. Cyclin D1-negative mantle cell lymphoma: a clinicopathologic study based on gene expression profiling. Blood 2005;106(13):4315–21.
85. Salaverria I, et al. Specific secondary genetic alterations in mantle cell lymphoma provide prognostic information independent of the gene expression-based proliferation signature. J Clin Oncol 2007;25(10):1216–22.
86. Du MQ. MALT lymphoma: recent advances in aetiology and molecular genetics. J Clin Exp Hematop 2007;47(2):31–42.
87. Remstein ED, James CD, Kurtin PJ. Incidence and subtype specificity of API2-MALT1 fusion translocations in extranodal, nodal, and splenic marginal zone lymphomas. Am J Pathol 2000;156(4):1183–8.
88. Remstein ED, et al. Primary pulmonary MALT lymphomas show frequent and heterogeneous cytogenetic abnormalities, including aneuploidy and translocations involving API2 and MALT1 and IGH and MALT1. Leukemia 2004;18(1):156–60.
89. Lucas PC, et al. Bcl10 and MALT1, independent targets of chromosomal translocation in malt lymphoma, cooperate in a novel NF-kappa B signaling pathway. J Biol Chem 2001;276(22):19012–9.
90. Ruefli-Brasse AA, French DM, Dixit VM. Regulation of NF-kappaB-dependent lymphocyte activation and development by paracaspase. Science 2003; 302(5650):1581–4.
91. Ruland J, et al. Differential requirement for Malt1 in T and B cell antigen receptor signaling. Immunity 2003;19(5):749–58.
92. Zhou H, et al. Bcl10 activates the NF-kappaB pathway through ubiquitination of NEMO. Nature 2004;427(6970):167–71.
93. Isaacson PG, Du MQ. MALT lymphoma: from morphology to molecules. Nat Rev Cancer 2004;4(8):644–53.
94. Streubel B, et al. T(3;14)(p14.1;q32) involving IGH and FOXP1 is a novel recurrent chromosomal aberration in MALT lymphoma. Leukemia 2005;19(4):652–8.
95. Hu H, et al. Foxp1 is an essential transcriptional regulator of B cell development. Nat Immunol 2006;7(8):819–26.
96. Du MQ, Isaccson PG. Gastric MALT lymphoma: from aetiology to treatment. Lancet Oncol 2002;3(2):97–104.
97. Chng WJ, et al. Gene expression profiling of pulmonary mucosa-associated lymphoid tissue lymphoma identifies new biologic insights with potential diagnostic and therapeutic applications. Blood 2009;113(3):635–45. doi: 10.1182/blood-2008-02-140996.
98. Blum KA, Lozanski G, Byrd JC. Adult Burkitt leukemia and lymphoma. Blood 2004;104(10):3009–20.
99. Hecht JL, Aster JC. Molecular biology of Burkitt's lymphoma. J Clin Oncol 2000; 18(21):3707–21.
100. Amati B, et al. Oncogenic activity of the c-Myc protein requires dimerization with Max. Cell 1993;72(2):233–45.
101. Haralambieva E, et al. Interphase fluorescence in situ hybridization for detection of 8q24/MYC breakpoints on routine histologic sections: validation in Burkitt lymphomas from three geographic regions. Genes Chromosomes Cancer 2004;40(1):10–8.
102. Boerma EG, et al. Translocations involving 8q24 in Burkitt lymphoma and other malignant lymphomas: a historical review of cytogenetics in the light of todays knowledge 2008;23(2):225–34.
103. Haralambieva E, et al. Clinical, immunophenotypic, and genetic analysis of adult lymphomas with morphologic features of Burkitt lymphoma. Am J Surg Pathol 2005;29(8):1086–94.

104. McClure RF, et al. Adult B-cell lymphomas with burkitt-like morphology are phenotypically and genotypically heterogeneous with aggressive clinical behavior. Am J Surg Pathol 2005;29(12):1652–60.

105. Chen W, et al. Heterologous promoters fused to BCL6 by chromosomal translocations affecting band 3q27 cause its deregulated expression during B-cell differentiation. Blood 1998;91(2):603–7.

106. Migliazza A, et al. Frequent somatic hypermutation of the 5' noncoding region of the BCL6 gene in B-cell lymphoma. Proc Natl Acad Sci U S A 1995;92(26):12520–4.

107. Dent AL, et al. Control of inflammation, cytokine expression, and germinal center formation by BCL-6. Science 1997;276(5312):589–92.

108. Ye BH, et al. The BCL-6 proto-oncogene controls germinal-centre formation and Th2-type inflammation. Nat Genet 1997;16(2):161–70.

109. Ohno H. Pathogenetic role of BCL6 translocation in B-cell non-Hodgkin's lymphoma. Histol Histopathol 2004;19(2):637–50.

110. Phan RT, et al. Genotoxic stress regulates expression of the proto-oncogene Bcl6 in germinal center B cells. Nat Immunol 2007;8(10):1132–9.

111. Saito M, et al. A signaling pathway mediating downregulation of BCL6 in germinal center B cells is blocked by BCL6 gene alterations in B cell lymphoma. Cancer Cell 2007;12(3):280–92.

112. De Paepe P, et al. ALK activation by the CLTC-ALK fusion is a recurrent event in large B-cell lymphoma. Blood 2003;102(7):2638–41.

113. Gascoyne RD, et al. ALK-positive diffuse large B-cell lymphoma is associated with Clathrin-ALK rearrangements: report of 6 cases. Blood 2003;102(7):2568–73.

114. Reichard KK, McKenna RW, Kroft SH. ALK-positive diffuse large B-cell lymphoma: report of four cases and review of the literature. Mod Pathol 2007; 20(3):310–9.

115. Alizadeh AA, et al. Distinct types of diffuse large B-cell lymphoma identified by gene expression profiling. Nature 2000;403(6769):503–11.

116. Rosenwald A, et al. The use of molecular profiling to predict survival after chemotherapy for diffuse large-B-cell lymphoma. N Engl J Med 2002;346(25): 1937–47. doi: 10.1056/NEJMoa012914.

117. Wright G, et al. A gene expression-based method to diagnose clinically distinct subgroups of diffuse large B cell lymphoma. Proc Natl Acad Sci U S A 2003; 100(17):9991–6. doi: 10.1073/pnas.1732008100.

118. de Jong D, et al. Immunohistochemical prognostic markers in diffuse large B-cell lymphoma: validation of tissue microarray as a prerequisite for broad clinical applications (a study from the Lunenburg Lymphoma Biomarker Consortium). J Clin Pathol 2009;62(2):128–38. doi: 10.1136/jcp.2008.057257.

119. Monti S, et al. Molecular profiling of diffuse large B-cell lymphoma identifies robust subtypes including one characterized by host inflammatory response. Blood 2005;105(5):1851–61. doi: 10.1182/blood-2004-07-2947.

120. Natkunam Y, et al. LMO2 protein expression predicts survival in patients with diffuse large b-cell lymphoma treated with anthracycline-based chemotherapy with and without rituximab. J Clin Oncol 2008;26(3):447–54. doi: 10.1200/JCO.2007.13.0690.

121. Damle RN, et al. Ig V gene mutation status and CD38 expression as novel prognostic indicators in chronic lymphocytic leukemia. Blood 1999;94(6):1840–7.

122. Hamblin TJ. Prognostic markers in chronic lymphocytic leukaemia. Best Pract Res Clin Haematol 2007;20(3):455–68.

123. Hamblin TJ, et al. Unmutated Ig V(H) genes are associated with a more aggressive form of chronic lymphocytic leukemia. Blood 1999;94(6):1848–54.

124. Moreno C, Montserrat E. New prognostic markers in chronic lymphocytic leukemia. Blood Rev 2008;22(4):211–9.

125. Oscier DG, et al. Multivariate analysis of prognostic factors in CLL: clinical stage, IGVH gene mutational status, and loss or mutation of the p53 gene are independent prognostic factors. Blood 2002;100(4):1177–84.

126. Rassenti LZ, et al. Relative value of ZAP-70, CD38, and immunoglobulin mutation status in predicting aggressive disease in chronic lymphocytic leukemia. Blood 2008;112(5):1923–30. doi: 10.1182/blood-2007-05-092882.

127. Seiler T, Dohner H, Stilgenbauer S. Risk stratification in chronic lymphocytic leukemia. Semin Oncol 2006;33(2):186–94.

128. Zent CS, et al. Update on risk-stratified management for chronic lymphocytic leukemia. Leuk Lymphoma 2006;47(9):1738–46.

129. Dicker F, et al. The detection of TP53 mutations in chronic lymphocytic leukemia independently predicts rapid disease progression and is highly correlated with a complex aberrant karyotype. 2008;23(1):117–24.

130. Fabris S, et al. Molecular and transcriptional characterization of 17p loss in B-cell chronic lymphocytic leukemia. Genes Chromosomes Cancer 2008; 47(9):781–93.

131. Zenz T, et al. Monoallelic TP53 inactivation is associated with poor prognosis in chronic lymphocytic leukemia: results from a detailed genetic characterization with long-term follow-up. Blood 2008;112(8):3322–9. doi: 10.1182/blood-2008-04-154070.

132. Rossi D, et al. The prognostic value of TP53 mutations in chronic lymphocytic leukemia is independent of Del17p13: implications for overall survival and chemorefractoriness. Clin Cancer Res 2009;15(3):995–1004. doi: 10.1158/1078-0432.CCR-08-1630.

133. Chiarle R, et al. The anaplastic lymphoma kinase in the pathogenesis of cancer. Nat Rev Cancer 2008;8(1):11–23.

134. Stein H, et al. CD30(+) anaplastic large cell lymphoma: a review of its histopathologic, genetic, and clinical features. Blood 2000;96(12):3681–95.

135. Falini B. Anaplastic large cell lymphoma: pathological, molecular and clinical features. Br J Haematol 2001;114(4):741–60.

136. Damm-Welk C, et al. Prognostic significance of circulating tumor cells in bone marrow or peripheral blood as detected by qualitative and quantitative PCR in pediatric NPM-ALK-positive anaplastic large-cell lymphoma. Blood 2007; 110(2):670–7. doi: 10.1182/blood-2007-02-066852.

137. Mussolin L, et al. Prevalence and clinical implications of bone marrow involvement in pediatric anaplastic large cell lymphoma. Leukemia 2005;19(9): 1643–7.

138. Krishnan B, Matutes E, Dearden C. Prolymphocytic leukemias. Semin Oncol 2006;33(2):257–63.

139. Pekarsky Y, Hallas C, Croce CM. The role of TCL1 in human T-cell leukemia. Oncogene 2001;20(40):5638–43.

140. De Schouwer PJ, et al. T-cell prolymphocytic leukaemia: antigen receptor gene rearrangement and a novel mode of MTCP1 B1 activation. Br J Haematol 2000; 110(4):831–8.

141. Pieters R, Carroll WL. Biology and treatment of acute lymphoblastic leukemia. Pediatr Clin North Am 2008;55(1):1–20, ix.

142. Heerema NA, et al. Hypodiploidy with less than 45 chromosomes confers adverse risk in childhood acute lymphoblastic leukemia: a report from the children's cancer group. Blood 1999;94(12):4036–45.

143. Pui CH, et al. Clinical heterogeneity in childhood acute lymphoblastic leukemia with 11q23 rearrangements. Leukemia 2003;17(4):700–6.

144. Dou Y, Hess J. Mechanisms of transcriptional regulation by MLL and its disruption in acute leukemia. Int J Hematol 2008;87(1):10–8.

145. Ford AM, et al. Origins of "late" relapse in childhood acute lymphoblastic leukemia with TEL-AML1 fusion genes. Blood 2001;98(3):558–64.

146. Schultz KR, et al. Risk- and response-based classification of childhood B-precursor acute lymphoblastic leukemia: a combined analysis of prognostic markers from the Pediatric Oncology Group (POG) and Children's Cancer Group (CCG). Blood 2007;109(3):926–35.

147. Szczepanski T. Why and how to quantify minimal residual disease in acute lymphoblastic leukemia? Leukemia 2007;21(4):622–6.

148. Campana D, Coustan-Smith E. Minimal residual disease studies by flow cytometry in acute leukemia. Acta Haematol 2004;112(1–2):8–15.

149. Borowitz MJ, et al. Minimal residual disease detection in childhood precursor-B-cell acute lymphoblastic leukemia: relation to other risk factors. A Children's Oncology Group study. Leukemia 2003;17(8):1566–72.

150. Cave H, et al. Clinical significance of minimal residual disease in childhood acute lymphoblastic leukemia. European Organization for Research and Treatment of Cancer–Childhood Leukemia Cooperative Group. N Engl J Med 1998; 339(9):591–8.

151. Flohr T, et al. Minimal residual disease-directed risk stratification using real-time quantitative PCR analysis of immunoglobulin and T-cell receptor gene rearrangements in the international multicenter trial AIEOP-BFM ALL 2000 for childhood acute lymphoblastic leukemia 2008;22(4):771–82.

152. Panzer-Grumayer ER, et al. Rapid molecular response during early induction chemotherapy predicts a good outcome in childhood acute lymphoblastic leukemia. Blood 2000;95(3):790–4.

153. van Dongen JJ, et al. Prognostic value of minimal residual disease in acute lymphoblastic leukaemia in childhood. Lancet 1998;352(9142):1731–8.

154. Mullighan CG, et al. Genome-wide analysis of genetic alterations in acute lymphoblastic leukaemia 2007;446(7137):758–64.

155. Mullighan CG, et al. Deletion of IKZF1 and prognosis in acute lymphoblastic leukemia. N Engl J Med 2009;360(5):470–80. doi: 10.1056/NEJMoa0808253.

156. Gondek LP, et al. Chromosomal lesions and uniparental disomy detected by SNP arrays in MDS, MDS/MPD, and MDS-derived AML. Blood 2008;111(3):1534–42.

157. Maciejewski JP, Mufti GJ. Whole genome scanning as a cytogenetic tool in hematologic malignancies. Blood 2008;112(4):965–74.

158. Wouters BJ, Lowenberg B, Delwel R. A decade of genome-wide gene expression profiling in acute myeloid leukemia: flashback and prospects. Blood 2009; 113(2):291–8.

159. Ley TJ, et al. DNA sequencing of a cytogenetically normal acute myeloid leukaemia genome. Nature 2008;456(7218):66–72.

160. He L, Hannon GJ. MicroRNAs: small RNAs with a big role in gene regulation. Nat Rev Genet 2004;5(7):522–31.

161. Lu J, et al. MicroRNA expression profiles classify human cancers. Nature 2005; 435(7043):834–8.

162. Calin GA, et al. A MicroRNA signature associated with prognosis and progression in chronic lymphocytic leukemia. N Engl J Med 2005;353(17):1793–801.

163. Marcucci G, et al. MicroRNA expression in cytogenetically normal acute myeloid leukemia. N Engl J Med 2008;358(18):1919–28.

Index

Note: Page numbers of article titles are in **boldface** type.

Hematol Oncol Clin N Am 23 (2009) 935–948
doi:10.1016/S0889-8588(09)00121-X
0889-8588/09/$ – see front matter © 2009 Elsevier Inc. All rights reserved.

hemonc.theclinics.com

Printed and bound by CPI Group (UK) Ltd, Croydon, CR0 4YY

03/10/2024

01040463-0008